Transcatheter Structural Heart Disease Interventions: Clinical Update

Transcatheter Structural Heart Disease Interventions: Clinical Update

Editors

Maurizio Taramasso
Ana Paula Tagliari

MDPI • Basel • Beijing • Wuhan • Barcelona • Belgrade • Manchester • Tokyo • Cluj • Tianjin

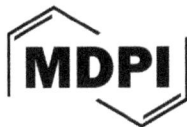

Editors
Maurizio Taramasso
HerzZentrum Hirslanden Zurich
Zürich, Switzerland

Ana Paula Tagliari
Universidade Federal do Rio Grande do Sul (UFRGS)
Porto Alegre, RS, Brazil

Editorial Office
MDPI
St. Alban-Anlage 66
4052 Basel, Switzerland

This is a reprint of articles from the Special Issue published online in the open access journal *Journal of Clinical Medicine* (ISSN 2077-0383) (available at: https://www.mdpi.com/journal/jcm/special_issues/Transcatheter-Structural-Heart-Disease-Interventions).

For citation purposes, cite each article independently as indicated on the article page online and as indicated below:

LastName, A.A.; LastName, B.B.; LastName, C.C. Article Title. *Journal Name* **Year**, *Volume Number*, Page Range.

ISBN 978-3-0365-5783-0 (Hbk)
ISBN 978-3-0365-5784-7 (PDF)

© 2022 by the authors. Articles in this book are Open Access and distributed under the Creative Commons Attribution (CC BY) license, which allows users to download, copy and build upon published articles, as long as the author and publisher are properly credited, which ensures maximum dissemination and a wider impact of our publications.

The book as a whole is distributed by MDPI under the terms and conditions of the Creative Commons license CC BY-NC-ND.

Contents

About the Editors vii

Ana Paula Tagliari and Maurizio Taramasso
The Heart in the Transcatheter Intervention Era: Where Are We?
Reprinted from: *J. Clin. Med.* **2022**, *11*, 5173, doi:10.3390/jcm11175173 1

Mohamed Salem, Christina Grothusen, Mostafa Salem, Derk Frank, Mohammed Saad, Markus Ernst, Thomas Puehler, Georg Lutter, Assad Haneya, Jochen Cremer and Jan Schoettler
Surgery after Failed Transcatheter Aortic Valve Implantation: Indications and Outcomes of a Concerning Condition
Reprinted from: *J. Clin. Med.* **2022**, *11*, 63, doi:10.3390/jcm11010063 5

Daniela Geisler, Piotr Nikodem Rudziński, Waseem Hasan, Martin Andreas, Ena Hasimbegovic, Christopher Adlbrecht, Bernhard Winkler, Gabriel Weiss, Andreas Strouhal, Georg Delle-Karth, Martin Grabenwöger and Markus Mach
Identifying Patients without a Survival Benefit following Transfemoral and Transapical Transcatheter Aortic Valve Replacement
Reprinted from: *J. Clin. Med.* **2021**, *10*, 4911, doi:10.3390/jcm10214911 15

Michał Chyrchel, Stanisław Bartuś, Artur Dziewierz, Jacek Legutko, Paweł Kleczyński, Rafał Januszek, Tomasz Gallina, Bernadeta Chyrchel, Andrzej Surdacki and Łukasz Rzeszutko
Safety and Efficacy of Four Different Diagnostic Catheter Curves Dedicated to One-Catheter Technique of Transradial Coronaro-Angiography—Prospective, Randomized Pilot Study. TRACT 1: Trans RAdial CoronaryAngiography Trial 1
Reprinted from: *J. Clin. Med.* **2021**, *10*, 4722, doi:10.3390/jcm10204722 29

Pawel Kleczynski, Aleksandra Kulbat, Piotr Brzychczy, Artur Dziewierz, Jaroslaw Trebacz, Maciej Stapor, Danuta Sorysz, Lukasz Rzeszutko, Stanislaw Bartus, Dariusz Dudek and Jacek Legutko
Balloon Aortic Valvuloplasty for Severe Aortic Stenosis as Rescue or Bridge Therapy
Reprinted from: *J. Clin. Med.* **2021**, *10*, 4657, doi:10.3390/10.3390/jcm10204657 39

Markus Mach, Thomas Poschner, Waseem Hasan, Tillmann Kerbel, Philipp Szalkiewicz, Ena Hasimbegovic, Martin Andreas, Christoph Gross, Andreas Strouhal, Georg Delle-Karth, Martin Grabenwöger, Christopher Adlbrecht and Andreas Schober
Transcatheter versus Isolated Surgical Aortic Valve Replacement in Young High-Risk Patients: A Propensity Score-Matched Analysis
Reprinted from: *J. Clin. Med.* **2021**, *10*, 3447, doi:10.3390/jcm10153447 51

Hatim Seoudy, Mohammed Saad, Mostafa Salem, Kassem Allouch, Johanne Frank, Thomas Puehler, Mohamed Salem, Georg Lutter, Christian Kuhn and Derk Frank
Calculated Plasma Volume Status Is Associated with Adverse Outcomes in Patients Undergoing Transcatheter Aortic Valve Implantation
Reprinted from: *J. Clin. Med.* **2021**, *10*, 3333, doi:10.3390/jcm10153333 63

Marco Gennari, Marta Rigoni, Giorgio Mastroiacovo, Piero Trabattoni, Maurizio Roberto, Antonio L. Bartorelli, Franco Fabbiocchi, Gloria Tamborini, Manuela Muratori, Laura Fusini, Mauro Pepi, Paola Muti, Gianluca Polvani and Marco Agrifoglio
Proper Selection Does Make the Difference: A Propensity-Matched Analysis of Percutaneous and Surgical Cut-Down Transfemoral TAVR
Reprinted from: *J. Clin. Med.* **2021**, *10*, 909, doi:10.3390/jcm10050909 73

Reprinted from: *J. Clin. Med.* **2020**, *9*, 4118, doi:10.3390/jcm9124118 . . . . **85**

Rodrigo Petersen Saadi, Ana Paula Tagliari, Eduardo Keller Saadi, Marcelo Haertel Miglioranza and Carisi Anne Polanczyck
Preoperative TAVR Planning: How to Do It
Reprinted from: *J. Clin. Med.* **2022**, *11*, 2582, doi:10.3390/jcm11092582 . . . . **95**

Diana R. Florescu, Denisa Muraru, Valentina Volpato, Mara Gavazzoni, Sergio Caravita, Michele Tomaselli, Pellegrino Ciampi, Cristina Florescu, Tudor A. Bălșeanu, Gianfranco Parati and Luigi P. Badano
Atrial Functional Tricuspid Regurgitation as a Distinct Pathophysiological and Clinical Entity: No Idiopathic Tricuspid Regurgitation Anymore
Reprinted from: *J. Clin. Med.* **2022**, *11*, 382, doi:10.3390/jcm11020382 . . . . **109**

Manuel Barreiro-Perez, Berenice Caneiro-Queija, Luis Puga, Rocío Gonzalez-Ferreiro, Robert Alarcon, Jose Antonio Parada, Andrés Iñiguez-Romo and Rodrigo Estevez-Loureiro
Imaging in Transcatheter Mitral Valve Replacement: State-of-Art Review
Reprinted from: *J. Clin. Med.* **2021**, *10*, 5973, doi:10.3390/jcm10245973 . . . . **123**

Ana Paula Tagliari, Rodrigo Petersen Saadi, Eduardo Ferreira Medronha and Eduardo Keller Saadi
The Use of BASILICA Technique to Prevent Coronary Obstruction in a TAVI-TAVI Procedure
Reprinted from: *J. Clin. Med.* **2021**, *10*, 5534, doi:10.3390/jcm10235534 . . . . **137**

Markus Mach, Sercan Okutucu, Tillmann Kerbel, Aref Arjomand, Sefik Gorkem Fatihoglu, Paul Werner, Paul Simon and Martin Andreas
Vascular Complications in TAVR: Incidence, Clinical Impact, and Management
Reprinted from: *J. Clin. Med.* **2021**, *10*, 5046, doi:10.3390/jcm10215046 . . . . **151**

About the Editors

Maurizio Taramasso

Specialist in cardiac surgery. Dr. Maurizio Taramasso completed his surgical training at San Raffaele University Hospital in Milan, Italy. He has carried out specific cross-training in interventional cardiology and transcatheter heart valve therapies (mitral and aortic) and completed a Fellowship in Aortic Surgery at the Hannover Medical School. His main areas of interest include surgical and transcatheter treatments of valvular heart diseases and heart failure.

Ana Paula Tagliari

Specialist in cardiac surgery. Dr. Ana Paula Tagliari completed her surgical training at Hospital de Clínicas de Porto Alegre and PhD at Federal University of Rio Grande do Sul in Porto Alegre, Brazil. She has carried out specific training in transcatheter heart valve interventions and completed a Fellowship at the University Hospital of Zurich. Her main areas of interest include surgical and transcatheter treatment of valvular heart diseases and arrhythmias...

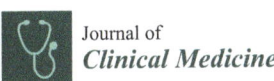

Editorial

The Heart in the Transcatheter Intervention Era: Where Are We?

Ana Paula Tagliari [1,2,3,*] and Maurizio Taramasso [4]

1. Post Graduate Program in Cardiology and Cardiovascular Science, Federal University of Rio Grande do Sul, Porto Alegre 90410-000, Brazil
2. Cardiovascular Surgery Department, Hospital São Lucas da PUC/RS, Porto Alegre 90619-900, Brazil
3. Cardiovascular Surgery Department, Hospital Mãe de Deus, Porto Alegre 90880-0481, Brazil
4. HerzZentrum Hirslanden Zurich Clinic of Cardiac Surgery, 8008 Zurich, Switzerland
* Correspondence: anapaulatagliari@gmail.com; Tel.: +55-(51)-33205186

It is so exciting to imagine that the heart, once considered an untouchable organ, is now routinely approached by so many different techniques and with a wide array of invasiveness. However, this evolution, or better said, revolution, took a lot of time and a great effort from bright inventors to become a reality.

The first percutaneous balloon angioplasty in 1977 can be considered one of the landmarks for the development of transcatheter structural heart interventions, which was driven by the first-in-man balloon aortic valvuloplasty accomplished in 1986 by Alain Cribier [1] and by the first transcatheter implantation of an artificial aortic valve in pigs carried out by Henning Rud Andersen in 1992 [2]. Nonetheless, only 10 years later, Alain Cribier performed the first-in-man transcatheter aortic valve implantation (TAVI) using a balloon-expandable stented aortic valve device. That day, 16 April 2002, was a turning point in the history of Cardiac Surgery [3].

The patient was an inoperable 57-year-old male with severe aortic stenosis, who presented cardiogenic shock, with a left ventricle ejection fraction (LVEF) of only 12%. Balloon aortic valvuloplasty had failed, and performing the first TAVI seemed the only option to save his life. Since the patient had no transfemoral arterial access available, the physicians proceeded with a transvenous and transseptal approach. The operators' main surprise was that, just a few minutes after the valve implantation, the patient's blood pressure returned to normal, and his grey complexion turned into a healthy pink color. In Cribier's own words: "we trusted in our idea, and our perseverance paid off. You can either give up, or you can find solutions, and that is what we did".

Undoubtedly, this first-in-man TAVI not only percutaneously treated that aortic valve stenosis but, most importantly, initiated the modern era of structural heart disease interventions. TAVI is now the standard-of-care treatment for inoperable and high-risk patients and a safe and effective option for those at intermediate and low risk [4–11]. It has been estimated that around 1.5 million patients in over 70 countries have had TAVI across these past 20 years.

In the mitral valve arena, transcatheter edge-to-edge repair (TEER) can be considered in cases of chronic primary mitral regurgitation in severely symptomatic patients (NYHA functional class III or IV) with high or prohibitive surgical risk provided that the mitral valve anatomy is favorable and the patient life expectancy is at least 1 year (class of indication IIa B according to the ACC/AHA Guidelines; class of indication IIb B according to the ESC/EACTS Guidelines). In the context of chronic severe secondary mitral regurgitation related to left ventricular systolic dysfunction (LVEF < 50%) and persistent symptoms (NYHA functional class II, III, or IV), TEER is reasonable if appropriate anatomy, LVEF between 20% and 50%, left ventricular end-systolic diameter (LVESD) ≤ 70 mm, and pulmonary artery systolic pressure ≤ 70 mmHg (class of indication IIa B according to the ACC/AHA Guidelines) are present. According to the ESC/EACTS Guidelines, if a patient has severe secondary mitral regurgitation and concomitant coronary artery disease

Citation: Tagliari, A.P.; Taramasso, M. The Heart in the Transcatheter Intervention Era: Where Are We? *J. Clin. Med.* **2022**, *11*, 5173. https://doi.org/10.3390/jcm11175173

Received: 24 August 2022
Accepted: 27 August 2022
Published: 1 September 2022

Publisher's Note: MDPI stays neutral with regard to jurisdictional claims in published maps and institutional affiliations.

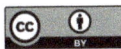

Copyright: © 2022 by the authors. Licensee MDPI, Basel, Switzerland. This article is an open access article distributed under the terms and conditions of the Creative Commons Attribution (CC BY) license (https://creativecommons.org/licenses/by/4.0/).

requiring treatment but is judged not appropriate for surgery, percutaneous coronary intervention, possibly followed by TTER (if persistent MR), should be considered (class of indication IIa C). On the other hand, if the patient had no concomitant coronary artery disease requiring treatment, TEER should be considered in selected symptomatic patients not eligible for surgery and fulfilling those criteria that suggest an increased chance of treatment response (class of indication IIa B). Lastly, for secondary tricuspid regurgitation, the transcatheter treatment may be considered in symptomatic inoperable patients (class of indication IIb C according to the ESC/EACTS Guidelines) [12,13].

Taking into consideration that every day new devices are developed and new indications for structural heart disease interventions are proposed, a high priority for the cardiovascular community must be to be engaged in this emerging area and to train the next generations of heart valve specialists, including surgeons, interventional and non-interventional cardiologists, heart failure and imaging specialists, anesthesiologists, geriatricians, nurse specialists, and researchers [14].

However, solid scientific evidence to support some of these new technological advancements is still lacking. Aiming to be part of this evidence generation process and present the most recent advances in transcatheter structural heart disease interventions, we provide this Special Issue.

This Special Issue of the *Journal of Clinical Medicine* (JCM) entitled "Transcatheter Structural Heart Disease Interventions: Clinical Update" offers eight original articles and four review articles. Ten articles focus on the transcatheter aortic valve approach, discussing all the relevant issues related to this technique, such as balloon aortic valvoplasty [15]; TAVI indications and patient selection [16]; pre-procedural planning [17]; access routes (open or percutaneous vascular access) [18]; potential access-related complications [19]; TAVI outcomes compared with surgery [20]; challenges of surgery after TAVI failure [21]; post-TAVI prognostic factors [22]; potential benefits of cerebral embolic protection devices [23]; and the BASILICA technique to prevent coronary obstruction [24]. Three additional articles discuss the state of the art in transcatheter mitral valve replacement images [25]; atrial functional tricuspid regurgitation [26]; and the use of different diagnostic catheters for transradial coronary angiography [27].

In summary, the articles presented in this Special Issue cover a broad spectrum of transcatheter heart interventions guiding readers through the best evidence-based approach.

Author Contributions: Conceptualization, writing—review and editing, visualization, supervision and project administration A.P.T. and M.T. All authors have read and agreed to the published version of the manuscript.

Funding: This research received no external funding.

Conflicts of Interest: Tagliari A.P. received a Research Grant from the Coordenação de Aperfeiçoamento de Pessoal de Nível Superior—Brasil (CAPES)—Finance Code 001. Taramasso has been a consultant or the recipient of consultancy fees from Abbott, Edwards Lifesciences, Boston Scientific, Shenqi Medical, CoreMedic, 4tech, Simulands, MTEx, Cardiovalve, and MEDIRA.

References

1. Cribier, A.; Savin, T.; Saoudi, N.; Rocha, P.; Berland, J.; Letac, B. Percutaneous transluminal valvuloplasty of acquired aortic stenosis in elderly patients: An alternative to valve replacement? *Lancet* **1986**, *1*, 63–67. [CrossRef]
2. Andersen, H.R.; Knudsen, L.L.; Hasenkam, J.M. Transluminal implantation of artificial heart valves. Description of a new expandable aortic valve and initial results with implantation by catheter technique in closed chest pigs. *Eur. Heart J.* **1992**, *13*, 704–708. [CrossRef] [PubMed]
3. Cribier, A.; Eltchaninoff, H.; Bash, A.; Borenstein, N.; Tron, C.; Bauer, F.; Derumeaux, G.; Anselme, F.; Laborde, F.; Leon, M.B. Percutaneous transcatheter implantation of an aortic valve prosthesis for calcific aortic stenosis: First human case description. *Circulation* **2002**, *106*, 3006–3008. [CrossRef]
4. Leon, M.B.; Smith, C.R.; Mack, M.; Miller, D.C.; Moses, J.W.; Svensson, L.G.; Tuzcu, E.M.; Webb, J.G.; Fontana, G.P.; Makkar, R.R.; et al. Transcatheter aortic-valve implantation for aortic stenosis in patients who cannot undergo surgery. *N. Engl. J. Med.* **2010**, *363*, 1597–1607. [CrossRef] [PubMed]

5. Smith, C.R.; Leon, M.B.; Mack, M.J.; Miller, D.C.; Moses, J.W.; Svensson, L.G.; Tuzcu, E.M.; Webb, J.G.; Fontana, G.P.; Makkar, R.R.; et al. Transcatheter versus surgical aortic-valve replacement in high-risk patients. *N. Engl. J. Med.* **2011**, *364*, 2187–2198. [CrossRef] [PubMed]
6. Adams, D.H.; Popma, J.J.; Reardon, M.J.; Yakubov, S.J.; Coselli, J.S.; Deeb, G.M.; Gleason, T.G.; Buchbinder, M.; Hermiller, J., Jr.; Kleiman, N.S.; et al. Transcatheter aortic-valve replacement with a self-expanding prosthesis. *N. Engl. J. Med.* **2014**, *370*, 1790–1798. [CrossRef] [PubMed]
7. Leon, M.B.; Smith, C.R.; Mack, M.J.; Makkar, R.R.; Svensson, L.G.; Kodali, S.K.; Thourani, V.H.; Tuzcu, E.M.; Miller, D.C.; Herrmann, H.C.; et al. Transcatheter or Surgical Aortic-Valve Replacement in Intermediate-Risk Patients. *N. Engl. J. Med.* **2016**, *374*, 1609–1620. [CrossRef]
8. Reardon, M.J.; Van Mieghem, N.M.; Popma, J.J.; Kleiman, N.S.; Søndergaard, L.; Mumtaz, M.; Adams, D.H.; Deeb, G.M.; Maini, B.; Gada, H.; et al. Surgical or Transcatheter Aortic-Valve Replacement in Intermediate-Risk Patients. *N. Engl. J. Med.* **2017**, *376*, 1321–1331. [CrossRef]
9. Mack, M.J.; Leon, M.B.; Thourani, V.H.; Makkar, R.; Kodali, S.K.; Russo, M.; Kapadia, S.R.; Malaisrie, S.C.; Cohen, D.J.; Pibarot, P.; et al. Transcatheter Aortic-Valve Replacement with a Balloon-Expandable Valve in Low-Risk Patients. *N. Engl. J. Med.* **2019**, *380*, 1695–1705. [CrossRef]
10. Popma, J.J.; Deeb, G.M.; Yakubov, S.J.; Mumtaz, M.; Gada, H.; O'Hair, D.; Bajwa, T.; Heiser, J.C.; Merhi, W.; Kleiman, N.S.; et al. Evolut Low Risk Trial Investigators. Transcatheter Aortic-Valve Replacement with a Self-Expanding Valve in Low-Risk Patients. *N. Engl. J. Med.* **2019**, *380*, 1706–1715. [CrossRef] [PubMed]
11. D'Ancona, G.; Pasic, M.; Buz, S.; Drews, T.; Dreysse, S.; Hetzer, R.; Unbehaun, A. TAVI for pure aortic valve insufficiency in a patient with a left ventricular assist device. *Ann. Thorac. Surg.* **2012**, *93*, e89–e91. [CrossRef] [PubMed]
12. Vahanian, A.; Beyersdorf, F.; Praz, F.; Milojevic, M.; Baldus, S.; Bauersachs, J.; Capodanno, D.; Conradi, L.; De Bonis, M.; De Paulis, R.; et al. ESC/EACTS Scientific Document Group. 2021 ESC/EACTS Guidelines for the management of valvular heart disease. *Eur. Heart J.* **2022**, *43*, 561–632. [CrossRef] [PubMed]
13. Otto, C.M.; Nishimura, R.A.; Bonow, R.O.; Carabello, B.A.; Erwin, J.P., 3rd; Gentile, F.; Jneid, H.; Krieger, E.V.; Mack, M.; McLeod, C.; et al. 2020 ACC/AHA Guideline for the Management of Patients With Valvular Heart Disease: Executive Summary: A Report of the American College of Cardiology/American Heart Association Joint Committee on Clinical Practice Guidelines. *Circulation* **2021**, *143*, e35–e71. [CrossRef] [PubMed]
14. Prendergast, B.D.; Baumgartner, H.; Delgado, V.; Gérard, O.; Haude, M.; Himmelmann, A.; Iung, B.; Leafstedt, M.; Lennartz, J.; Maisano, F.; et al. Transcatheter heart valve interventions: Where are we? Where are we going? *Eur. Heart J.* **2019**, *40*, 422–440. [CrossRef]
15. Kleczynski, P.; Kulbat, A.; Brzychczy, P.; Dziewierz, A.; Trebacz, J.; Stapor, M.; Sorysz, D.; Rzeszutko, L.; Bartus, S.; Dudek, D.; et al. Balloon Aortic Valvuloplasty for Severe Aortic Stenosis as Rescue or Bridge Therapy. *J. Clin. Med.* **2021**, *10*, 4657. [CrossRef]
16. Geisler, D.; Rudziński, P.N.; Hasan, W.; Andreas, M.; Hasimbegovic, E.; Adlbrecht, C.; Winkler, B.; Weiss, G.; Strouhal, A.; Delle-Karth, G.; et al. Identifying Patients without a Survival Benefit following Transfemoral and Transapical Transcatheter Aortic Valve Replacement. *J. Clin. Med.* **2021**, *10*, 4911. [CrossRef]
17. Saadi, R.P.; Tagliari, A.P.; Saadi, E.K.; Miglioranza, M.H.; Polanczyck, C.A. Preoperative TAVR Planning: How to Do It. *J. Clin. Med.* **2022**, *11*, 2582. [CrossRef]
18. Gennari, M.; Rigoni, M.; Mastroiacovo, G.; Trabattoni, P.; Roberto, M.; Bartorelli, A.L.; Fabbiocchi, F.; Tamborini, G.; Muratori, M.; Fusini, L.; et al. Proper Selection Does Make the Difference: A Propensity-Matched Analysis of Percutaneous and Surgical Cut-Down Transfemoral TAVR. *J. Clin. Med.* **2021**, *10*, 909. [CrossRef]
19. Mach, M.; Okutucu, S.; Kerbel, T.; Arjomand, A.; Fatihoglu, S.G.; Werner, P.; Simon, P.; Andreas, M. Vascular Complications in TAVR: Incidence, Clinical Impact, and Management. *J. Clin. Med.* **2021**, *10*, 5046. [CrossRef]
20. Mach, M.; Poschner, T.; Hasan, W.; Kerbel, T.; Szalkiewicz, P.; Hasimbegovic, E.; Andreas, M.; Gross, C.; Strouhal, A.; Delle-Karth, G.; et al. Transcatheter versus Isolated Surgical Aortic Valve Replacement in Young High-Risk Patients: A Propensity Score-Matched Analysis. *J. Clin. Med.* **2021**, *10*, 3447. [CrossRef]
21. Salem, M.; Grothusen, C.; Salem, M.; Frank, D.; Saad, M.; Ernst, M.; Puehler, T.; Lutter, G.; Haneya, A.; Cremer, J.; et al. Surgery after Failed Transcatheter Aortic Valve Implantation: Indications and Outcomes of a Concerning Condition. *J. Clin. Med.* **2022**, *11*, 63. [CrossRef] [PubMed]
22. Seoudy, H.; Saad, M.; Salem, M.; Allouch, K.; Frank, J.; Puehler, T.; Salem, M.; Lutter, G.; Kuhn, C.; Frank, D. Calculated Plasma Volume Status Is Associated with Adverse Outcomes in Patients Undergoing Transcatheter Aortic Valve Implantation. *J. Clin. Med.* **2021**, *10*, 3333. [CrossRef] [PubMed]
23. Tagliari, A.P.; Ferrari, E.; Haager, P.K.; Schmiady, M.O.; Vicentini, L.; Gavazzoni, M.; Gennari, M.; Jörg, L.; Khattab, A.A.; Blöchlinger, S.; et al. Feasibility and Safety of Cerebral Embolic Protection Device Insertion in Bovine Aortic Arch Anatomy. *J. Clin. Med.* **2020**, *9*, 4118. [CrossRef] [PubMed]
24. Tagliari, A.P.; Petersen Saadi, R.; Medronha, E.F.; Keller Saadi, E. The Use of BASILICA Technique to Prevent Coronary Obstruction in a TAVI-TAVI Procedure. *J. Clin. Med.* **2021**, *10*, 5534. [CrossRef]
25. Barreiro-Perez, M.; Caneiro-Queija, B.; Puga, L.; Gonzalez-Ferreiro, R.; Alarcon, R.; Parada, J.A.; Iñiguez-Romo, A.; Estevez-Loureiro, R. Imaging in Transcatheter Mitral Valve Replacement: State-of-Art Review. *J. Clin. Med.* **2021**, *10*, 5973. [CrossRef]

26. Florescu, D.R.; Muraru, D.; Volpato, V.; Gavazzoni, M.; Caravita, S.; Tomaselli, M.; Ciampi, P.; Florescu, C.; Bălșeanu, T.A.; Parati, G.; et al. Atrial Functional Tricuspid Regurgitation as a Distinct Pathophysiological and Clinical Entity: No Idiopathic Tricuspid Regurgitation Anymore. *J. Clin. Med.* **2022**, *11*, 382. [CrossRef]
27. Chyrchel, M.; Bartuś, S.; Dziewierz, A.; Legutko, J.; Kleczyński, P.; Januszek, R.; Gallina, T.; Chyrchel, B.; Surdacki, A.; Rzeszutko, Ł. Safety and Efficacy of Four Different Diagnostic Catheter Curves Dedicated to One-Catheter Technique of Transradial Coronaro-Angiography—Prospective, Randomized Pilot Study. TRACT 1: Trans RAdial CoronaryAngiography Trial 1. *J. Clin. Med.* **2021**, *10*, 4722. [CrossRef]

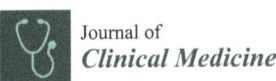

Journal of
Clinical Medicine

Article

Surgery after Failed Transcatheter Aortic Valve Implantation: Indications and Outcomes of a Concerning Condition

Mohamed Salem [1,*], Christina Grothusen [1], Mostafa Salem [2], Derk Frank [2,3], Mohammed Saad [2], Markus Ernst [1], Thomas Puehler [1,3], Georg Lutter [1,3], Assad Haneya [1], Jochen Cremer [1] and Jan Schoettler [1]

1. Department of Cardiovascular Surgery, Campus Kiel, University Hospital Schleswig-Holstein, 24105 Kiel, Germany; christina.grothusen@uksh.de (C.G.); markus.ernst@uksh.de (M.E.); Thomas.Puehler@uksh.de (T.P.); Georg.Lutter@uksh.de (G.L.); assad.haneya@uksh.de (A.H.); Jochen.Cremer@uksh.de (J.C.); Jan.Schoettler@uksh.de (J.S.)
2. Department of Cardiology and Angiology, Campus Kiel, University Hospital Schleswig-Holstein, 24105 Kiel, Germany; mostafa.salem@uksh.de (M.S.); derk.frank@uksh.de (D.F.); Mohammed.Saad@uksh.de (M.S.)
3. DZHK (German Centre for Cardiovascular Research), Partner Site Hamburg/Kiel/Lübeck, Potsdamer Str. 58, 10785 Berlin, Germany
* Correspondence: Mohamed.salem@uksh.de; Tel.: +49-(0431)-5002-2002 (ext. 67089); Fax: +49-(0431)-5002-2004

Abstract: Objectives: The number of transcatheter aortic valve implantations (TAVI) has increased enormously in recent decades. Transcatheter valve prosthesis failure and the requirement of conventional surgical replacement are expected to attract more focus in the near future. Indeed, given the scarcity of research in this field, the next decade will likely represent the beginning of a period of meaningful exploration of the degenerative changes that occur with transcatheter valves. The current study represents—through a series of consecutive cases—one of the first analyses of the underlying causes of TAVI failure, i.e., degenerative, functional and infective, followed by surgical aortic valve replacement (SAVR) and postoperative outcome. Methods: Between October 2008 and March 2021, 2098 TAVI procedures, including 1423 with transfemoral, 309 with transapical, and 366 with transaortic access, were performed in our institution. Among these, 0.5% (number(n) = 11) required acute SAVR (n = 6) within 7 days (n = 3) or later (n = 2), and were included in the study. Results: Valve stent dislocation was the most common cause of replacement (83%). Causes of replacement within 7 days after TAVI were multifactorial. In the later course, endocarditis was the sole indication for SAVR after TAVI. TAVI with transapical or transaortic approach had a higher EuroSCORE II (10.9 (7.2–35.3) vs. 3.5 (1.8–7.8)). Their 30-day mortality after surgical conversion was higher (67% vs. 20%), when compared to those who underwent a transfemoral procedure. The longest documented survival beyond 30 days was 58 months. Conclusions: The causes of SAVR after TAVI failure are multifactorial, and include biological, physical and infectious factors. An acceptable midterm prognosis may be expected in patients with physical causes when dislocation of the catheter prosthesis is observed; in such cases, emergency conversion is required. Conversion due to infection, as in cases of endocarditis, had the worst outcome. Prognosis after conversion due to degeneration is still problematic, due to a lack of autopsies and the recent history of prosthetic implantations.

Keywords: TAVI degeneration; SAVR after TAVI; long-term outcome of TAVI

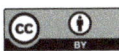

1. Introduction

Due to demographic changes, the incidence of aortic valve stenosis requiring treatment is increasing. While approximately 15,000 isolated aortic valve procedures were performed in Germany in 2010, nearly 25,000 were performed in 2019 [1]. For decades, the gold standard for the treatment of symptomatic aortic valve stenosis was conventional surgical aortic valve replacement (SAVR) alone [2]. Since 2006, transcatheter aortic valve implantation (TAVI) has been considered a well-established alternative technique [3]. In 2017, for the first time, more than half of isolated aortic valve procedures in Germany were performed as TAVI, and in 2019, the TAVI proportion was already around 60% [1].

According to current recommendations, TAVI is the procedure of choice for older and sicker patients, i.e., those aged 75 years and older with a Society of Thoracic Surgeons Score (STS Score) or EuroSCORE II of at least 4% [4]. TAVI application in younger patients with fewer comorbidities is still being investigated in clinical trials [5,6]. If possible, TAVI is performed via the transfemoral approach (TF-TAVI) [4]. In cases of small diameters of femoral arteries, peripheral arterial occlusive disease and severe atherosclerosis or marked kinking of the descending aorta, TAVI can also be applied via the left ventricular apex (TA-TAVI) or the ascending aorta (TAO-TAVI), as well as transsubclavian and transcarotid, each using a minimally invasive technique [7,8].

The results after TAVI are promising. The increasing expertise of heart teams and ongoing improvements of catheter valve implants have made TAVI safer as a low-complication procedure. Even the number of paravalvular leaks, which were seen more frequently in the past, is decreasing [9]. The durability of the implants appears to be sufficient, despite initial concerns [10]. However, the degenerative, biomedical and infectious factors leading to TAVI dysfunction have not yet been thoroughly investigated. Until now, TAVI durability data are based on the absence of reintervention or post-TAVI-SAVR in populations of elderly patients with an already a low survival rate of 30% at 5 y [11,12]. This is due to the recent history of prosthetic implantation. Moreover, the criteria of choosing TAVI patients such as old age and high comorbidities, and thus, the associated higher mortality rate, do not facilitate accurate analyses of the causes of the degenerative changes and failure of transcatheter prostheses.

In this paper, we report our experience regarding the various factors leading to TAVI dysfunction and the need for subsequent surgical replacement.

2. Materials and Methods

2.1. Patients

Between October 2008 and March 2021, 2098 consecutive TAVI procedures, including 1423 with transfemoral, 309 with transapical, and 366 with transaortic access, were performed in the cardiovascular department of the University Hospital of Schleswig-Holstein, Campus Kiel. TAVI was performed either through balloon-expandable or self-expandable valves. Retrospectively, we reviewed all patients who underwent surgical replacement of aortic valve following TAVI. The study population was defined as any SAVR after TAVI due to any form of deterioration of the primary implanted transcatheter aortic valve (TAV). The causes included malposition or dislocation of the TAV, paravalvular regurgitation, degeneration of TAV, annulus and ventricular perforation or infective endocarditis. SAVR were done either as an emergency procedure after unsuccessful primary TAVI or due to a prosthesis failure after successful TAVI. The cases were diagnosed either through transthoracic echocardiography or transesophageal echocardiography intra- or postoperative or through postoperative computer tomography. Data were collected and extracted from the institution's database and from medical records. The study protocol was approved by the local ethics committee in Kiel (D 415/21), and patient consent was obtained prior to and during hospital stay.

2.2. Statistical Analysis and Definitions

Descriptive statistics are reported as mean $\pm$ SD for normally distributed continuous variables or otherwise as median and 25th–75th percentile (interquartile range). Absolute and relative frequencies are reported for categorical variables. A univariate comparison between the groups for categorical variables was made using the x^2 and the Fisher's exact test. A survival analysis was performed with the Kaplan–Meier method through extraction from the city database. The normality of continuous variables was assessed by Kolmogorov-Smirnow-Test. A statistical analysis was performed using the SPSS Statistics software (Version 18.0) and Stata 10 SE (Stata Corp., College Station, TX, USA). The primary endpoint was 30-day mortality. Secondary endpoints were intraoperative variables and postoperative course (e.g., ventilation time, bleeding, acute renal failure, neurological complications and late mortality).

2.3. Surgical Technology

All operations were done either as emergency procedures (such in cases of dislocation of the TAV, annulus rupture or coronary ostium occlusion during the primary TAVI procedure), or either on an urgent or elective basis (such in cases of late deterioration of valve function due to high grade paravalvular leak or endocarditis). Surgery was performed via median sternotomy using cardiopulmonary bypass and cardioplegic cardiac arrest. Salvage of the dislocated valve stents into the distal ascending aorta or the aortic arch sometimes required circulatory arrest and deep hypothermia. A transverse supracoronary aortic incision was made to remove dislocated valve stents and to visualize the aortic root. In SAVR cases after initially successful TAVI, the deployed wire meshes of the transcatheter valve were separated from the aortic wall with a dissector, and the prosthetic stent was then removed piece by piece, using a wire cutter if necessary. Finally, after excision of the aortic valve leaflets and careful decalcification of the aortic valve annulus, implantation of a biological prosthetic heart valve was performed in the usual manner. In cases of annulus rupture, a biological patch was used to strengthen the aortic wall.

3. Results

3.1. Demographic Data and Preoperative Variables

Between October 2008 and March 2021, 2098 TAVI procedures, including 1423 with transfemoral, 309 with transapical, and 366 with transaortic access, were performed in our institution. Among these, 0.52% (n = 11; five patients (45%) transfemoral TAVI (TF-TAVI), six patients (55%) transaortal or apical TAVI (TA/TAO-TAVI)) of patients underwent SAVR after TAVI failure, of which six were done on an emergency basis, three within 7 days, and two at a later time. The clinical characteristics of this population are shown in Table 1. The median age was 79 years (interquartile range (64–85) and four (36%) were female. The mean EuroSCORE II was 7.8 (1.8–35.3). Ten patients (91%) suffered from coronary heart disease with previous coronary stenting. Four patients (36%) required dialysis and seven (64%) presented with peripheral arterial disease (PAD). When comparing the preoperative demographic data between TF-TAVI und TA/TAO TAVI, we found that patients with surgical TAVI were more often male (83% vs. 40%), had a higher EuroSCORE II (median 10.9 (7.2–35.3) vs. 3.5 (1.8–7.8)), and tended to have more chronic obstructive lung disease (83% vs. 20%), renal insufficiency with dialysis (50% vs. 20%), and peripheral artery disease (83% vs. 40%), Table 1.

Table 1. Preoperative variables.

	Total (n = 11)	TF-TAVI (n = 5)	TA/TAO-TAVI (n = 6)
Male gender (n)	7 (64%)	2 (40%)	5 (83%)
Age (years)	79 (64–85)	78 (76–79)	83 (64–85)
EuroSCORE II	7.8 (1.8–35.3)	3.5 (1.8–7.8)	10.9 (7.2–35.3)
Previous cerebral insult (n)	2 (18%)	1 (20%)	1 (17%)
Coronary artery disease (n)	10 (91%)	5 (100%)	5 (83%)
Previous coronary stenting (n)	10 (91%)	5 (100%)	5 (83%)
Previous cardiac surgery (n)	0	0	0
Obstructive lung disease (n)	6 (55%)	1 (20%)	5 (83%)
Dialysis (n)	4 (36%)	1 (20%)	3 (50%)
Peripheral artery disease (n)	7 (64%)	2 (40%)	5 (83%)
Implant size (mm)	26 (23–34)	26 (23–34)	27.5 (23–34)

TF-TAVI: transfemoral transcatheter aortic valve implantation, TA/TAO-TAVI: transapical/transaortal transcatheter aortic valve implantation.

3.2. Pro-Procedual TAVI-Metrics

TAVI valve sizing and design were based on annulus dimension (mainly diameter), as well as the distance between aortic valve annulus and both sinotubular junction and the right and left ostia. The important measurements are represented in Table 2. Calcium score was mainly assessed as ordinary CAC-Score, and in recent cases, was assessed through absolute Agatston—Score, Table 2.

Table 2. TAVI-Metrics.

Patient	CAC-Score (Agatston Units)	Aortic Annulus (mm)	Sinotubular Junction (mm)	Distance between RCA Ostia to Annulus	Distance between LM Ostia to Annulus
Patient 1 (m, 80Y)	Mild	23 × 29 mm	n.m	20 mm	17 mm
Patient 2 (f, 78Y)	Severe	20 × 22 mm	n.m	14 mm	12 mm
Patient 3 (f, 76Y)	Extensive (2461)	20 × 25 mm	30 mm	20 mm	16 mm
Patient 4 (m, 83Y)	High	22 × 28 mm	29 mm	7 mm	16 mm
Patient 5 (m, 65Y)	High	23 × 34 mm	21 mm	13 mm	11 mm
Patient 6 (f, 83Y)	Mild	19 × 23 mm	22 mm	6 mm	13 mm
Patient 7 (m, 85Y)	Extensive (1955)	18 × 24 mm	29 mm	21 mm	16 mm
Patient 8 (m, 78Y)	Extensive (3028)	26 × 33 mm	29 mm	15 mm	8 mm
Patient 9 (f, 76Y)	Mild	17 × 24 mm	26 mm	15 mm	13 mm
Patient 10 (m, 83Y)	Extensive (2460)	25 × 29 mm	25 mm	17 mm	14 mm
Patient 11 (m, 79Y)	Extensive (1485)	22 × 28 mm	27 mm	16 mm	15 mm

CAC-Score: Coronary Artery Calcium score, n.m: no measurement, RCA: right coronary artery, LM: left main, f: Female, m: Male.

3.3. Type of Prosthesis and Sizes of Implanted TAV

The ratio between self-expanding to balloon-expanding prostheses was 55% vs. 45%. The sizes ranged from 23 to 34 mm with no noticeable difference between the groups. Table 3 provides information on the prosthesis types and sizes used in previous TAVI procedures.

Table 3. TAVI prosthesis types and sizes.

	Total ($n = 11$)	TF-TAVI ($n = 5$)	TA/TAO-TAVI ($n = 6$)
Sapien XT® (n)	2 (18%)	1 (20%)	1 (17%)
Sapien 3® (n)	3 (27%)	1 (20%)	2 (33%)
CoreValve® (n)	5 (45%)	2 (40%)	3 (50%)
Symetis® (n)	1 (9%)	1 (20%)	0

3.4. Core Data and Indication of SAVR

An analysis of the core data of the 11 patients showed that all subjects received a biological prosthetic heart valve, i.e., 64% received a porcine aortic valve and 36% a bovine pericardial tissue heart valve. One patient was stabilized with an extracorporeal circulatory support system (ECLS) even before SAVR. In another patient, closure of a newly formed ventricular septal defect (VSD) was required in addition to SAVR. The indication for surgical intervention SAVR was dislocation of TAV in five patients, either in LVOT or in the ascending aorta or aortic arch. One patient suffered from moderate to severe paravalvular leakage. Endocarditis as the cause of intravalvular regurgitation was documented in two patients. Two patients suffered from annulus perforation (one with VSD). Occlusion of the coronary left main trunk was a reason for SAVR in one patient. Late TAV degeneration was recognized at scheduled echocardiographic or computer tomography follow-up; see Table 4.

Table 4. Core Data and Indications for Intervention.

Patient	TAVI	Problem	SAVR	30-Day Mortality
Patient 1 (m, 80Y)	TA-TAVI 26 mm Sapien XT	Dislocation into left ventricular outflow tract	Single-stage 27 mm Hancock II	no
Patient 2 (f, 78Y)	TF-TAVI 23 mm Sapien XT	Annulus perforation	≤7 days 21 mm PERIMOUNT	no
Patient 3 (f, 76Y)	TF-TAVI 26 mm CoreValve	Dislocation into ascending aorta	Single-stage 23 mm Hancock II circulatory arrest	no
Patient 4 (m, 83Y)	TAO-TAVI 29 mm CoreValve	Occlusion of the coronary left main trunk	Single-stage 21 mm Trifecta	yes
Patient 5 (m, 65Y)	TAO-TAVI 34 mm CoreValve	Paravalvular leakage	≤7 days 25 mm Hancock II ECLS before SAVR	yes
Patient 6 (f, 83Y)	TA-TAVI 26 mm Sapien 3	Annulus perforation with VSD	≤7 days 21 mm Trifecta closure of VSD	yes
Patient 7 (m, 85Y)	TAO-TAVI 29 mm CoreValve	Endocarditis	>3 months 25 mm Hancock II	no
Patient 8 (m, 78Y)	TF-TAVI 34 mm CoreValve	Dislocation into LVOT	Single-stage 29 mm Hancock II ECLS after SAVR	no
Patient 9 (f, 76Y)	TF-TAVI 25 mm Symetis	Dislocation into ascending aorta	Single-stage 25 mm Hancock II circulatory arrest	yes
Patient 10 (m, 83Y)	TA-TAVI 23 mm Sapien 3	Endocarditis	>3 months 21 mm Hancock II	yes
Patient 11 (m, 79Y)	TF-TAVI 26 mm Sapien 3	Dislocation into aortic arch	Single-stage 23 mm PERIMOUNT circulatory arrest	no

f: Female, m: Male., SAVR: surgical aortic valve replacement, ECLS: Extracorporeal Life Support System

3.5. Timing of Surgery

In six cases (55%), a single-stage conversion was required. Three patients (27%) underwent SAVR at 7 days after the TAVI procedure, and two (18%) at an interval of more than 3 months after TAVI. Single-stage surgery (80% vs. 33%) and dislocation of the catheter valve (80% vs. 17%) were observed more frequently in the group which had undergone transfemoral procedure, Table 5.

Table 5. Timing of Surgery.

	Total (n = 11)	TF-TAVI (n = 5)	TA/TAO-TAVI (n = 6)
Single-stage operation (n)	6 (55%)	4 (80%)	2 (33%)
Two-stage ≤ 7 days (n)	3 (27%)	1 (20%)	2 (33%)
Two-stage > 3 months (n)	2 (18%)	0	2 (33%)
Catheter valve dislocation (n)	5 (45%)	4 (80%)	1 (17%)
Annulus perforation (n)	2 (18%)	1 (20%)	1 (17%)
Paravalvular leakage (n)	1 (9%)	0	1 (17%)
Ventricular septal defect (n)	1 (9%)	0	1 (17%)
Left main trunk occlusion (n)	1 (9%)	0	1 (17%)
Catheter valve endocarditis (n)	2 (18%)	0	2 (33%)

3.6. Intraoperative Variables

Procedual durations in cases of transfemoral or surgical TAVI did not differ significantly. A preference for a specific biological valve prosthesis could not be determined. Implant sizes did not differ in our comparison; see Table 6.

Table 6. Intraoperative Variables.

	Total (n = 11)	TF-TAVI (n = 5)	TA/TAO-TAVI (n = 6)
Bypass time (min)	122 (74–187)	122 (74–140)	127.5 (106–187)
Cross-clamp-time (min)	83 (49–143)	84 (49–102)	80 (72–143)
Circulatory arrest (n)	3 (27%)	2 (40%)	1 (17%)
Hancock II (n)	7 (64%)	3 (60%)	4 (67%)
PERIMOUNT® (n)	2 (18%)	2 (40%)	0
Trifecta® (n)	2 (18%)	0	2 (33%)
Implant size (mm)	23 (21–39)	23 (21–29)	23 (21–27)

3.7. Postoperative Variables

Patients who underwent SAVR after a failed surgical TAVI had a longer duration of mechanical ventilation (median 121 (48–283) vs. 28 (15–125)) and appeared to require more frequent postoperative dialysis (67% vs. 20%), associated with a longer stay in the intensive care unit (median 9.5 (2–26) vs. 3 (2–6)). Their 30-day mortality was higher than that of the group which had undergone the primary transfemoral procedure (67% vs. 20%), Table 7.

Table 7. Postoperative Variables.

	Total (n = 11)	TF-TAVI (n = 5)	TA/TAO-TAVI (n = 6)
Stay on ICU (d)	5 (2–26)	3 (2–6)	9.5 (2–26)
Hospital length of stay (d)	15 (2–45)	15 (5–20)	17.5 (2–45)
Ventilation duration (h)	100 (15–283)	28 (15–125)	121 (48–283)
Tracheostomy (n)	2 (18%)	0	2 (33%)
Rethoracotomy (n)	2 (18%)	1 (20%)	1 (17%)
Delirium (n)	3 (27%)	0	3 (50%)

Table 7. Cont.

	Total (n = 11)	TF-TAVI (n = 5)	TA/TAO-TAVI (n = 6)
Cerebral Insult (n)	2 (18%)	1 (20%)	1 (17%)
Atrial fibrillation (n)	6 (55%)	3 (60%)	3 (50%)
Atrioventricular block (n)	4 (36%)	2 (40%)	2 (33%)
Pacemaker dependence (n)	1 (9%)	1 (20%)	0
Dialysis (n)	5 (45%)	1(20%)	4 (67%)
Wound infection (n)	1 (9%)	1 (20%)	0
30-day mortality (n)	5 (45%)	1 (20%)	4 (67%)

Survival at the time of follow-up ranged from 1 to 58 months. Two patients are currently still alive. In total, a cumulative survival of nearly 10 patient-years has been achieved to date.

4. Discussion

At present, the use of TAVI is increasing in comparison to SAVR. TAVI is currently more applicable in medium- and in lower-risk patients, rather than only high-risk patients. This brings about a need for more adequate studies and strategies to be implemented, as not taking action regarding these young patients—as opposed to older, multimorbid patients—is no longer an option. The circumstances of TAVI failure, including etiology, incidence, management and outcome, are still under analysis. The causes of these failures should be more thoroughly analyzed in the near future. Thus, our study aimed to analyze the various early and late factors leading to TAVI failure.

Moreover, it is not clear whether patients after TAVI should undergo SAVR in emergency unsuccessful TAVI or in the course after primarily successful TAVI. In this context, there are only registry data for emergency cardiac surgical procedures during TF-TAVI [13,14]. Both TAVI surgeries with transapical or transaortic access and two-stage surgeries later in the course were not considered in this registry. Furthermore, these registries did not focus in detail on the factors leading to TAVI failure.

The present study considers almost 13 years of TAVI experience. From 28 October 2008 to 31 January 2021, 2098 TAVI procedures were performed in Kiel, including 1423 TF-TAVI and 675 surgical TAVI, of which 309 were transapical and 366 were transaortic. During this time, a total of only 11 patients (0.5%), i.e., six with primarily unsuccessful TAVI and five after primarily successful TAVI, underwent SAVR early-postoperatively for prosthesis-associated complications or because of subsequent prosthesis failure.

The causes of TAVI failure are multifactorial. According to the literature, during TF-TAVI, left ventricular perforation by the guidewire, annulus rupture, embolization or migration of the transcatheter valves, and aortic dissection are prominent as emergency indications for conversion to cardiac surgery [13]. These problems are generally associated with the TAVI, and consequently, are also observed in surgical implantations. In our work, a performed SAVR was considered an inclusion criterion, regardless of whether there the transfemoral or surgical approach was applied. Cases in which cardiac perforations were treated using a heart–lung machine, or even other cardiac surgical procedures without explantation of the TAVI prosthesis, such as isolated replacement of the ascending aorta for Stanford type A aortic dissection, were not included in our work. Therefore, the reason for primary failure of the TAVI procedure in our collective was mainly dislocations of the catheter valve. Only one of our patients required emergency conversion to SAVR for a different reason, namely, occlusion of the main left coronary trunk by the implanted valve stent.

Indication for cardiac surgery in the early-postoperative phase was due to to a periannular rupture, an annulus-near ventricular septal defect, and a catheter valve that was not fully deployed with increasing paravalvular leakage. All procedures in the early course after primary successful TAVI were required within 7 days of the procedure. The complications observed during this period were among the known intraprocedural complications. It is plausible that there are TAVI-associated problems that present with a latency of days in individual cases. According to the European Registry on Emergency Cardiac Surgery during TAVI, more than 90% of complications still occur during the TAVI procedure. Only about 3% of TAVI patients manifest problems requiring emergency cardiac surgery with a median sternotomy after more than 24 h [13].

Later, only two patients underwent SAVR because of manifest endocarditis of the valve stent. Endocarditis is not a TAVI-specific problem. In general, patients undergoing valve replacement are at higher than average risk of endocarditis. Prognoses of prosthetic endocarditis are compromised not only by local findings, but also by the inflammatory effects on the whole organism. Using a multicenter registry, Amat-Santos et al. demonstrated that the incidence of infective endocarditis 1 year after TAVI is 0.5%. The majority of affected patients from this registry were treated conservatively, and overall hospital mortality was approximately 47%, [14].

Overall, SAVR was associated with significant mortality in the patients included in our study, as expected. Even though none of the patients died on the operating table, i.e., the procedures were technically successful, the 30-day mortality was 45%. In 2013, Hein et al. published an almost identical 30-day mortality of 45.8% in patients who were converted from TAVI procedure to emergency cardiac surgery [15]. However, those authors studied only patients who required cardiac surgery immediately after TAVI; cardiac surgery at a later stage after TAVI was not considered in their publication. Furthermore, in contrast to our study, SAVR was not an explicit inclusion criterion in their registry analysis, and TAVI procedures with a primarily surgical approach were excluded from the outset.

Compared with data reported by Hein et al., our directly converted TAVI patients had a lower 30-day mortality of 33%. Two-stage procedures within 7 days of TAVI had a 30-day mortality of 67% in our collective, and we observed a 30-day mortality of 50% in subsequent valve surgeries after primary successful TAVI due to prosthetic endocarditis.

In our comparison of transfemoral and surgical TAVI procedures, we found that patients in whom the transfemoral approach was chosen had a better prognosis after SAVR. Indeed, only one patient with TF-TAVI access died within 30 days after SAVR. The remaining decedents had surgical access, i.e., two of them via the left ventricular apex and two via the ascending aorta. Extrapolating from these facts, our patients had an 80% 30-day survival after SAVR for subjects with primary TF-TAVI and of approximately 33% for those with primary surgical TAVI access. The lower survival of SAVR after surgical TAVI is certainly not due to the transapical or transaortic approach itself. Instead, it may be due to the fact that surgical TAVI patients have a different risk profile than those that are eligible for TF-TAVI [16]. In our collective, surgical TAVI patients had a higher EuroSCORE II, and findings requiring SAVR intraprocedurally or early in the course were more complex in such cases. Thus, only one patient required acute conversion after surgical TAVI because of a less complex prosthesis dislocation without concomitant cardiac problems. The failure of these interventions may be attributed to a wide range of factors.

According to our results, acute emergency surgery for primary unsuccessful TAVI is feasible with a reasonable risk, depending on the reason for conversion to SAVR. In cases of severe complications, such as circulatory collapse due physical occlusion of the left coronary main trunk that cannot be treated interventionally, the prognosis is very bad. In such cases, it may therefore be justified not to escalate treatment further. In contrast, in cases with only dislocated valve stent and existing circulatory stability, emergency SAVR may be carried out safely, because in this constellation, postoperative outcome seems to be acceptable, regardless of TAVI access. The 30-day mortality of these patients in our study was only 20%, and in individual cases, we observed survival times of 1 to almost 5 years.

In our experience, two-stage SAVR for early postoperative cardiac complications after primary successful TAVI is unpromising with regard to the mid-term prognosis.

In cases of late degenerative damage due to endocarditis of valve stents, we showed that SAVR is still associated with high risk. We also predict an acceptable chance for surgery on degenerated valvular stents, despite not having been assigned a patient with such characteristics for SAVR to date. Even if younger patients will more commonly undergo the TAVI procedure in the future, a significant number of such referrals is probably not to be expected, because, at most, mild and hemodynamically insignificant degeneration is observed on catheter valves 5 years after TAVI [16]. Moreover, subsequent problems not related to endocarditis, such as hemodynamically relevant degeneration or valvular and paravalvular insufficiencies, can, in principle, also be resolved by a repeat TAVI, [17].

5. Conclusions

Cases requiring emergency surgical intervention are most often those with improper TAV sizing and selection. Mostly, emergency cases may be attributed to valve dislocation either in the ascending aorta, aortic arch or LVOT. Such displacements either block the coronary ostia when moved in the direction of blood flow or lead to extensive aortic valve insufficiency when moved in the other direction. Those patients require an emergency thoracotomy and should be connected to a heart and lung machine. Also, TAV sizing mismatches play a significant role in cases requiring revision due to annulus rupture with or without VSD, sometimes even leading to the need for aortic dissection. Such cases must be also treated as life-threatening. In the study population, patients who presented in the late course with infective endocarditis also suffered from recurrent attacks of postoperative high-grade fever and shivering. Blood culture tests were mostly positive, and echocardiography proved the above diagnoses, and thus, the need for revision. The causes of SAVR after TAVI failure are multifactorial, including degenerative, physical or infectious factors. Acceptable mid-term prognoses were observed in patients with symptoms associated with the dislocation of the catheter prosthesis, for whom emergency conversions were required. Conversion due to infection, e.g., endocarditis, had the worst outcome. Prognoses after conversion due to degenerative causes are still lacking. This is due to a lack of enough autopsies and the recent history of prosthetic implantation. A proportion of affected patients can be saved by SAVR, both acute and subsequent. In cases of acute complications, rapid cardiac surgical intervention is required; in such instances, TAVI procedures must be performed at specialized centers with a broad cardiac surgical infrastructure. Cardiac surgery after TAVI should also be performed at TAVI centers with high levels of expertise, as these operations can be equally demanding.

Limitations

Only patients who had undergone a TAVI procedure in our hospital and received a SAVR during the procedure or at a later stage were included. Since such operations are a rarity, very few patients could be studied. Therefore, the conclusions drawn here should be considered with caution.

Author Contributions: Conceptualization, M.S. (Mohamed Salem) and J.S.; methodology, all authors.; software, M.S. (Mohamed Salem), J.S. and M.E.; validation, M.S. (Mohamed Salem), J.S.; formal analysis, M.S. (Mohamed Salem), J.S., M.E.; investigation, M.S. (Mohamed Salem) and J.S.; resources, M.S. (Mohamed Salem), J.S., A.H., D.F., M.S. (Mohammed Saad), and J.C.; data curation, M.S. (Mohamed Salem) and J.S.; writing—original draft preparation, M.S. (Mohamed Salem) and J.S.; writing—review and editing, M.S. (Mohamed Salem) and J.S.; visualization, all authors; writing—review and editing, all authors.; project administration, M.S. (Mohamed Salem) and J.S.; funding acquisition, none. All authors have read and agreed to the published version of the manuscript.

Funding: We acknowledge financial support by DFG within the funding programme Open Access Publizieren.

Institutional Review Board Statement: The study was conducted according to the guidelines of the Declaration of Helsinki, and approved by local Ethics Committee in Kiel (D 415/21).

Informed Consent Statement: Informed consent was obtained from all subjects involved in the study.

Conflicts of Interest: The authors declare no conflict of interest.

References

1. Beckmann, A.; Meyer, R.; Lewandowski, J.; Markewitz, A.; Gummert, J. German heart surgery report 2019: The annual updated registry of the German society for thoracic and cardiovascular surgery. *Thorac. Cardiovasc. Surg.* **2020**, *68*, 263–276. [CrossRef] [PubMed]
2. Cribier, A.; Eltchaninoff, H.; Tron, C.; Bauer, F.; Agatiello, C.; Sebagh, L.; Bash, A.; Nusimovici, D.; Litzler, P.Y.; Bessou, J.P.; et al. Early experience with percutaneous transcatheter implantation of heart valve prothesis for the treatment of end-stage inoperable patients with calcific aortic stenosis. *J. Am. Coll. Cardiol.* **2001**, *43*, 698–703. [CrossRef] [PubMed]
3. Hörte, L.G.R.; Stahle, E. Observed and relative survival after aortic valve replacement. *J. Am. Coll. Cardiol.* **2000**, *35*, 747–756.
4. Baumgartner, H.; Falk, V.; Bax, J.J.; De Bonis, M.; Hamm, C.; Holm, P.J.; Iung, B.; Lancellotti, P.; Lansac, E.; Rodriguez Muñoz, D.; et al. 2017 ESC/EACTS Guidelines for the management of valvular heart disease. *Eur. Heart J.* **2017**, *38*, 2739–2791. [CrossRef]
5. Baron, S.J.; Arnold, S.V.; Wang, K.; Magnuson, E.A.; Chinnakondepali, K.; Makkar, R.; Herrmann, H.C.; Kodali, S.; Thourani, V.H.; Kapadia, S.; et al. Health status benefits of transcatheter vs surgical aortic valve replacement in patients with serve aortic stenosis at intermediate surgical risk: Results from the PARTNER 2 randomized clinical trial. *JAMA Cardiol.* **2017**, *2*, 837–845. [CrossRef] [PubMed]
6. Mack, M.J.; Leon, M.B.; Thourani, V.H.; Makkar, R.; Kodali, S.K.; Russo, M.; Kapadia, S.R.; Malaisrie, S.C.; Cohen, D.J.; Pibarot, P.; et al. Transcatheter Aortic-Valve Replacement with a Balloon-Expandaable Valve in Low-Risk Patients. *N. Eng. J. Med.* **2019**, *380*, 1695–1705. [CrossRef] [PubMed]
7. Reents, W.; Barth, S.; Griese, D.P.; Winkler, S.; Babin-Ebell, J.; Kerber, S.; Diegeler, A.; Zacher, M.; Hamm, K. Transfemoral versus transapical transcatheter aortic valve implantation: A single-centre experience. *Eur. J. Cardio-Thorac. Surg.* **2019**, *55*, 744–750. [CrossRef] [PubMed]
8. Dunne, B.; Tan, D.; Chu, D.; Yau, V.; Xiao, J.; Ho, K.M.; Yong, G.; Larbalestier, R. Transapical versus transaortic transcatheter aortic valve implantation: A systematic review. *Ann. Thorac. Surg.* **2015**, *100*, 354–361. [CrossRef] [PubMed]
9. Arai, T.; Lefèvre, T.; Hovasse, T.; Morice, M.-C.; Garot, P.; Benamer, H.; Unterseeh, T.; Hayashida, K.; Watanabe, Y.; Bouvier, E.; et al. Comparison of Edwards SAPIEN 3 versus SAPIEN XT in transfemoral transcatheter aortic valve implantation: Difference of valve selection in the real world. *J. Cardiol.* **2017**, *69*, 565–569. [CrossRef] [PubMed]
10. Mack, M.J.; Leon, M.B.; Smith, C.R.; Miller, D.C.; Moses, J.W.; Tuzcu, E.M.; Webb, J.G.; Douglas, P.S.; Anderson, W.N.; Blackstone, E.H.; et al. 5-Year outcomes of trancatheter aortic valve replacement or surgical aortic valve replacement for high surgical risk patients with aortic stenosis (PARTNER 1): A randomised controlled trial. *Lancet* **2015**, *385*, 2477–2484. [CrossRef]
11. Schmidt, T.; Frerker, C.; Alessandrini, H.; Schlüter, M.; Kreidel, F.; Schäfer, U.; Thielsen, T.; Kuck, K.-H.; Jose, J.; Holy, E.W.; et al. Redo TAVI: Initial experience at two German centres. *EuroIntervention* **2016**, *12*, 875–882. [CrossRef] [PubMed]
12. Haussig, S.; Pleissner, C.; Mangner, N.; Woitek, F.; Zimmer, M.; Kiefer, P.; Schlotter, F.; Stachel, G.; Leontyev, S.; Holzhey, D.; et al. Long-term follow-up after transcatheter aortic valve replacement. *CJC Open* **2021**, *3*, 845–853. [CrossRef] [PubMed]
13. Eggebrecht, H.; Vaquerizo, B.; Moris, C.; Bossone, E.; Lämmer, J.; Czerny, M.; Zierer, A.; Schröfel, H.; Kim, W.K.; Walther, T.; et al. Incidence and outcomes of emergent cardiac surgery during transfemoral transcatheter aortic valve implantation (TAVI): Insights from the European Registry on Emergent Cardiac Surgery during TAVI (EuRECS-TAVI). *Eur. Heart J.* **2018**, *39*, 676–684. [CrossRef] [PubMed]
14. Amat-Santos, I.J.; Messika-Zeitoun, D.; Eltchaninoff, H. Infective endocardotis after transcatheter aortic valve implantation. *Circulation* **2015**, *131*, 1566–1574. [CrossRef] [PubMed]
15. Hein, R.; Abdel-Wahab, M.; Sievert, H.; Kuck, K.-H.; Voehringer, M.; Hambrecht, R.; Sack, S.; Hauptmann, K.E.; Senges, J.; Zahn, R.; et al. Outcome of patients after emergency conversion from transcatheter aortic valve implantation to surgery. *EuroIntervention* **2013**, *9*, 446–451. [CrossRef] [PubMed]
16. Ferrari, E.; Eeckhout, E.; Keller, S.; Muller, O.; Tozzi, P.; Berdajs, D.; von Segesser, L.K. Transfemoral versus transapical approach for transcatheter aortic valve implantation: Hospital outcome and risk factor analysis. *J. Cardiothorac. Surg.* **2017**, *12*, 78. [CrossRef] [PubMed]
17. Sulženko, J.; Toušek, P.; Kočka, V.; Bednář, F.; Línková, H.; Petr, R.; Laboš, M.; Widimský, P. Degenerative changes and immune response after transcatheter aortic valve implantation. Comparison with surgical aortic valve replacement. *J. Cardiol.* **2017**, *69*, 483–488. [CrossRef] [PubMed]

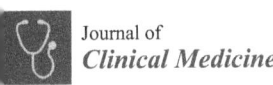

Article

Identifying Patients without a Survival Benefit following Transfemoral and Transapical Transcatheter Aortic Valve Replacement

Daniela Geisler [1], Piotr Nikodem Rudziński [2,3], Waseem Hasan [4], Martin Andreas [3], Ena Hasimbegovic [3,5], Christopher Adlbrecht [6], Bernhard Winkler [1], Gabriel Weiss [7,8], Andreas Strouhal [9], Georg Delle-Karth [9], Martin Grabenwöger [1,8] and Markus Mach [3,*]

1. Department of Cardio-Vascular Surgery, Klinik Floridsdorf and Karl Landsteiner Institute for Cardio-Vascular Research, 1210 Vienna, Austria; daniela.geisler@gesundheitsverbund.at (D.G.); bernhard.winkler@gesundheitsverbund.at (B.W.); martin.grabenwoeger@gesundheitsverbund.at (M.G.)
2. Department of Coronary and Structural Heart Diseases, The Cardinal Stefan Wyszyński Institute of Cardiology, 04-628 Warsaw, Poland; piotr.rudzinski@ikard.pl
3. Department of Cardiac Surgery, Medical University Vienna, 1090 Vienna, Austria; martin.andreas@meduniwien.ac.at (M.A.); ena.hasimbegovic@meduniwien.ac.at (E.H.)
4. Imperial College London, London SW7 2AZ, UK; waseem.hasan15@imperial.ac.uk
5. Department of Internal Medicine II, Division of Cardiology, Vienna General Hospital, 1090 Vienna, Austria
6. Imed19-Privat, Private Clinical Research Center, Chimanistrasse 1, 1190 Vienna, Austria; c.adlbrecht@imed19.at
7. Department of Vascular Surgery, Klinik Ottakring, 1160 Vienna, Austria; gabriel.weiss@gesundheitsverbund.at
8. Medical Faculty, Sigmund Freud University, 1020 Vienna, Austria
9. Department of Cardiology, Klinik Floridsdorf and the Karl Landsteiner Institute for Cardiovascular & Intensive Care Research Vienna, 1210 Vienna, Austria; andreas.strouhal@gesundheitsverbund.at (A.S.); georg.delle-karth@gesundheitsverbund.at (G.D.-K.)
* Correspondence: markus.mach@meduniwien.ac.at; Tel.: +43-1-40400-52620

Abstract: Transcatheter aortic valve replacement (TAVR) offers a novel treatment option for patients with severe symptomatic aortic valve stenosis, particularly for patients who are unsuitable candidates for surgical intervention. However, high therapeutical costs, socio-economic considerations, and numerous comorbidities make it necessary to target and allocate available resources efficiently. In the present study, we aimed to identify risk factors associated with futile treatment following transfemoral (TF) and transapical (TA) TAVR. Five hundred and thirty-two consecutive patients (82 ± 9 years, female 63%) who underwent TAVR between June 2009 and December 2016 at the Vienna Heart Center Hietzing were retrospectively analyzed to identify predictors of futility, defined as all-cause mortality at one year following the procedure for the overall patient cohort, as well as the TF and TA cohort. Out of 532 patients, 91 (17%) did not survive the first year after TAVR. A multivariate logistic model identified cerebrovascular disease, home oxygen dependency, wheelchair dependency, periinterventional myocardial infarction, and postinterventional renal replacement therapy as the factors independently associated with an increased one-year mortality. Our findings underscore the significance of a precise preinterventional evaluation, as well as illustrating the subtle differences in baseline characteristics in the TF and TA cohort and their impact on one-year mortality.

Keywords: futility; TAVI; TAVR; SAVR

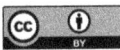

1. Introduction

Although transcatheter aortic valve replacement (TAVR) has made it possible to treat patients that were deemed high- or extremely high-risk in the context of conventional heart surgery, the central question that still has not been sufficiently explored is whether certain risk factors will preclude the patients from benefiting from the procedure.

In the last few years, TAVR has become a mainstay in the treatment of severe symptomatic aortic stenosis, yet optimizing the periinterventional management through adequate patient selection and preventing complications associated with poor outcome remains pivotal. The number of TAVR procedures is expected to keep rising due to the growing elderly population but also as a result of an increase in the number of TAVR interventions in the low-risk and intermediate-risk population, as well as the increased number of centers performing the procedures at higher volumes. This increase is attributable to the results of the randomized-controlled PARTNER3 and EVOLUT low-risk trials that managed to demonstrate a non-inferiority of TAVR in the low-risk patient collective, with regard to both safety and efficacy [1–5].

However, the ever-expanding role of TAVR in the treatment of severe symptomatic aortic stenosis, combined with the high costs to the healthcare system and the high level of expertise required, will inevitably bring the issue of cost-effectiveness to the forefront in the coming years [6–8]. Optimizing patient selection and preventing complications associated with a poor outcome will be crucial steps in ensuring the ideal allocation of scarce healthcare resources to patients who are most likely to benefit from their use.

While commonly used risk scores have proved their utility in identifying low-risk patients eligible for cardiac surgery, they are associated with numerous limitations in accurately predicting outcomes after TAVR, including an inability to adequately account for co-morbidities, frailty, and predicted mortality [2,9–13].

Thus, the objective of this study was to identify clinically relevant predictors of futility within the first year after TAVR, with an underlying aim of improving the effectiveness of preinterventional screening and enhancing the vigilance for certain risk factors to further improve survival and reduce the financial strain on the healthcare system.

2. Methods

2.1. Design and Patients

Between June 2009 and December 2016, 532 consecutive patients (female 63%) undergoing TAVR for symptomatic aortic valve stenosis at the Heart Center Hietzing in Vienna were prospectively enrolled in the Vienna Cardiothoracic Aortic Valve Registry (VICTORY). The mean age was 82 ± 9 years. As an early adopter of TAVR and national referral center for transapical (TA) procedures, the TAVR procedure was performed equally via the transfemoral (TF; $n = 266$) or the TA access route ($n = 266$). Operative mortality risk was calculated using the logistic European System for Cardiac Operative Risk Evaluation (EuroSCORE) and the EuroSCORE II [14,15]. The eligibility for TAVR was assessed by a multi-disciplinary heart team consisting of cardiothoracic surgeons, cardiologists, anesthesiologists, and radiologists. The institutional diagnostic protocol for patients with aortic valve stenosis follows the general recommendations stated in the current ESC/EACTS guidelines for the management of valvular heart disease [2].

The study was approved by the Ethics Committee of Vienna (EK18-027-VK). All recruited patients signed an informed consent prior to the enrollment in the registry. Subsequently, a retrospective analysis of the patient characteristics including medical history, length of hospital stay, echocardiographic information, clinical and interventional data, and mortality was carried out in order to identify independent predictors of 1-year mortality. Mortality data, including the cause of death, was obtained by examining hospital records and via an inquiry to the Federal Institute for Statistics Austria.

2.2. Procedure

The preinterventional assessment included preinterventional echocardiography as well as multislice computed tomography examinations for all patients. The interventions were performed in a standard fashion by the institution's heart team and have been described in detail before [16]. Balloon pre- and post-dilatation was performed at the operator's discretion. Different generations of transcatheter heart valves (THV) by Edwards Lifesciences (Edwards Lifesciences, Irvine, CA, USA), Medtronic (Medtronic, Minneapolis,

MN, USA), JenaValve (JenaValve Technology GmbH, Munich, Germany), and Symetis (Symetis SA, a Boston Scientific company, Ecublens, Switzerland) were used for TAVR procedures. The choice of valve size was based on a multislice computed tomography scan and echocardiography performed prior to the intervention. General anesthesia was used for all TA-TAVR procedures and for TF procedures performed before September 2014. Following a change in the institutional standard operating procedures, TF-TAVR was performed under conscious sedation after this time, whenever applicable.

2.3. Endpoints

The primary endpoint of this analysis was futility, defined as all-cause mortality at one year following TAVR, regardless of the patient's subjective quality of life indicators or functional parameter improvement. The secondary endpoints, as determined by the Valve Academic Research Consortium (VARC)-2 document, were compared between survivors and non-survivors at one year following TAVR [17]. Cerebrovascular disease (CVD) was diagnosed using preinterventional doppler, and cerebrovascular accident was diagnosed according to VARC-2 criteria.

2.4. Statistical Analysis

The study population was separated into two cohorts: patients for whom treatment with TAVR was futile, i.e., who did not survive the first year, and patients who lived past the one-year post-TAVR timepoint. Further stratification has been performed according to the chosen access strategy. Dichotomous parameters were expressed as absolute and relative frequencies and continuous variables as median and median deviation of the median (MAD). A univariate Cox regression analysis was used to identify preinterventional, peri-interventional, and postinterventional factors, which were associated with a change in the hazard ratio. Significant preinterventional factors were finally included in a multivariate Cox regression analysis to identify those with a true impact on futile TAVR treatment.

Statistical analysis was completed using RStudio (Version 1.4.1717, 2009–2021 RStudio PBC), the reported *p*-values are 2-sided with an alpha level set at <0.05 for statistical significance.

3. Results

3.1. Baseline Characteristics

A detailed comparison of the baseline characteristics is presented in Table 1.

Table 1. Baseline clinical characteristics of futile and non-futile TAVR procedures.

	Combined Access		TF-TAVR				TA-TAVR			
			Futile		Non-Futile		Futile		Non-Futile	
Demographics										
	n = 532		n = 32		n = 234		n = 59		n = 207	
Age, median (MAD)	82	(5.9)	84.5	(5.2)	83	(5.9)	83	(7.4)	80	(7.4)
Female, n (%)	335	(63)	19	(59.4)	153	(65.4)	33	(55.9)	130	(62.8)
Body mass index kg/m2, median (MAD)	25.8	(4.7)	26.2	(5.4)	25.9	(4.4)	24.8	(4.9)	26.1	(4.9)
Risk profile										
Logistic EuroSCORE, median (MAD)	15.1	(9.2)	13.6	(6.5)	14.5	(8.4)	19.3	(11.8)	15.5	(10.4)
EuroSCORE II, median (MAD)	4.6	(3.2)	4.8	(2.3)	4.3	(2.9)	6.6	(3.7)	4.6	(3.5)
Incremental risk score, median (MAD)	6	(8.9)	9.5	(9.6)	6.2	(9.1)	7	(10.4)	5	(7.4)
Chronic health conditions and risk factors ordered by its frequency										
Hypertension, n (%)	467	(87.8)	30	(93.8)	205	(87.6)	53	(89.8)	179	(86.5)
Dyslipidaemia, n (%)	320	(60.2)	19	(59.4)	123	(52.6)	43	(72.9)	135	(65.2)
Renal impairment eGFR < 60 mL/min/1.73 m², n (%)	296	(55.6)	16	(50)	129	(55.1)	34	(57.6)	117	(56.5)
Coronary artery disease, n (%)	267	(50.2)	14	(43.8)	115	(49.1)	33	(55.9)	105	(50.7)
Prior PCI, n (%)	165	(31)	10	(31.2)	70	(29.9)	20	(33.9)	65	(31.4)

Table 1. Cont.

	Combined Access		TF-TAVR				TA-TAVR			
			Futile		Non-Futile		Futile		Non-Futile	
Atrial fibrillation, n (%)	163	(30.6)	11	(34.4)	67	(28.6)	17	(28.8)	68	(32.9)
Peripheral vascular disease, n (%)	106	(19.9)	3	(9.4)	24	(10.3)	24	(40.7)	55	(26.6)
Diabetes mellitus (IDDM), n (%)	91	(17.1)	5	(15.6)	38	(16.2)	13	(22)	35	(16.9)
Prior myocardial infarction, n (%)	89	(16.7)	5	(15.6)	29	(12.4)	13	(22)	42	(20.3)
Permanent pacemaker, n (%)	85	(16)	7	(21.9)	48	(20.5)	10	(16.9)	20	(9.7)
Previous CABG, n (%)	84	(15.8)	5	(15.6)	30	(12.8)	11	(18.6)	38	(18.4)
Cerebrovascular disease, n (%)	83	(15.6)	4	(12.5)	27	(11.5)	20	(33.9)	32	(15.5)
Cerebrovascular accident, n (%)	70	(13.2)	4	(12.5)	34	(14.5)	9	(15.3)	23	(11.1)
COPD, n (%)	66	(12.4)	4	(12.5)	15	(6.4)	14	(23.7)	33	(15.9)
Previous valve surgery, n (%)	50	(9.4)	1	(3.1)	26	(11.1)	5	(8.5)	18	(8.7)
Liver cirrhosis, n (%)	28	(5.3)	3	(9.4)	7	(3)	4	(6.8)	14	(6.8)
Home oxygen dependence, n (%)	8	(1.5)	1	(3.1)	4	(1.7)	3	(5.1)	0	(0)
Wheel chair dependency, n(%)	5	(0.9)	2	(6.2)	3	(1.3)	0	(0)	0	(0)
Renal replacement therapy, n (%)	4	(0.8)	0	(0)	0	(0)	1	(1.7)	3	(1.4)
Creatinine mg/dL, median (MAD)	1.1	(0.4)	1.2	(0.5)	1.1	(0.4)	1.2	(0.4)	1.1	(0.3)
Preinterventional echocardiographic data										
Low-flow–low-gradient stenosis, n (%)	77	(14.5)	6	(18.8)	29	(12.4)	12	(20.3)	30	(14.5)
Aortic valve area, median (MAD)	0.7	(0.1)	0.7	(0.1)	0.7	(0.1)	0.7	(0.3)	0.7	(0.1)
Mean pressure gradient, median (MAD)	45	(14.8)	43	(11.9)	45.5	(13.3)	43.5	(15.6)	45	(17.8)
Max. pressure gradient, median (MAD)	69	(20.8)	67	(16.3)	71	(19.3)	68.2	(25.6)	69	(22.2)
Peak velocity m/sec, median (MAD)	4.1	(0.6)	4	(0.5)	4.1	(0.6)	4	(0.6)	4	(0.7)
LVEF %, median (MAD)	55	(7.4)	60	(0)	60	(0)	55	(7.4)	55	(7.4)

CABG—coronary artery bypass graft; COPD—chronic obstructive pulmonary disease; eGFR—estimated glomerular filtration rate; EuroSCORE—European System for Cardiac Operative Risk Evaluation; IDDM—insulin-dependent diabetes mellitus; MAD—median deviation of the median; LVEF—left ventricular ejection fraction; PCI—percutaneous coronary intervention; TA—transapical; TAVR—transcatheter aortic valve replacement; TF—transfemoral.

3.2. Preinterventional Parameters of Survival in the First Year

In a univariate Cox regression analyses, the TA approach, EuroSCORE II, chronic obstructive pulmonary disease (COPD), peripheral vascular disease (PVD), CVD, home oxygen dependence, and the mean and maximum pressure gradient across the aortic valve demonstrated to be of significant influence on the primary study endpoint in the overall patient cohort, respectively (Table 2). In the TF subgroup, only wheelchair dependence was a significant negative factor of survival in the first year (Table 2). In the TA subgroup, the logistic EuroSCORE, the EuroSCORE II, peripheral vascular disease, CVD, and home oxygen dependence showed significantly increased hazard ratios (Table 2).

CVD remained associated with futile treatment following TAVR in the multivariate Cox regression analyses (Supplementary Table S1) in the combined access cohort as well as the TA subgroup. Home oxygen dependence remained statistically significant in the TA subgroup.

3.3. Interventional Factors of Survival in the First Year

Conversion to open surgery, total hours in the intensive care unit (ICU), total hours ventilated, and length of stay after TAVR showed to be significant in the combined access cohort in the univariate Cox regression analysis (Table 3).

Table 2. Univariate Cox regression analyses of futile events based on patients' baseline characteristics of preinterventional factors. A hazard ratio (HR) above 1 increases the risk, below 1 decreases the risk of futility.

	Combined Access			TF-TAVR			TA-TAVR		
	HR	95% CI	p-Value	HR	95% CI	p-Value	HR	95% CI	p-Value
Demographics									
Transapical access	1.9	1.2 2.9	0.003						
Age	1.014	0.985 1.045	0.345	1.019	0.961 1.08	0.535	1.027	0.991 1.064	0.145
Male gender	1.29	0.852 1.954	0.23	1.26	0.622 2.552	0.52	1.266	0.757 2.116	0.369
Body mass index	0.988	0.948 1.03	0.56	1.019	0.955 1.088	0.565	0.967	0.916 1.021	0.227
Risk profile									
Logistic EuroSCORE	1.014	0.999 1.029	0.075	0.985	0.953 1.019	0.384	1.024	1.007 1.041	0.006
EuroSCORE II	1.039	1.002 1.078	0.039	0.972	0.894 1.058	0.514	1.069	1.024 1.116	0.003
Incremental risk score	1.008	0.986 1.03	0.5	1.003	0.966 1.042	0.876	1.011	0.985 1.038	0.414
Chronic health conditions and risk factors ordered by its frequency as in Table 1									
Hypertension	1.468	0.711 3.034	0.299	1.991	0.476 8.331	0.346	1.324	0.569 3.08	0.515
Dyslipidaemia	1.455	0.936 2.262	0.095	1.312	0.648 2.656	0.451	1.348	0.759 2.393	0.308
Renal impairment	0.962	0.636 1.453	0.853	0.82	0.41 1.639	0.574	1.033	0.616 1.731	0.903
Coronary artery disease	1.06	0.703 1.6	0.779	0.793	0.395 1.595	0.516	1.229	0.735 2.054	0.433
Prior PCI	1.091	0.705 1.689	0.696	1.023	0.484 2.16	0.953	1.122	0.655 1.924	0.675
Atrial fibrillation	1.008	0.646 1.573	0.973	1.259	0.607 2.612	0.535	0.861	0.49 1.512	0.602
Peripheral vascular disease	1.765	1.126 2.768	0.013	0.906	0.276 2.975	0.871	1.719	1.022 2.89	0.041
Diabetes mellitus	1.223	0.730 2.049	0.444	0.979	0.377 2.542	0.965	1.315	0.711 2.435	0.383
Prior myocardial infarction	1.245	0.743 2.085	0.406	1.236	0.476 3.208	0.664	1.114	0.602 2.061	0.732
Permanent pacemaker	1.215	0.717 2.058	0.47	1.101	0.476 2.545	0.822	1.591	0.806 3.142	0.181
Previous CABG	1.141	0.665 1.958	0.632	1.229	0.473 3.191	0.672	1.01	0.525 1.945	0.976
Cerebrovascular disease	2.042	1.281 3.256	0.003	1.076	0.377 3.066	0.892	2.322	1.354 3.982	0.002
Cerebrovascular accident	1.132	0.629 2.035	0.68	0.855	0.3 2.439	0.77	1.417	0.697 2.882	0.336
COPD	1.744	1.041 2.921	0.035	1.862	0.653 5.31	0.245	1.432	0.786 2.609	0.241
Previous valve surgery	0.63	0.275 1.441	0.274	0.27	0.037 1.977	0.197	0.889	0.356 2.222	0.801
Liver cirrhosis	1.545	0.715 3.34	0.269	2.564	0.781 8.417	0.121	1.057	0.383 2.917	0.915
Home oxygen dependence	3.294	1.208 8.983	0.020	1.695	0.231 12.415	0.604	6.334	1.963 20.438	0.002
Wheel chair dependency	3.402	0.838 13.818	0.087	4.976	1.188 20.844	0.028			
Renal replacement therapy	1.614	0.225 11.584	0.634				1.235	0.171 8.914	0.835
Creatinine mg/dL	1.221	0.959 1.555	0.105	1.184	0.634 2.212	0.596	1.186	0.917 1.534	0.193
Preinterventional echocardiographic data									
Aortic valve area	2.798	0.812 9.64	0.103	3.07	0.408 23.085	0.276	2.219	0.454 10.839	0.325
Mean pressure gradient	0.986	0.974 0.998	0.020	0.983	0.959 1.008	0.175	0.989	0.977 1.003	0.113
Max. pressure gradient	0.988	0.979 0.997	0.009	0.987	0.97 1.005	0.156	0.99	0.98 1	0.051
Peak velocity m/sec	0.841	0.659 1.072	0.161	0.871	0.576 1.316	0.511	0.841	0.621 1.139	0.262
LVEF %	0.988	0.971 1.006	0.186	1.003	0.974 1.034	0.826	0.981	0.959 1.004	0.107
Low-flow-low-gradient stenosis	1.509	0.901 2.528	0.118	1.581	0.651 3.842	0.312	1.397	0.741 2.633	0.302

CABG—coronary artery bypass graft; COPD—chronic obstructive pulmonary disease; EuroSCORE—European System for Cardiac Operative Risk Evaluation; LVEF—left ventricular ejection fraction; PCI—percutaneous coronary intervention; TA—transapical; TAVR—transcatheter aortic valve replacement; TF—transfemoral.

Table 3. Univariate Cox regression analyses of futile events based on interventional parameters. A hazard ratio (HR) above 1 increases the risk, below 1 decreases the risk of futility.

	Combined Access			TF-TAVR			TA-TAVR		
	HR	95% CI	p-Value	HR	95% CI	p-Value	HR	95% CI	p-Value
Dichotomic parameters									
Predilatation necessary	1.469	0.909 2.374	0.116	1.448 0.508 4.127		0.489	2.046	1.175 3.561	0.011
Balloon expanding valve	1.091	0.723 1.647	0.677	1.085 0.502 2.346		0.835	0.629	0.367 1.079	0.092
Postdilatation necessary	1.322	0.805 2.171	0.271	0.872 0.336 2.265		0.779	1.61	0.896 2.893	0.111
Conversion to open surgery	7.023	3.066 16.083	<0.001	0 0 Inf		0.998	7.166	3.075 16.697	<0.001
Unplanned V-i-V implantation	0	0 Inf	0.995	0 0 Inf		0.996	0	0 Inf	0.995
Interval scaled parameters									
Prosthesis size	0.955	0.872 1.046	0.319	0.981 0.839 1.148		0.811	1.045	0.911 1.199	0.53
Absorbed radiation	1	1 1	0.196	1 1 1		0.844	1	1 1	0.888
Contrast medium dosage	1	0.999 1.001	0.521	1.002 1.001 1.003		<0.001	1	0.998 1.002	0.776
Procedure time	1.003	1 1.006	0.072	0.999 0.989 1.01		0.885	1.003	1 1.006	0.037
Max. creatinine in 72 h	1.126	0.874 1.451	0.359	1.026 0.587 1.793		0.927	1.124	0.839 1.506	0.434
Total hours in the ICU	1.004	1.002 1.005	<0.001	1.006 1.002 1.009		0.001	1.003	1.002 1.004	<0.001
Total hours ventilated	1.007	1.005 1.009	<0.001	1.001 0.988 1.013		0.936	1.008	1.006 1.011	<0.001
Length of hospital stay	1.028	1.015 1.042	<0.001	1.019 0.993 1.046		0.151	1.038	1.019 1.058	<0.001

ICU—intensive care unit; MAD—median deviation of the median; TA—transapical; TAVR—transcatheter aortic valve replacement; TF—transfemoral, V-i-V—valve in valve.

In the TF subgroup, applied contrast medium dosage and total ICU hours were significantly associated with futile TAVR treatment. In the TA subgroup, predilatation, conversion to open surgery, total ICU hours, total hours ventilated, and length of in-hospital stay after TAVR showed significantly increased hazard ratios (Table 3).

After multivariate Cox regression analysis total hours in the ICU and length of stay after TAVR remained independently associated with futile treatment in the TF and the TA groups, respectively (Supplementary Table S2)

3.4. Adverse Events

In the combined access cohort, the VARC-2 composite endpoints of device success and the 30-day combined safety endpoint as well as acute kidney injury, new atrial fibrillation, reoperation for non-cardiac problems, reoperation for bleeding/tamponade, major bleeding complications, new renal replacement therapy, neurological adverse events, and peri- or postinterventional myocardial infarction were associated with futile treatment within the first year after TAVR following univariate Cox regression analysis (Table 4).

Major bleeding complications, neurological adverse events, and the maximum pressure gradient across the TAVR prosthesis were significantly associated with futile TAVR treatment in the TF subgroup in the univariate regression model (Table 4).

Device success, the 30-day combined safety endpoint, acute kidney injury, new atrial fibrillation, reoperation for non-cardiac problems, reoperation for bleeding/tamponade, pneumonia under antibiotic treatment, major bleeding complications, new renal replacement therapy, major vascular complication, neurological adverse events, reoperation for valvular dysfunction, and myocardial infarction showed to be negative factors of survival within the first year after TA-TAVR (Table 4).

Multivariate Cox regression analysis identified an increased risk of futility with new renal replacement therapy in the combined access cohort. Major bleeding complication and myocardial infarction were independently associated with futility following TA-TAVR (Supplementary Table S3).

Table 4. Univariate Cox regression analyses of futile events based on postinterventional adverse events. A hazard ratio (HR) above 1 increases the risk, below 1 decreases the risk of futility.

	Combined access				TF-TAVR				TA-TAVR			
	HR	95% CI		p-Value	HR	95% CI		p-Value	HR	95% CI		p-Value
Dichotomic parameters												
Device success	0.528	0.294	0.95	0.033	0.65	0.267	1.579	0.341	0.219	0.099	0.482	<0.001
30-day combined safety endpoint	0.117	0.078	0.178	<0.001	0.095	0.047	0.19	<0.001	0.135	0.081	0.226	<0.001
Acute kidney injury	1.764	1.083	2.873	0.023	1.413	0.611	3.267	0.419	2.196	1.205	4.003	0.01
New pacemaker implanted	0.619	0.299	1.28	0.196	0.833	0.32	2.17	0.709	0.553	0.173	1.77	0.318
New AV-block III	0.526	0.23	1.205	0.129	0.448	0.107	1.877	0.272	0.603	0.218	1.667	0.33
New atrial fibrillation	1.927	1.122	3.309	0.017	1.389	0.422	4.569	0.589	1.905	1.029	3.528	0.04
Major bleeding complication	4.267	2.657	6.852	<0.001	6.289	2.82	14.024	<0.001	3.133	1.742	5.634	<0.001
Reoperation for bleeding/tamponade	2.788	1.548	5.021	0.001	2.268	0.689	7.46	0.178	2.772	1.402	5.479	0.003
Reoperation for other cardiac problems	1.659	0.903	3.047	0.103	1.893	0.776	4.614	0.161	1.822	0.783	4.24	0.164
Reoperation for non-cardiac problems	2.453	1.387	4.339	0.002	1.809	0.432	7.584	0.417	2.267	1.202	4.276	0.011
Pneumonia under antibiotic treatment	1.843	0.926	3.669	0.082	0.374	0.051	2.739	0.333	5.042	2.378	10.688	<0.001
New renal replacement therapy	6.319	3.352	11.91	<0.001	2.914	0.696	12.201	0.143	9.582	4.636	19.808	<0.001
Major vascular complication	1.952	0.716	5.319	0.191	0	0	Inf	0.997	5.513	1.996	15.225	0.001
Neurological adverse event	3.576	1.45	8.818	0.006	4.086	1.243	13.432	0.02	4.486	1.091	18.455	0.038
Reoperation for valvular dysfunction	3.491	0.859	14.194	0.081	0	0	Inf	0.998	4.237	1.03	17.434	0.045
Myocardial infarction	8.152	2.003	33.17	0.003	0	0	Inf	0.998	41.535	9.121	189.135	<0.001
Interval scaled parameters post-implant												
Mean gradient aortic valve	0.955	0.872	1.046	0.319	0.981	0.839	1.148	0.811	1.045	0.911	1.199	0.53
Max. gradient aortic valve	1	1	1	0.196	1	1	1.003	0.844	1	1	1	0.888
Max. flow velocity aortic valve	1	0.999	1.001	0.521	1.002	1.001	1.003	<0.001	1	0.998	1.002	0.776

AV—atrioventricular; MAD—median deviation of the median; TA—transapical; TAVR—transcatheter aortic valve replacement; TF—transfemoral.

4. Discussion

The reported 1-year mortality rates following TAVR range between 1% and 14.5%, depending on whether the patients belong to the low or intermediate risk group [3,5,18,19]. This suggests that, although this treatment option is not as invasive as surgical aortic valve replacement (SAVR) and carries many associated benefits, a considerable number of patients will fail to show signs of clinical improvement and are at an increased risk of dying shortly after the procedure. Depending on the patient's comorbidities and further clinical factors, the choice of access is most often made between the TF and the TA access site. The latter remains the main alternative access route in most hospitals worldwide despite other potentially less invasive access route strategies. The respective patient cohorts differ both in their preclinical makeup and in the range of postinterventional adverse events and outcomes. Thus, in our study, we attempted to highlight some of the most important risk factors for futility for the combined access patient collective, on the one hand, but more importantly, we considered these factors for both access sites independently in order help optimize patient selection, access site allocation, promote a fast-track post-operative course, early discharge, and thus, improve overall survival. Thus, in our work, we were not only able to validate certain parameters that have been demonstrated to be significant predictors for futility in existing research, but based on our extensive database structure, we were also able to identify several new parameters that have received little attention in the past and have not yet found their way into clinical trials.

4.1. Clinical Baseline Characteristics

Our study has been able to confirm that TA access is an independent predictor of 1-year mortality following TAVR, which has been demonstrated by Mohr et al. [20]. Whilst in the TF-TAVR group, the 1-year mortality was 12.0%; in the TA-TAVR group, the 1-year mortality showed to be 22.2%. Expectedly, the logistic EuroSCORE and the EuroSCORE II correlated well with the risk of futile treatment following TA-TAVR in the first year, a mean EuroSCORE II of 4.6 means a hazard ratio (HR) of 1.4 (=$1.069^{4.6}$), a EuroSCORE of 10 a HR of 1.9 (=1.069^{10}), and a EuroSCORE II of 15 a HR of 2.7 (=1.069^{15}). Therefore, they need to be interpreted with due caution especially in combination with the identified risk factors of futility during the preinterventional assessment.

The major indications for a TA approach are primarily the inability to perform the valve replacement through a TF approach due to small vessel size or their prominent tortuosity or calcification, a history of previous vascular interventions in the aorta, the iliac or femoral arteries, or a pronounced obesity with deep vessels and, thus, a high risk of vascular complications [21–26]. In contrast, the list of contraindications for a TA access procedure is rather short and mostly revolves around a reduced ejection fraction or thrombotic material in the apex area [21–23].

We identified PVD to occur in one fifth of the patients in the combined access cohort with a HR of 1.7 for futile treatment. Interestingly, patients with pronounced PVD were also found to be less likely to benefit from the TA access. Since atherosclerosis is known to be a systemic disease, it is mostly not limited to a single artery territory, but spread to the whole organism. CVD, on the other hand, puts the patient at a 2.3-fold higher risk of undergoing futile TA-TAVR treatment and affects every sixth patient. After multivariate Cox regression analysis, CVD remained the strongest predictor for 1-year mortality following TAVR in the combined access cohort and the TA access group. Thus, we advocate that patients with a combination of CVD and pronounced PVD be subjected to a more stringent risk–benefit analysis prior to undergoing TA-TAVR.

One of the most prominent novel findings in our TF-TAVR cohort is wheelchair use as a predictor of TF-TAVR futility that is currently not regularly considered and evaluated when planning TAVR interventions and choosing the access site. It should also be questioned whether and to what extent this patient collective is likely to subjectively benefit from an increase in their physical resilience. Thus, this finding warrants further studies in this particular patient collective.

Although it is well established in the recent literature that COPD as a concomitant risk factor does not necessarily lead to a worse outcome after TA-TAVR, our study demonstrated that pronounced pulmonary oxygenation impairment resulting in home oxygen dependence is significantly associated with futile treatment after TA-TAVR [27]. However, it has to be pointed out that home oxygen dependence is a very rare clinical condition with an overall incidence of less than 2%, yet should be incorporated in the preinterventional decision making process when present.

Additionally, a lower preinterventional mean and maximum pressure gradient across the aortic valve such as is often encountered in patients with low-flow–low-gradient aortic stenosis were associated with futile TAVR treatment in the overall TAVR group. This finding is consistent with evidence from the recent literature [PMID: 31000012, PMID: 33289422] and emphasizes the importance of correctly interpreting long-term myocardial sequelae rather than assessing LVEF alone in preinterventional risk assessment. As the overall incidence paradoxical low-flow–low-gradient aortic stenosis was rather low (<1% in the entire cohort), our finding supports the hypothesis that patients with a low LVEF and consecutively low pressure gradients across the aortic valve display worse postinterventional outcome after TAVR than patients with a low LVEF that can nevertheless generate high gradients across the aortic valve [28–30]. The absence of the binary variable low-flow–low-gradient aortic stenosis in our cohort as a significant predictor of futile treatment at 1 year indicates that pressure gradients are likely to have a higher sensitivity due to the relatively high cut-off value of 50% for LVEF in the current guidelines. Substratification within this patient population based on their LVEF could potentially provide new, important conclusions in future analyses.

4.2. Interventional Factors

Although technical procedure-related problems are diverse and hard to predict, our results once again underpin the importance of avoiding a conversion to open heart surgery, most importantly through a precise preinterventional risk assessment. The severity of this rare complication is perhaps best illustrated by the fact that only three of the nine patients who underwent a conversion to SAVR survived past the 1-year timepoint. The procedures documented in this study were all undertaken in either a cardiac catheterization laboratory or a standard operating room (OR). The implementation of TAVR in a hybrid OR may provide distinct advantages such as prompt treatment of unplanned procedures or procedures requiring circulatory support, as well as the optimal infrastructural background for the collaboration between cardiologists and cardiothoracic surgeons. At our institution, all TAVR procedures are now performed in the hybrid OR. This approach seems to be the optimal way to maximize the safety and comfort of the patient and enable the staff to perform the most complex bail-out procedures at maximum speed and efficiency. In line with already available data, some of the more prominent drivers were increased ventilation times, prolonged ICU and hospital stay in the combined access cohort [12], and total hours at the ICU in the TF-TAVR group, respectively. However, the factor time must not be regarded as a cause rather than effect and relates to severely ill patients. Consequently, our data further indicate that a prolonged procedure time was associated with a worse outcome in the TA access cohort, with this increase generally attributable to either increased difficulty of the surgical procedure itself (due to patient-specific anatomic conditions) or intraoperative complications.

With respect to the choice of anesthesia, opting for conscious sedation rather than general anesthesia has gained popularity over the last couple of years, especially in patients with ventilatory disorders and difficult airways. Patients with chronic lung disease are particularly prone to prolonged ventilation times, which negatively impact the weaning process and extend the length of their ICU and hospital stay [31]. Thus, ventilation times must be interpreted as a surrogate parameter for several clinical factors including preinterventional morbidity, interventional complexity, and postinterventional complications, as well as frailty. Another important contributing factor towards a prolonged postinterventional course is the increased risk of pneumonia requiring antibiotic treatment in the transapical cohort. Furthermore, home oxygen dependence as a predictor of futility in the TA-TAVR group is likely to result in longer ventilation times and a correspondingly prolonged ICU stay. It is important to point out that the TF patients whose data were collected for this study were not routinely treated under conscious sedation, a standard in our institution since 2014.

4.3. Success Factors and Adverse Events

As expected, the VARC-2 composite endpoints of device success and safety at thirty days are closely related to the risk of futility after TAVR. Other adverse events that were identified as significant predictors of TAVR futility include acute kidney injury, postinterventional renal replacement therapy, major bleeding complications, new-onset atrial fibrillation reoperation for non-cardiac problems or reoperation for bleeding or cardiac tamponade, neurological adverse events, and myocardial infarction [32]. Acute kidney injury is one of the most recognized complications following TAVR and plays a key role in short- and long-term mortality. New renal replacement therapy was associated with a six-fold increased risk of futility in the combined access cohort and a nearly 10-fold increase in risk in the TA-TAVR group. This finding particularly stresses the importance of future research being directed towards preventive strategies to reduce the incidence of acute kidney injury following TAVR. While major bleeding complications occurred in both the transfemoral and transapical cohorts, they resulted in an associated hazard ratio of 4.2 in the combined access cohort, highlighting the importance of careful postinterventional hemostasis. Neurological adverse events following TAVR displayed as one of the overarching risk factors for futile procedures in both cohorts, and thus, we have to emphasize the importance of developing and expanding periinterventional neuroprotection protocols and improving the preinterventional risk assessment in patients with a history of cerebrovascular disease with regard to stroke prevention. These findings are in line with results presented in the recent literature [24,33]. However, in the multivariate analysis, major bleeding complications and neurological adverse events were outperformed by the 30-day composite safety endpoint.

Although periinterventional myocardial infarction occurred with an overall incidence of only 0.6%, it should be noted that this pivotal clinical event was associated with a 40-fold increased risk of futile treatment in the TA-TAVR cohort and, hence, warrants special consideration in high-risk settings such as valve-in-valve procedures in failed bioprostheses with outside-mounted leaflets.

As the volume of data available on the topic of TF-TAVR is high due to the increasing number of conducted interventions, it is important to point out that a standardized tool to identify patients for whom a futile intervention seems likely is still not available, and many futility predictors might not yet have been identified. In this respect, and with the ever-increasing number of TAVR patients and indications, it is important, both in order to optimize resource distribution in the healthcare system and to avoid unnecessary interventions, to work towards identifying comorbidities that might make a futile TAVR highly likely. The proportion of patients treated through a TA access site in our cohort is relatively high because of the high referral rate of patients ineligible for a TF approach, and the TF-TAVR route remains the first-choice treatment for most patients, due to its low invasiveness and good outcomes. However, it is important to recognize that the results of side-by-side comparisons of TF- and TA-TAVR are often skewed by the makeup of the patient collective [34]. To summarize, the choice of access site is more than a purely technical consideration, and it is paramount that all patients undergo a detailed preinterventional evaluation in order to choose the optimal access point and plan the intervention depending on the patient's anatomy [21–23,35]. Further research should be directed towards exploring the possibility that the poor TA-TAVR-associated outcome might be improved by identifying patient subgroups that might have a high futility risk and might benefit from an entirely different access point.

5. Study Limitations

Futility has not yet been defined in any of the current valvular heart disease guidelines. Furthermore, there is no common agreement on which the quality of life (QOL) assessment tool should be used before and after TAVR and how "improvement" is defined. Due to the wide range of symptoms and the varying clinical state of the patients, different QOL indicators might only be applicable to or disproportionately subjectively valued by certain patient subgroups. Inherent limitations of this study are the retrospective single-center design and the fact that the assessment was based solely on clinical endpoints and available registry data. This is mostly a direct consequence of the fact that the patient collective stems from multiple regions of Austria, and further follow-up examinations mostly take place in the referring institution. The number of events in each group is small, which should be considered when establishing statistical comparisons. Technical advances, the implementation of new generation THV devices, and an inherent learning curve could have biased outcomes. Furthermore, there is currently an ever-increasing shift towards performing TAVR in a hybrid OR, whilst the interventions described in the study took place in a cardiac catheterization laboratory or a standard OR.

6. Conclusions

In our study, we attempted to highlight some of the most important risk factors for futility for TAVR patients on the one hand, but more importantly we considered these factors for both access sites, TF and TA, independently in order help optimize patient selection, access site allocation, promote a fast-track post-operative course, early discharge, and thus, improve overall survival. Factors were addressed in three groups according to their timely order (pre-, intra-, and post-procedure).

Our findings suggest reevaluating and expanding neuroprotection protocols for all patients following TAVR, but particularly for patients with a history of cerebrovascular disease. Furthermore, strategies to prevent major bleeding complications are of particular importance, especially in the patients treated via transapical access. With an almost two-fold increase in risk for futility after TAVR, the transapical access should be strictly restricted to patients with no viable option for percutaneous transfemoral treatment. A more detailed risk assessment of oxygen and wheelchair-dependent patients seems warranted in patients treated via transapical and transfemoral access pathways, respectively.

Supplementary Materials: The following are available online at https://www.mdpi.com/article/10.3390/jcm10214911/s1, Supplementary Table S1: Multivariate Cox regression analyses of futile events based on patients' baseline characteristics of preoperative factors. Supplementary Table S2: Multivariate Cox regression analyses of futile events based on patients' interventional characteristics. Supplementary Table S3: Multivariate Cox regression analyses of futile events based on patients' VARC-2 adverse events.

Author Contributions: Conceptualization: M.M. and C.A.; methodology, M.M.; validation, M.A., M.G. and G.D.-K.; formal analysis, M.M.; investigation, A.S.; resources, M.G.; writing—original draft preparation, D.G.; data curation and writing—review and editing, P.N.R., W.H., E.H., and M.A.; visualization, G.W.; supervision, A.S. and M.M.; project administration, B.W. All authors have read and agreed to the published version of the manuscript.

Funding: This research received no external funding.

Institutional Review Board Statement: The study was conducted according to the guidelines of the Declaration of Helsinki and approved by the Institutional Ethics Committee of the City of Vienna (EK18-027-VK; 1 March 2018).

Informed Consent Statement: Patient consent was waived due to the retrospective nature of the analysis.

Data Availability Statement: The data presented in this study are available on reasonable request from the corresponding author.

Acknowledgments: The authors would like to express their special gratitude to Francesco Maisano, Maurizio Taramasso, Carlos Mestres, Barbara Jenny, and the extended CAS Cardiac Structural Interventions Faculty for creating an immensely inspiring environment that supported the clinical, academic, and scientific pillars of our field of work and helped us to transcend traditional boundaries into a new, modern, and pioneering era of structural heart interventions.

Conflicts of Interest: Markus Mach has received institutional grants from Symetis, Edwards Lifesciences, and JenaValve. Martin Andreas is a proctor for Edwards Lifesciences and Abbott and an advisor for Medtronic. Martin Andreas has received institutional grants from LSI, Edwards Lifesciences, Medtronic, and Abbott. All other authors have reported that they have no relationships to disclose that would be relevant to the contents of this paper.

References

1. Braghiroli, J.; Kapoor, K.; Thielhelm, T.P.; Ferreira, T.; Cohen, M.G. Transcatheter aortic valve replacement in low risk patients: A review of PARTNER 3 and Evolut low risk trials. *Cardiovasc. Diagn. Ther.* **2020**, *10*, 59–71. [CrossRef]
2. Falk, V.; Baumgartner, H.; Bax, J.J.; De Bonis, M.; Hamm, C.; Holm, P.J.; Iung, B.; Lancellotti, P.; Lansac, E.; Muñoz, D.R.; et al. 2017 ESC/EACTS Guidelines for the Management of Valvular Heart Disease. *Rev. Esp. Cardiol.* **2018**, *71*, 110. [CrossRef]
3. Mack, M.J.; Leon, M.B.; Thourani, V.H.; Makkar, R.; Kodali, S.K.; Russo, M.; Kapadia, S.R.; Malaisrie, S.C.; Cohen, D.J.; Pibarot, P.; et al. Transcatheter Aortic-Valve Replacement with a Balloon-Expandable Valve in Low-Risk Patients. *N. Engl. J. Med.* **2019**, *380*, 1695–1705. [CrossRef]
4. Mack, M.J.; Leon, M.B.; Smith, C.R.; Miller, D.C.; Moses, J.W.; Tuzcu, E.M.; Webb, J.G.; Douglas, P.S.; Anderson, W.N.; Blackstone, E.H.; et al. 5-year outcomes of transcatheter aortic valve replacement or surgical aortic valve replacement for high surgical risk patients with aortic stenosis (PARTNER 1): A randomised controlled trial. *Lancet* **2015**, *385*, 2477–2484. [CrossRef]
5. Popma, J.J.; Deeb, G.M.; Yakubov, S.J.; Mumtaz, M.; Gada, H.; O'Hair, D.; Bajwa, T.; Heiser, J.C.; Merhi, W.; Kleiman, N.S.; et al. Transcatheter Aortic-Valve Replacement with a Self-Expanding Valve in Low-Risk Patients. *N. Engl. J. Med.* **2019**, *380*, 1706–1715. [CrossRef]
6. Orlando, R.; Pennant, M.; Rooney, S.; Khogali, S.; Bayliss, S.; Hassan, A.; Moore, D.; Barton, P. Cost-effectiveness of transcatheter aortic valve implantation (TAVI) for aortic stenosis in patients who are high risk or contraindicated for surgery: A model-based economic evaluation. *Heal. Technol. Assess.* **2013**, *17*, 1–86. [CrossRef] [PubMed]
7. Baron, S.J.; Wang, K.; House, J.A.; Magnuson, E.A.; Reynolds, M.R.; Makkar, R.; Herrmann, H.C.; Kodali, S.; Thourani, V.H.; Kapadia, S.; et al. Cost-Effectiveness of Transcatheter Versus Surgical Aortic Valve Replacement in Patients with Severe Aortic Stenosis at Intermediate Risk. *Circulation* **2019**, *139*, 877–888. [CrossRef]
8. Geisler, B.P.; Jørgensen, T.H.; Thyregod, H.G.H.; Pietzsch, J.B.; Søndergaard, L. Cost-effectiveness of transcatheter versus surgical aortic valve replacement in patients at lower surgical risk: Results from the NOTION trial. *EuroIntervention* **2019**, *15*, e959–e967. [CrossRef] [PubMed]
9. Van Mourik, M.S.; Vendrik, J.; Abdelghani, M.; van Kesteren, F.; Henriques, J.P.; Driessen, A.H.; Wykrzykowska, J.J.; de Winter, R.J.; Piek, J.J.; Tijssen, J.G.; et al. Guideline-defined futility or patient-reported outcomes to assess treatment success after TAVI: What to use? Results from a prospective cohort study with long-term follow-up. *Open Heart* **2018**, *5*, e000879. [CrossRef]

10. Martin, G.P.; Sperrin, M.; Ludman, P.F.; De Belder, M.A.; Gale, C.P.; Toff, W.D.; Moat, N.E.; Trivedi, U.; Buchan, I.; Mamas, M.A. Inadequacy of existing clinical prediction models for predicting mortality after transcatheter aortic valve implantation. *Am. Hear J.* **2016**, *184*, 97–105. [CrossRef] [PubMed]
11. Conradi, L.; Seiffert, M.; Schnabel, R.; Schön, G.; Blankenberg, S.; Reichenspurner, H.; Diemert, P.; Treede, H.; Silaschi, M. Predicting Risk in Transcatheter Aortic Valve Implantation: Comparative Analysis of EuroSCORE II and Established Risk Stratification Tools. *Thorac. Cardiovasc. Surg.* **2014**, *63*, 472–478. [CrossRef]
12. Amrane, H.; Deeb, G.M.; Popma, J.J.; Yakubov, S.J.; Gleason, T.G.; Van Mieghem, N.M.; Reardon, M.J.; Williams, M.R.; Mumtaz, M.; Kappetein, A.P.; et al. Causes of death in intermediate-risk patients: The Randomized Surgical Replacement and Transcatheter Aortic Valve Implantation Trial. *J. Thorac. Cardiovasc. Surg.* **2019**, *158*, 718–728.e3. [CrossRef]
13. Dewey, T.M.; Brown, D.; Ryan, W.H.; Herbert, M.A.; Prince, S.L.; Mack, M.J. Reliability of risk algorithms in predicting early and late operative outcomes in high-risk patients undergoing aortic valve replacement. *J. Thorac. Cardiovasc. Surg.* **2008**, *135*, 180–187. [CrossRef] [PubMed]
14. Nashef, S.A.; Roques, F.; Sharples, L.D.; Nilsson, J.; Smith, C.; Goldstone, A.R.; Lockowandt, U.; Euroscore, i.i. EuroSCORE II. *Eur. J. Cardiothorac Surg.* **2012**, *41*, 734–744. [CrossRef]
15. Roques, F.; Michel, P.; Goldstone, A.; Nashef, S. The logistic EuroSCORE. *Eur. Hear J.* **2003**, *24*, 882–883. [CrossRef]
16. Mach, M.; Wilbring, M.; Winkler, B.; Alexiou, K.; Kappert, U.; Delle-Karth, G.; Grabenwöger, M.; Matschke, K. Cut-down outperforms complete percutaneous transcatheter valve implantation. *Asian Cardiovasc. Thorac. Ann.* **2018**, *26*, 107–113. [CrossRef]
17. Kappetein, A.P.; Head, S.J.; Généreux, P.; Piazza, N.; Van Mieghem, N.M.; Blackstone, E.H.; Brott, T.G.; Cohen, D.J.; Cutlip, D.E.; Van Es, G.-A.; et al. Updated standardized endpoint definitions for transcatheter aortic valve implantation: The Valve Academic Research Consortium-2 consensus document (VARC-2). *Eur. J. Cardio-Thoracic Surg.* **2012**, *42*, S45–S60. [CrossRef]
18. Reardon, M.J.; Van Mieghem, N.M.; Popma, J.J.; Kleiman, N.S.; Søndergaard, L.; Mumtaz, M.; Adams, D.H.; Deeb, G.M.; Maini, B.; Gada, H.; et al. Surgical or Transcatheter Aortic-Valve Replacement in Intermediate-Risk Patients. *N. Engl. J. Med.* **2017**, *376*, 1321–1331. [CrossRef] [PubMed]
19. Leon, M.B.; Smith, C.R.; Mack, M.J.; Makkar, R.R.; Svensson, L.G.; Kodali, S.K.; Thourani, V.H.; Tuzcu, E.M.; Miller, D.C.; Herrmann, H.C.; et al. Transcatheter or Surgical Aortic-Valve Replacement in Intermediate-Risk Patients. *N. Engl. J. Med.* **2016**, *374*, 1609–1620. [CrossRef]
20. Mohr, F.W.; Holzhey, D.; Möllmann, H.; Beckmann, A.; Veit, C.; Figulla, H.R.; Cremer, J.; Kuck, K.-H.; Lange, R.; Zahn, R.; et al. The German Aortic Valve Registry: 1-year results from 13 680 patients with aortic valve disease. *Eur. J. Cardio-Thoracic Surg.* **2014**, *46*, 808–816. [CrossRef] [PubMed]
21. Biasco, L.; Ferrari, E.; Pedrazzini, G.; Faletra, F.; Moccetti, T.; Petracca, F.; Moccetti, M. Access Sites for TAVI: Patient Selection Criteria, Technical Aspects, and Outcomes. *Front. Cardiovasc. Med.* **2018**, *5*, 88. [CrossRef] [PubMed]
22. Madigan, M.; Atoui, R. Non-transfemoral access sites for transcatheter aortic valve replacement. *J. Thorac. Dis.* **2018**, *10*, 4505–4515. [CrossRef]
23. Bleiziffer, S.; Krane, M.; Deutsch, M.; Elhmidi, Y.; Piazza, N.; Voss, B.; Lange, R. Which way in? The Necessity of Multiple Approaches to Transcatheter Valve Therapy. *Curr. Cardiol. Rev.* **2014**, *9*, 268–273. [CrossRef] [PubMed]
24. Gaasch, W.H.; D'Agostino, R.S. Transcatheter aortic valve implantation: The transfemoral versus the transapical approach. *Ann. Cardiothorac. Surg.* **2012**, *1*, 200–205. [CrossRef] [PubMed]
25. Ramlawi, B.; Anaya-Ayala, J.E.; Reardon, M.J. Transcatheter Aortic Valve Replacement (TAVR): Access Planning and Strategies. *Methodist DeBakey Cardiovasc. J.* **2012**, *8*, 22–25. [CrossRef]
26. Mach, M.; Poschner, T.; Hasan, W.; Szalkiewicz, P.; Andreas, M.; Winkler, B.; Geisler, S.; Geisler, D.; Rudziński, P.N.; Watzal, V.; et al. The Iliofemoral tortuosity score predicts access and bleeding complications during transfemoral transcatheter aortic valve replacement: DataData from the VIenna Cardio Thoracic aOrtic valve registrY (VICTORY). *Eur. J. Clin. Investig.* **2021**, *51*, e13491.
27. Mach, M.; Koschutnik, M.; Wilbring, M.; Winkler, B.; Reinweber, M.; Alexiou, K.; Kappert, U.; Adlbrecht, C.; Delle-Karth, G.; Grabenwöger, M.; et al. Impact of COPD on Outcome in Patients Undergoing Transfemoral versus Transapical TAVI. *Thorac. Cardiovasc. Surg.* **2019**, *67*, 251–256. [CrossRef]
28. Conrotto, F.; D'Ascenzo, F.; D'Amico, M.; Moretti, C.; Pavani, M.; Scacciatella, P.; Omedè, P.; Montefusco, A.; Biondi-Zoccai, G.; Gaita, F.; et al. Outcomes of patients with low-pressure aortic gradient undergoing transcatheter aortic valve implantation: A Meta-analysis. *Catheter. Cardiovasc. Interv.* **2017**, *89*, 1100–1106. [CrossRef]
29. Conrotto, F.; D'Ascenzo, F.; Stella, P.; Pavani, M.; Rossi, M.L.; Brambilla, N.; Napodano, M.; Covolo, E.; Saia, F.; Tarantini, G.; et al. Transcatheter aortic valve implantation in low ejection fraction/low transvalvular gradient patients: The rule of 40. *J. Cardiovasc Med. (Hagerstown)* **2017**, *18*, 103–108. [CrossRef]
30. Penso, M.; Pepi, M.; Fusini, L.; Muratori, M.; Cefalù, C.; Mantegazza, V.; Gripari, P.; Ali, S.; Fabbiocchi, F.; Bartorelli, A.; et al. Predicting Long-Term Mortality in TAVI Patients Using Machine Learning Techniques. *J. Cardiovasc. Dev. Dis.* **2021**, *8*, 44. [CrossRef]
31. Afshar, A.H.; Pourafkari, L.; Nader, N.D. Periprocedural considerations of transcatheter aortic valve implantation for anesthesiologists. *J. Cardiovasc. Thorac. Res.* **2016**, *8*, 49–55. [CrossRef] [PubMed]

32. Conrotto, F.; Salizzoni, S.; Andreis, A.; D'Ascenzo, F.; D'Onofrio, A.; Agrifoglio, M.; Chieffo, A.; Colombo, A.; Rapetto, F.; Santini, F.; et al. Transcatheter Aortic Valve Implantation in Patients with Advanced Chronic Kidney Disease. *Am. J. Cardiol.* **2017**, *119*, 1438–1442. [CrossRef] [PubMed]
33. Van Der Boon, R.M.; Marcheix, B.; Tchetche, D.; Chieffo, A.; Van Mieghem, N.M.; Dumonteil, N.; Vahdat, O.; Maisano, F.; Serruys, P.W.; Kappetein, A.P.; et al. Transapical versus transfemoral aortic valve implantation: A multicenter collaborative study. *Ann. Thorac. Surg.* **2014**, *97*, 22–28. [CrossRef] [PubMed]
34. Schymik, G.; Würth, A.; Bramlage, P.; Herbinger, T.; Heimeshoff, M.; Pilz, L.; Schymik, J.S.; Wondraschek, R.; Süselbeck, T.; Gerhardus, J.; et al. Long-Term Results of Transapical Versus Transfemoral TAVI in a Real World Population of 1000 Patients With Severe Symptomatic Aortic Stenosis. *Circ. Cardiovasc. Interv.* **2015**, *8*, e000761. [CrossRef]
35. Pascual, I.; Carro, A.; Avanzas, P.; Hernandez-Vaquero, D.; Díaz, R.; Rozado, J.; Lorca, R.; Martín, M.; Silva, J.; Morís, C. Vascular approaches for transcatheter aortic valve implantation. *J. Thorac. Dis.* **2017**, *9*, S478–S487. [CrossRef]

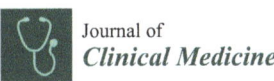

Article

Safety and Efficacy of Four Different Diagnostic Catheter Curves Dedicated to One-Catheter Technique of Transradial Coronaro-Angiography—Prospective, Randomized Pilot Study. TRACT 1: Trans RAdial CoronaryAngiography Trial 1

Michał Chyrchel [1,2], Stanisław Bartuś [1,2], Artur Dziewierz [1,2], Jacek Legutko [3], Paweł Kleczyński [3], Rafał Januszek [1,2], Tomasz Gallina [4], Bernadeta Chyrchel [2], Andrzej Surdacki [1,2] and Łukasz Rzeszutko [1,2,*]

[1] Department of Cardiology and Cardiovascular Interventions, University Hospital, 2 Jakubowskiego Street, 30-688 Cracow, Poland; mchyrchel@gmail.com (M.C.); stanislaw.bartus@uj.edu.pl (S.B.); artur.dziewierz@uj.edu.pl (A.D.); jaanraf@interia.pl (R.J.); andrzej.surdacki@uj.edu.pl (A.S.)

[2] Second Department of Cardiology, Faculty of Medicine, Institute of Cardiology, Jagiellonian University Medical College, 30-688 Cracow, Poland; chyrchelb@gmial.com

[3] Department of Interventional Cardiology, Institute of Cardiology, Jagiellonian University Medical College, John Paul II Hospital, 31-202 Krakow, Poland; jacek.legutko@uj.edu.pl (J.L.); kleczu@interia.pl (P.K.)

[4] Students' Scientific Group, Second Department of Cardiology, Jagiellonian University Medical College, 2 Jakubowskiego Street, 30-688 Krakow, Poland; tomasz.gallina@student.uj.edu.pl

* Correspondence: lrzeszutko@cathlab.krakow.pl; Tel.: +48-12-400-2250; Fax: +48-12-400-2256

Citation: Chyrchel, M.; Bartuś, S.; Dziewierz, A.; Legutko, J.; Kleczyński, P.; Januszek, R.; Gallina, T.; Chyrchel, B.; Surdacki, A.; Rzeszutko, Ł. Safety and Efficacy of Four Different Diagnostic Catheter Curves Dedicated to One-Catheter Technique of Transradial Coronaro-Angiography—Prospective, Randomized Pilot Study. TRACT 1: Trans RAdial CoronaryAngiography Trial 1. *J. Clin. Med.* **2021**, *10*, 4722. https://doi.org/10.3390/jcm10204722

Academic Editor: Fabio Mangiacapra

Received: 28 September 2021
Accepted: 12 October 2021
Published: 14 October 2021

Publisher's Note: MDPI stays neutral with regard to jurisdictional claims in published maps and institutional affiliations.

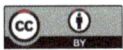

Copyright: © 2021 by the authors. Licensee MDPI, Basel, Switzerland. This article is an open access article distributed under the terms and conditions of the Creative Commons Attribution (CC BY) license (https://creativecommons.org/licenses/by/4.0/).

Abstract: Transradial coronaro-angiography (TRA) can be performed with one catheter. We investigate the efficacy of four different DxTerity catheter curves dedicated to the single-catheter technique and compare this method to the standard two-catheter approach. For this prospective, single-blinded, randomized pilot study, we enrolled 100 patients. In groups 1, 2, 3, and 4, the DxTerity catheters Trapease, Ultra, Transformer and Tracker Curve, respectively, were used. In group 5 (control), standard Judkins catheters were used. The study endpoints were the percentage of optimal stability, proper ostial artery engagement and a good quality angiogram, the duration of each procedure stage, the amount of contrast, and the radiation dose. The highest rate of optimal stability was observed in groups 2 (90%) and 5 (95%). Suboptimal results with at least one episode of catheter fallout from the ostium were most frequent in group 1 (45%). The necessity of using another catheter was observed most frequently in group 4. The analysis of time frames directly depending on the catheter type revealed that the shortest time for catheter introduction and for searching coronary ostia was achieved in group 2 (Ultra). There were no differences in contrast volume and radiation dose between groups. DxTerity catheters are suitable tools to perform TRA coronary angiography. The Ultra Curve catheter demonstrated an advantage over other catheters in terms of its ostial stability rate and procedural time.

Keywords: transradial coronaro-angiography; single-catheter technique; coronary artery disease

1. Introduction

Coronary angiography is still the method of choice in the diagnosis of coronary artery disease. For many years, it was performed mainly from the femoral artery. The radial approach is currently recommended as the first choice for vascular access for this purpose [1]. Transradial coronary angiography (TRA) was introduced by Campeau in 1989 [2] and Kiemeneij in 1992 [3]. In contrast to transfemoral access, TRA reduces major bleeding, access site-related vascular complications, and major adverse cardiac events and enables faster patient mobilization after the procedure [4–6]. TRA can be performed using two standard Judkins diagnostic catheter curves: left and right dedicated to homonymous arteries. Alternatively, TRA can be performed with one catheter designed for a single-catheter technique. Although, comparative data on the performance of different catheters are limited. Thus, in the present study, we sought to investigate the efficacy of four different catheter curves dedicated to a single-catheter technique of TRA and compare the results to the standard two-catheter approach.

2. Materials and Methods

This is a prospective, single-blinded, randomized pilot study. From March 2019 to December 2020, 103 patients were screened in the Second Department of Cardiology, Jagiellonian University in Krakow. Inclusion criteria were as follows: written informed consent, stable coronary artery disease, and qualification for invasive diagnostic angiography, age >18 years, and a good pulse above the radial artery confirmed by physical examination. Exclusion criteria comprised a diagnosis of acute coronary syndrome, cardiogenic shock, previous coronary artery by-pass grafting, pregnancy, renal replacement therapy—hemodialysis with active fistula in forearm, hyperthyroidism, and previous failure of TRA. Before coronary angiography, patients were randomized using a computer-generated list into five groups. In groups 1, 2, 3, and 4, DxTerity TRA diagnosticcCatheters dedicated to the single-catheter technique of TRA angiography from Medtronic (Medtronic, Santa Rosa, CA, USA) were used. Each DxTerity catheter differs in the shape of the tip. The groups used the following catheters: group 1: Trapease Curve catheter 6F $n = 20$; group 2: Ultra Curve catheter 6F $n = 20$; group 3: Transformer Curve catheter 6F $n = 20$; group 4: Tracker Curve catheter 6F $n = 20$. Finally, in group 5 (control, standard two catheter, group), Judkins right 4.0 and Judkins left 3.5 diagnostic catheters were used, 6F $n = 20$ (Figure 1).

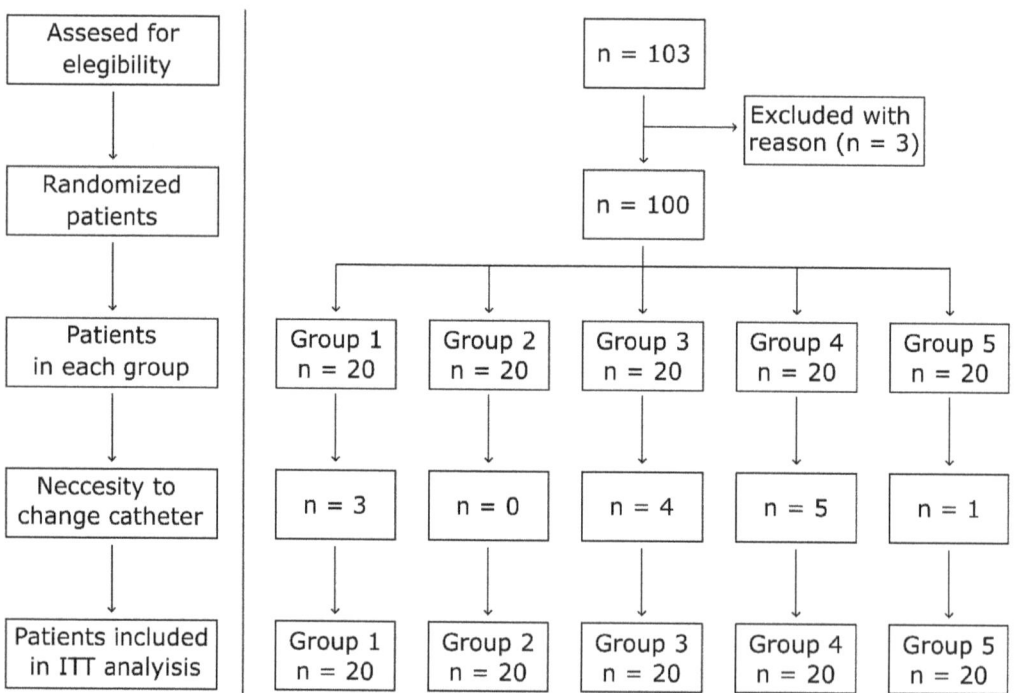

Figure 1. Randomization scheme. ITT—intention to treat; n—number of patients.

All procedures in the study were performed by physicians experienced in the TRA approach. TRA was successfully performed in 100 patients. Three patients were excluded from the study due to ineffective radial artery puncture and radial sheath insertion. In all excluded patients, the procedure was safely completed from the femoral artery without further complications.

Procedures were performed in a standard fashion from the right radial artery using 6F vascular sheaths. After sheath insertion, 5000 IU of unfractionated heparin was injected. Study endpoints included the percentage of catheter stability and proper engagement of coronary artery ostia during contrast injection. Ostial stability was assessed as optimal with grade 1, with proper ostial artery engagement and a good quality angiogram. Suboptimal stability was shown with grade 2, which was determined when at least one diagnostic catheter fell out from the coronary ostium and the catheter position had to be corrected. Finally, the worst stability of grade 3 was determined when ostial engagement was not achieved, and another catheter had to be introduced. The duration of each procedure stage was calculated from catheterization reports prepared by the study technician or nonoperating physician accompanying each procedure:

T1: time of beginning the procedure;

T2: time needed to introduce the diagnostic catheter, from entering the vascular sheath to reaching the ascending aorta;

T3: time needed to properly engage the ostium of the first coronary artery by the catheter positioned in the ascending aorta;

T4: time of fluoroscopy during recording the angiography of the first coronary artery;

T5: time needed to properly engage the ostium of the other coronary artery by the catheter positioned in the ascending aorta. In the standard group, the time for T5 was separated into T5a (changing Judkins catheters) and T5b (time needed to properly engage the ostium of the other coronary artery);

T6: time of fluoroscopy during recording the angiography of the second coronary artery;

T7: total procedural time.

Standard angiography projections were used: four for the left coronary artery (LCA) and two for the right coronary artery (RCA). The amount of contrast needed to find and record each coronary artery was evaluated. The total amount of contrast used during the whole procedure was measured. In all cases, contrast was injected manually. The radiation dose applied during the assessment of each coronary artery (mGy) and the total radiation dose for the whole procedure were assessed. Before angiography, the operator was obliged to declare which coronary artery would cannulated first. The frequency of change of the initial operator's intention was assessed. The rate of necessity of using another catheter due to coronary ostium cannulation failure was also calculated. Complications related to the catheter insertion, passage through the arteries, and maneuvers in the aorta were recorded, including radial artery spasm, pain during catheter introduction, hematoma at the puncture site, upper limb hematoma, coronary artery dissection, catheter malfunction, and fracture. The serious adverse event rate was calculated, including myocardial infarction (MI), death, and repeated angiography. Basic echocardiography parameters including the left ventricular ejection fraction (EF; %); ascending aorta diameter (mm), and left ventricle maximum diameter (mm) were collected.

Statistical analysis was performed using jamovi 1.2.27 software. First, a baseline analysis, including the mean, median, standard deviation (SD) value, and assumption of normality (Shapiro–Wilk normality test), was performed. Second, to assess the statistical significance of the results, appropriate statistical tests were used. Generally, an intention-to-treat analysis was performed. Continuous variables were assessed using a one-way ANOVA (for parametric variables) or U-Mann–Whitney test, and a Kruskal–Wallis one-way ANOVA (for non-parametric variables) with post-hoc analysis was performed between each group. Nominal variables were assessed with the Chi-square test. The significance level was set at $p < 0.05$.

The study protocol was approved by the Institutional Review Board of the Jagiellonian University (approval No: 1072.6120.101.2019 issued on 24 April 2019).

3. Results

3.1. Baseline Characteristics

There was no difference among the groups with regard to age, basic anthropometric parameters, and basic echocardiographic parameters, except for the higher EF in groups 2 and 5 in compared to group 4—see Table 1.

Table 1. Baseline and echocardiographic characteristics.

Characteristics	Group 1	Group 2	Group 3	Group 4	Group 5	p Value
Age (years)	65.1 ± 7.8	63.1 ± 11.3	66 ± 10.1	68 ± 8.6	69.3 ± 9	0.28
Weight (kg)	84.6 ± 16.2	78.3 ± 10.1	88.5 ± 17.4	82.6 ± 20.9	77.6 ± 14.3	0.22
Height (cm)	173 ± 9.3	170 ± 9.2	171 ± 9.3	166 ± 9.2	168 ± 6.6	0.08
BMI (kg/m^2)	28.3 ± 4.5	27.1 ± 3.1	30 ± 4.7	29.8 ± 7	27.4 ± 4.6	0.39
Men (n (%))	15 (75)	17 (85)	16 (80)	12 (60)	13 (65)	0.36
Diameter of aorta (mm)	35.8 ± 4.5	33.9 ± 4.0	36.1 ± 4.3	35.9 ± 6.4	35.8 ± 4.8	0.48
Left ventricle diameter (mm)	55.6 ± 9.1	50.5 ± 7.1	53.8 ± 8.2	56.7 ± 8.5	51.0 ± 7.9	0.07
EF (%)	43.6 ± 13.0	52.8 ± 12.7	46.3 ± 12.9	42.5 ± 12.0	51.8 ± 11.2	0.012 [a]
Diabetes (n (%))	4 (20)	3 (15)	5 (25)	4 (20)	6 (30)	0.82
Hypertension (n (%))	14 (70)	13 (65)	18 (90)	15 (75)	17 (85)	0.30
PAD (n (%))	1 (5)	2 (10)	1 (5)	2 (10)	3 (15)	0.78
CKD (n (%))	2 (10)	1 (5)	3 (15)	3 (15)	5 (25)	0.45

BMI—Body Mass Index; EF—ejection fraction; PAD—peripheral artery disease; CKD—chronic kidney disease. [a] Kruskal–Wallis one-way ANOVA (in post-hoc analysis significant difference in group 4 vs. 2 $p = 0.041$ and group 4 vs. 5 $p = 0.035$).

3.2. Ostial Stability and Engagement in Investigated Groups

The highest rate of optimal stability was observed in group 2 (90%) and group 5 (95%). Suboptimal results with at least one episode of a catheter falling out from the ostium were most frequent in group 1 (45%). The necessity of usage of another catheter was observed most frequently in group 4. All results concerning catheter stability and the rate of necessity to change the catheter are presented in Figure 2 and Table S1 (Supplementary Materials).

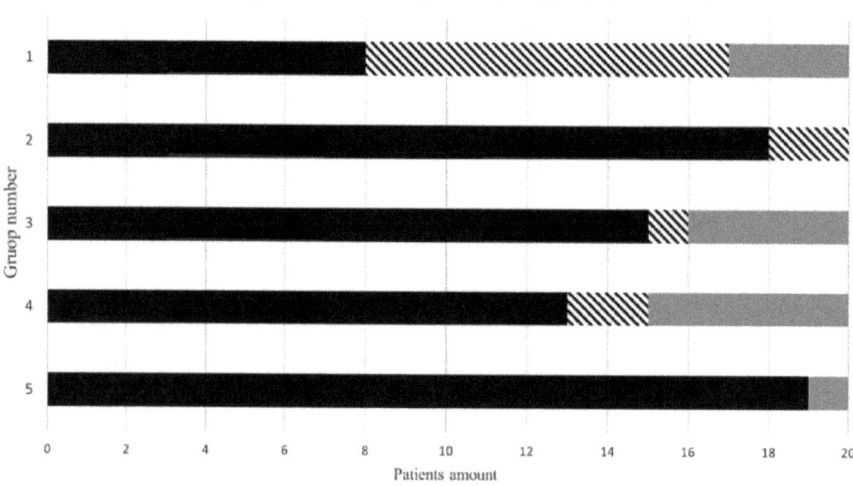

Figure 2. Ostial stability assessment among investigated groups. Figure legend: black—optimal stability; striped—suboptimal stability; gray—necessity to change catheter.

Generally, the rate of catheter instability or necessity of catheter change was more frequently observed during the cannulation of the left coronary artery (LCA) in comparison to the right coronary artery (RCA), especially in group 1. Details are presented in Table 2.

Table 2. Rate of catheter ostial instability and rate of need for the usage of another catheter among study groups in LCA and RCA arteries.

Group	Suboptimal Ostial Stability during Cannulation of LCA and RCA (n)	Necessity of Catheter Change during Cannulation of LCA and RCA (n)
1	LCA: 8	LCA: 3
	RCA: 1	RCA: 0
2	LCA: 1	LCA: 0
	RCA: 1	RCA: 0
3	LCA: 1	LCA: 2
	RCA: 1	RCA: 2
4	LCA: 2	LCA: 2
	RCA: 1	RCA: 3
5	LCA: 0	LCA: 0
	RCA: 0	RCA: 1

LCA—left coronary artery; RCA—right coronary artery.

3.3. Procedural Characteristic

In all groups, TRA was performed from the right radial artery. The intention to cannulate the RCA first was declared in the majority of patients irrespective of the catheter type. The exact proportions of the declared order of the cannulation of coronary arteries (right/left) among study groups were as follows: group 1: 13/7; group 2: 15/5; group 3: 14/6; group 4: 15/5; group 5: 20/0. The necessity of changing the original intention was most frequent in group 3, at four times (three times from right to left and one from left to right). In group 1 and group 4, the original intention was changed once.

3.4. Duration of Each Procedural Step

Time frames of each procedural stage are presented in Tables S2 and S3.

Comparing all groups, T2 was significantly shorter in group 2, with $p = 0.005$. Among particular groups, T2 was significantly shorter in group 2 then in group 4, with $p = 0.001$, and shorter in group 3 in comparison to group 4, with $p = 0.059$. Regarding T3, there were no significant differences between groups, with $p = 0.11$. There were no significant differences between groups in T4, with $p = 0.90$. T5 was shorter in group 1 (difference 43.5 s) and significantly shorter in group 2 (difference 44.1 s) in comparison to control group 5 with $p = 0.07$ and $p = 0.023$, respectively. There were no significant differences between groups in T6, with $p = 0.11$. There were also no significant differences between groups in T7, with $p = 0.15$. Analysis of timeframes directly depending on the catheter type (T2 + T3 + T5 (a + b)) revealed that the shortest time for catheter introduction and searching for coronary ostia was achieved in group 2, as shown in Figure 3.

3.5. Contrast Volume and Radiation Dose

Angiography of the RCA: There were no differences between study groups in terms of the contrast volume and radiation dose. Angiography of the LCA: there were no differences between study groups in contrast volume. In the post hoc analysis, the lowest radiation dose was observed in group 2, with $p = 0.045$. All results are summarized in Table 3.

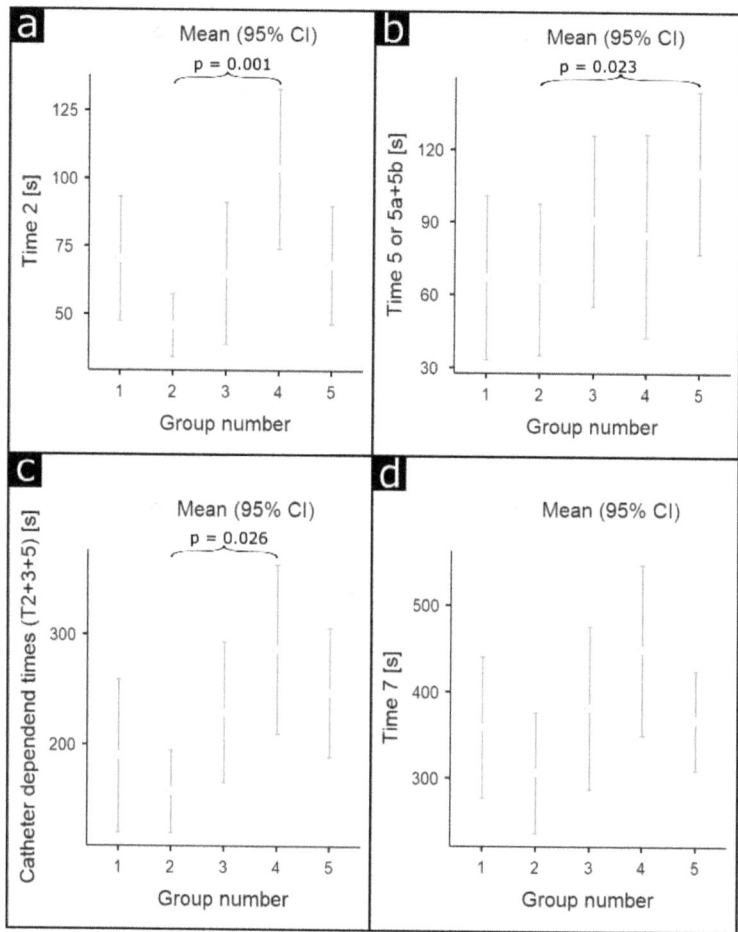

Figure 3. Differences in timeframes among groups. (a) T2 [s]: time needed to introduce the diagnostic catheter, from entering the vascular sheath to reaching the ascending aorta; (b) T5 [s]: time needed to properly engage the ostium of the other coronary artery by the catheter positioned in the ascending aorta. In the standard group, the time for T5 was separated into T5a (changing Judkins catheters) and T5b (time needed to properly en-gage the ostium of the other coronary artery); (c) T2 + T3 + T5 [s]—sum of time that directly associated with catheter type; (d) T7 [s]: total procedural time.

Table 3. Summary of contrast volume and radiation dose during the procedure in all groups.

Amount of Contrast and Radiation	Group 1	Group 2	Group 3	Group 4	Group 5	p Value
RCA contrast volume (mL)	15.9 11.3	18.1 ± 9.2	23.1 ± 18.6	26.7 ± 21.3	19 ± 10.4	0.19
RCA radiation dose (mGy)	38.1 ± 25.1	29.4 ± 23.7	47 ± 27.1	41 ± 31	40.1 ± 36.6	0.23
LCA contrast volume (mL)	36.8 ± 11.3	38 ± 18.2	39.2 ± 17.5	45 ± 20.8	38.2 ± 14.4	0.71
Total radiation dose (mGy)	115 ± 71.4	67 ± 45.2	108 ± 58.5	86.9 ± 78.5	80.5 ± 40.7	0.045 [a]
Total contrast volume (mL)	60.4 ± 32.1	57.4 ± 22.4	64.8 ± 31.4	71.8 ± 31.6	63.3 ± 30.6	0.39

LCA—left coronary artery; RCA—right coronary artery; [a] Kruskal–Wallis one-way ANOVA ± without significant differences between subgroups in post-hoc analysis).

3.6. Periprocedural Complications

Complications in all study groups were rare. There was no hematoma, coronary dissections caused by diagnostic catheters, periprocedural MI, re-PCI ± percutaneous coronary intervention), death, or catheter fracture or malfunction. Radial artery spasm was observed in one patient in group 3 and one patient in group 4—the spasm of the vessel subsided after i.a. (intra-arterial) the injection of nitroglycerin. Pain during catheter insertion was observed in one patient from groups 2, 3, and 4. In group 5, pain during catheter exchange ± from right Judkins to left one) was observed in three patients.

3.7. Treatment Pathway after Diagnostic Catheterization

All patients after diagnostic catheterization received optimal treatment based on the diagnostic catheterization results, patient symptoms, and preferences. Furthermore, Heart Team consultations were also taken into account, if necessary. Most of the patients received optimal pharmacological treatment—OMT ± optimal medical therapy). If invasive treatment was required, PCI ± percutaneous coronary intervention) was more often performed than CABG ± coronary artery by-pass graft). Particular information is presented in Table 4.

Table 4. Treatment pathway after diagnostic catheterization.

Treatment Pathway	Group 1	Group 2	Group 3	Group 4	Group 5	p Value
OMT ± n ± %	13 ± 65	6 ± 30	10 ± 50	13 ± 65	10 ± 50	0.16
PCI ± n ± %	4 ± 20	11 ± 55	9 ± 45	4 ± 20	9 ± 45	0.065
CABG ± n ± %	3 ± 15	3 ± 15	1 ± 5	3 ± 15	1 ± 5	0.71

OMT—optimal medical therapy; PCI—percutaneous coronary intervention; CABG—coronary artery by-pass graft.

4. Discussion

Trans radial vascular access is currently the preferred access method for coronary interventions in most cathlabs [7,8]. The wide range of TRA applications in everyday practice results in a significant reduction of major bleeding and access site complications and a reduction of adverse cardiac events, and finally allows for faster patient mobilization and shorter hospitalization compared to femoral and other vascular accesses [9,10]. The main goal for introducing the single-catheter method of TRA was to avoid catheter exchange, reduce upper limb vessel mechanical irritation, and finally achieve shorter procedural times, less contrast use, and smaller radiation exposure. Chronologically, research attention was focused on the Tiger diagnostic catheter, which was designed for the one-catheter TRA concept. Originally it was assessed in a small study by Kim et al. and proved to be effective in the perfect ostial engagement of the RCA in 100% of cases and less effective in LCA ostium engagement, in 91% of cases [11]. Later, the effectiveness of the Tiger catheter was confirmed in a large study, especially in terms of engaging RCA ostium. However, almost 33% instability during left coronary angiography was demonstrated with the necessity to switch to a regular Judkins catheter to complete the procedure [12]. In the following years, the one-catheter TRA concept was investigated using TIGER II and Judkins left modified catheters [13–15]. In the present study, the newer generation of four different curves of DxTerity TRA diagnostic catheters from Medtronic ± Trapease, Ultra, Transformer and Tracker) dedicated to the TRA one-catheter concept were evaluated. In the study, we also observed a higher rate of successful cannulation and stability during RCA angiography in comparison with LCA for all investigated catheters ± Figure 4a–c). In previous studies, catheter instability also predominantly affected LCA. In our study, ostial stability among investigated catheters was the best for the Ultra catheter group in comparison to standard catheters ± Figure 4d). Moreover, the worst stability and highest rate of the necessity of making a catheter switch was observed in the Tracker catheter group. It is worthwhile to underline that some catheters, especially Transformer Curve, tend to deeply intubate RCA, which could increase the risk of artery dissection and require special attention from the operator ± Figure 4e). The poor stability in the present study was observed in the Trapease group ± Figure 4f). Ostial catheter stability is a very important condition for optimal performance and the adequate estimation of the angiogram. In the past, even experienced operators using the one-catheter technique complained of relatively frequent difficulties with proper catheter stable position in ostium ± non-co-axial) which was associated with frequent fall-out or poor arterial visualization during dye injection. Stability is also crucial during fractional flow reserve assessment, which is performed by some operators through diagnostic catheters.

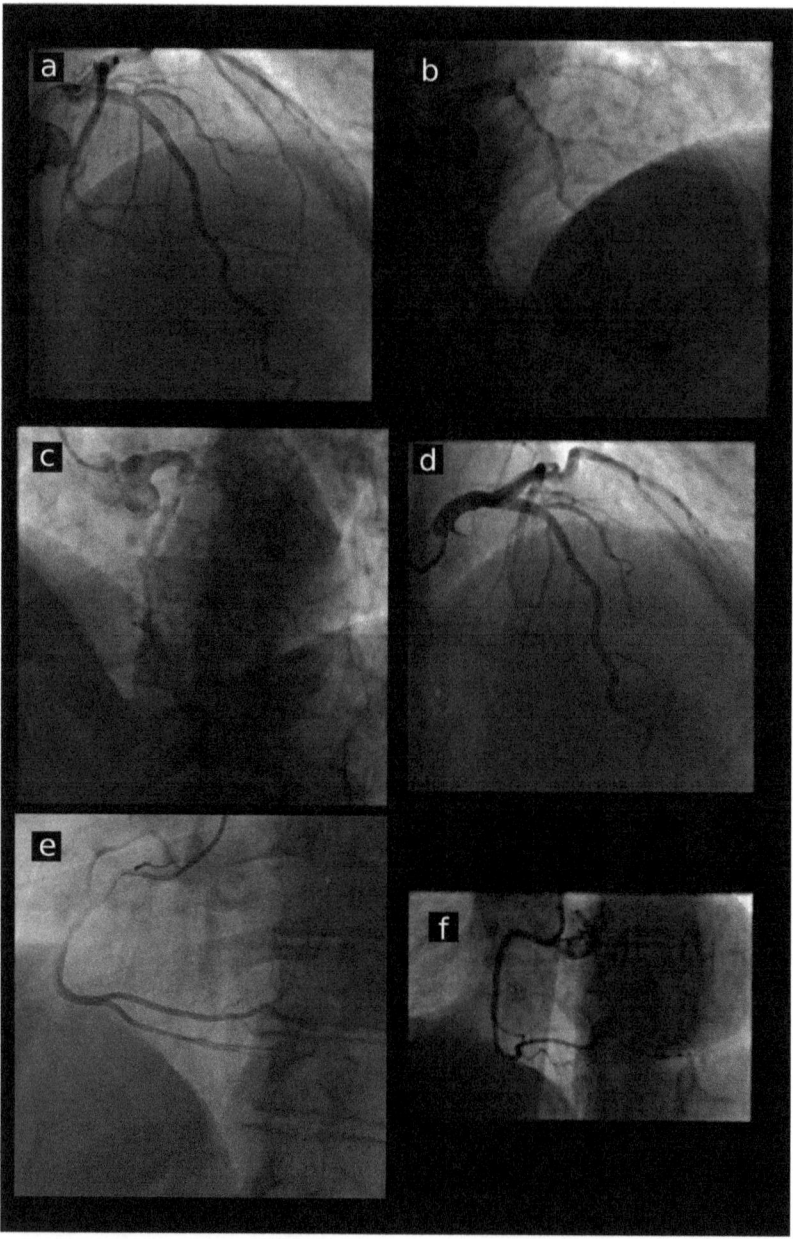

Figure 4. Examples of ostial stability among investigated catheters. (**a**–**c**) Instability and fall-out of investigated catheters during LCA cannulation. (**d**) Optimal stability of Ultra catheter during contrast injection to LCA, (**e**) unintentional deep intubation of RCA with Transformer catheter, (**f**) poor stability of Trapease catheter during RCA angiography. LCA—left coronary artery; RCA—right coronary artery.

Generally, one of the potential targets for the TRA one-catheter concept was to reduce procedural time. In the present study, we did not observe a significant difference in the total procedural time ± T7) among investigated groups. However, when times directly associated with catheter curves were analyzed ± T2, T3, T5) the shortest time periods were observed in the Ultra group. Potentially, the prolongation of the procedure through the radial artery may intensify radial spasm, reduce patient comfort, and increase the risk of complications [16,17].

According to our observations, the contrast volume was similar in all groups ± between 57–70 mL) and comparable to the study with Tiger catheters ± 65 mL), and lower than a past study with Amplatzer left catheters ± 103 mL) [18]. In other studies, the amount of contrast saved by the one-catheter strategy compared to the standard method was very small [14,15].

In cases with the one-technique catheter, pain during catheter insertion was observed very rarely. However, during TRA procedures, radial spasm can be very painful. The continuation of the procedure despite the pain could result in radial or brachial artery rupture or cross-over to the femoral artery and, in consequence, increase the risk of further complications [19]. In the present study, the rate of complications concerning radial artery reactions, hematoma rate, serious adverse events, and catheter malfunction was rare.

The major limitation of the study is the relatively small sample size. However, this is a pilot study, and investigation will be continued with a larger number of participants. Another obvious limitation is the different vascular anatomy in patients and the fact that TRA angiography was not performed in each patient using all investigated catheters. Procedures were performed by four operators, and the only vascular access site was the right radial artery. For this reason, the results cannot be automatically referenced to the procedures performed from the left radial artery.

5. Conclusions

DxTerity catheters dedicated to the one-catheter concept of TRA are suitable tools for performing TRA coronary angiography with a low rate of procedural complications. Different curves of diagnostic catheters seem not to be equal in terms of the effectiveness of TRA. Among the investigated catheters, the Ultra Curve catheter has demonstrated an advantage over other catheters in terms of the ostial stability rate and procedural time. Parameters which could identify the best diagnostic catheter for TRA in a single patient are still to be determined.

Supplementary Materials: The following are available online at https://www.mdpi.com/article/10.3390/jcm10204722/s1, Table S1: Ostial stability assessment among investigated groups ± $p < 0.001$). Table S2: Comparison of time frames between single catheter groups and control group. And Table S3: Comparison of time frames in each group.

Author Contributions: Conceptualization, Ł.R. and M.C.; methodology, Ł.R.; software, T.G.; validation, A.D., R.J. and B.C.; formal analysis, M.C.; T.G.; investigation, M.C., Ł.R., A.D.; resources M.C.; data curation, R.J., P.K., J.L.; writing—M.C.; writing—review and editing, S.B., A.D., J.L., P.K., R.J., T.G., B.C., A.S., Ł.R.; visualization, M.C., A.D. supervision, A.S., S.B., J.L. project administration, M.C.; funding acquisition, Ł.R. All authors have read and agreed to the published version of the manuscript.

Funding: The APC was covered by the Jagiellonian University Medical College (Cracow, Poland) (grant No. N41/DBS/000467).

Institutional Review Board Statement: The study was conducted according to the guidelines of the Declaration of Helsinki, and approved by the Institutional Review Board of the Jagiellonian University, (approval No.: 1072.6120.101.2019 issued on 24 April 2019).

Informed Consent Statement: Informed consent was obtained from all subjects involved in the study.

Conflicts of Interest: The authors declare no conflict of interest.

References

1. Dworeck, C.; Redfors, B.; Völz, S.; Haraldsson, I.; Angerås, O.; Råmunddal, T.; Ioanes, D.; Myredal, A.; Odenstedt, J.; Hirlekar, G.; et al. Radial artery access is associated with lower mortality in patients undergoing primary PCI: A report from the SWEDEHEART registry. *Eur. Heart J. Acute. Cardiovasc. Care* **2020**, *9*, 323–332. [CrossRef] [PubMed]
2. Campeau, L. Percutaneous radial artery approach for coronary angiography. *Cathet. Cardiovasc. Diagn.* **1989**, *16*, 3–7. [CrossRef] [PubMed]
3. Kiemeneij, F.; Laarman, G.J. Percutaneous transradial artery approach for coronary Palmaz-Schatz stent implantation. *Am. Heart J.* **1994**, *128*, 167–174. [CrossRef]
4. Mamas, M.A.; Anderson, S.G.; Car, M.; Ratib, K.; Buchan, I.; Sirker, A.; Fraser, D.G.; Hildick-Smith, D.; de Belder, M.; Ludman, F.P. Baseline bleeding risk and arterial access site practice in relation to procedural outcomes following percutaneous coronary intervention. *J. Am. Coll. Cardiol.* **2014**, *64*, 1554–1564. [CrossRef] [PubMed]
5. Mamas, M.A.; Anderson, S.G.; Ratib, K.; Routledge, H.; Neyses, L.; Fraser, D.G.; Buchan, I.; de Belder, M.A.; Ludman, P.; Nolan, J. Arterial access site utilization in cardiogenic shock in the United Kingdom: Is radial access feasible? *Am. Heart J.* **2014**, *167*, 900–908. [CrossRef] [PubMed]
6. Cooper, C.J.; El-Shiekh, R.A.; Cohen, D.J.; Blaesing, L.; Burket, M.W.; Basu, A.; Moore, J.A. Effect of transradial access on quality of life and coast of cardiac catheterization: A randomized comparison. *Am. Heart J.* **1999**, *138*, 430–436. [CrossRef]
7. Anderson, S.G.; Ratib, K.; Myint, P.K.; Keavney, B.; Kwok, C.S.; Zaman, A.; Dm, B.B.K.; de Belder, M.A.; Nolan, J.; Mamas, M.A.; et al. Impact of age on access site-related outcomes in 469,983 percutaneous coronary intervention procedures: Insights from the British Cardiovascular Intervention Society. *Catheter. Cardiovasc. Interv.* **2015**, *86*, 965–972. [CrossRef] [PubMed]
8. Feldman, D.N.; Swaminathan, R.V.; Kaltenbach, L.A.; Baklanov, D.V.; Kim, L.K.; Wong, S.C.; Minutello, R.M.; Messenger, J.C.; Moussa, I.; Garratt, K.N. Adoption of radial access and comparison of outcomes to femoral access in percutaneous coronary intervention: An updated report from the National Cardiovascular Data Registry ± 2007–2012). *Circulation* **2013**, *127*, 2295–2306. [CrossRef] [PubMed]
9. Bartrand, O.F.; Bernat, I. Radial artery occlusion: Still the Achille's heel of transradial approach or is it? *Coron. Artery Dis.* **2015**, *26*, 97–98. [CrossRef] [PubMed]
10. Mitchell, M.D.; Hong, J.A.; Lee, B.Y.; Umscheid, C.A.; Bartsch, S.M.; Don, C.W. Systematic Review and Cost–Benefit Analysis of Radial Artery Access for Coronary Angiography and Intervention. *Circ. Cardiovasc. Qual. Outcomes* **2012**, *5*, 454–462. [CrossRef] [PubMed]
11. Kim, S.-M.; Kim, D.-K.; Kim, O.-I.; Kim, N.-S.; Joo, S.-J.; Lee, J.-W. Novel diagnostic catheter specifically designed for both coronary arteries via the right transradial approach. *Int. J. Cardiovasc. Imaging* **2005**, *22*, 295–303. [CrossRef] [PubMed]
12. Langer, C.; Riehle, J.; Wuttig, H.; Dürrwald, S.; Lange, H.; Samol, A.; Frey, N.; Wiemer, M. Efficacy of a one-catheter concept for transradial coronary angiography. *PLoS ONE* **2018**, *13*, e0189899. [CrossRef] [PubMed]
13. Turan, B.; Erkol, A.; Mutlu, A.; Daşlı, T.; Erden, I. Effectiveness of Left Judkins Catheter as a Single Multipurpose Catheter in Transradial Coronary Angiography From Right Radial Artery: A Randomized Comparison With Conventional Two-Catheter Strategy. *J. Interv. Cardiol.* **2016**, *29*, 257–264. [CrossRef] [PubMed]
14. Chen, O.; Goel, S.; Acholonu, M.; Kulbak, G.; Verma, S.; Travlos, E.; Casazza, R.; Borgen, E.; Malik, B.; Friedman, M.; et al. Comparison of Standard Catheters Versus Radial Artery–Specific Catheter in Patients Who Underwent Coronary Angiography Through Transradial Access. *Am. J. Cardiol.* **2016**, *118*, 357–361. [CrossRef] [PubMed]
15. Xanthopoulou, I.; Stavrou, K.; Davlouros, P.; Tsigkas, G.; Koufou, E.-E.; Almpanis, G.; Koutouzis, M.; Tsiafoutis, I.; Perperis, A.; Moulias, A.; et al. Randomised comparison of JUDkins vs. tiGEr catheter in coronary angiography via the right radial artery: The JUDGE study. *EuroIntervention* **2018**, *13*, 1950–1958. [CrossRef] [PubMed]
16. Abdelaal, E.; Brousseau-Provencher, C.; Montminy, S.; Plourde, G.; MacHaalany, J.; Bataille, Y.; Molin, P.; Déry, J.-P.; Barbeau, G.; Roy, L.; et al. Risk Score, Causes, and Clinical Impact of Failure of Transradial Approach for Percutaneous Coronary Interventions. *JACC Cardiovasc. Interv.* **2013**, *6*, 1129–1137. [CrossRef] [PubMed]
17. De-an, I.A.; Zhou, Y.; Shi, D.; Liu, Y.; Wang, J.; Liu, X.; Wang, Z.; Yang, S.; Ge, H.; Hu, B. Incidence and predictors of radial artery spasm during transradial coronary angi-ography and intervention. *Chin. Med. J.* **2010**, *123*, 843–847.
18. Sanmartin, M.; Esparza, J.; Moxica, J.; Baz, J.A.; Iñiguez-Romo, A. Safety and efficacy of a multipurpose coronary angiography strategy using the transradial technique. *J. Invasive Cardiol.* **2005**, *17*, 594–597. [PubMed]
19. Trilla, M.; Freixa, X.; Regueiro, A.; Fernández-Rodriguez, D.; Brugaletta, S.; Martin-Yuste, V.; Jiménez, M.; Betriu, A.; Sabaté, M.; Masotti, M. Impact of Aging on Radial Spasm during Coronary Catheterization. *J. Invasive Cardiol.* **2015**, *27*, E303–E3037. [PubMed]

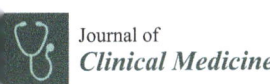

Journal of Clinical Medicine

Article

Balloon Aortic Valvuloplasty for Severe Aortic Stenosis as Rescue or Bridge Therapy

Pawel Kleczynski [1,*], Aleksandra Kulbat [2], Piotr Brzychczy [2], Artur Dziewierz [3], Jaroslaw Trebacz [1], Maciej Stapor [1], Danuta Sorysz [3], Lukasz Rzeszutko [3], Stanislaw Bartus [3], Dariusz Dudek [3] and Jacek Legutko [1]

1. Department of Interventional Cardiology, Institute of Cardiology, Jagiellonian University Medical College, John Paul II Hospital, Pradnicka 80 Street, 31-202 Krakow, Poland; jartrebacz@gmail.com (J.T.); maciej.stapor@gmail.com (M.S.); jacek.legutko@uj.edu.pl (J.L.)
2. Students' Scientific Group at the Department of Interventional Cardiology, Jagiellonian University Medical College, John Paul II Hospital, Pradnicka 80 Street, 31-202 Krakow, Poland; alexandra.kulbat@gmail.com (A.K.); piotrbrzy@gmail.com (P.B.)
3. 2nd Department of Cardiology, Institute of Cardiology, Jagiellonian University Medical College, University Hospital, Jakubowskiego 2 Street, 30-688 Krakow, Poland; adziewierz@gmail.com (A.D.); dtsorysz@op.pl (D.S.); lrzeszutko@cathlab.krakow.pl (L.R.); mbbartus@cyf-kr.edu.pl (S.B.); mcdudek@cyfronet.pl (D.D.)
* Correspondence: kleczu@interia.pl

Abstract: The study aimed to assess procedural complications, patient flow and clinical outcomes after balloon aortic valvuloplasty (BAV) as rescue or bridge therapy, based on data from our registry. A total of 382 BAVs in 374 patients was performed. The main primary indication for BAV was a bridge for TAVI (n = 185, 49.4%). Other indications included a bridge for AVR (n = 26, 6.9%) and rescue procedure in hemodynamically unstable patients (n = 139, 37.2%). The mortality rate at 30 days, 6 and 12 months was 10.4%, 21.6%, 28.3%, respectively. In rescue patients, the death rate raised to 66.9% at 12 months. A significant improvement in symptoms was confirmed after BAV, after 30 days, 6 months, and in survivors after 1 year ($p < 0.05$ for all). Independent predictors of 12-month mortality were baseline STS score [HR (95% CI) 1.42 (1.34 to 2.88), $p < 0.0001$], baseline LVEF <20% [HR (95% CI) 1.89 (1.55–2.83), $p < 0.0001$] and LVEF <30% at 1 month [HR (95% CI) 1.97 (1.62–3.67), $p < 0.0001$] adjusted for age/gender. In everyday clinical practice in the TAVI era, there are still clinical indications to BAV a standalone procedure as a bridge to surgery, TAVI or for urgent high risk non-cardiac surgical procedures. Patients may improve clinically after BAV with LV function recovery, allowing to perform final therapy, within limited time window, for severe AS which ameliorates long-term outcomes. On the other hand, in patients for whom an isolated BAV becomes a destination therapy, prognosis is extremely poor.

Keywords: aortic stenosis; balloon aortic valvuloplasty; bridge therapy; destination therapy; heart failure

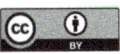

1. Introduction

At present, management of severe aortic valve stenosis (AS) offers surgical or endovascular therapy depending on a patients' risk profile and severity of clinical symptoms [1,2]. Endovascular treatment includes transcatheter aortic valve implantation (TAVI) or balloon aortic valvuloplasty (BAV). There are also patients who are too sick to benefit from invasive treatment and thus scheduled to conservative therapy with the worst prognosis. Balloon aortic valvuloplasty has gained importance in recent years, especially in patients who were recognized as in not optimal clinical condition for any definitive treatment due to severe comorbidities. Baloon valvuloplasty can either serve as a standalone palliative procedure performed in haemodynamicaly unstable patients or as a bridge to final therapy [1–3]. Furthermore, BAV allows AS patients to undergo an urgent non-cardiac surgery with its good immediate hemodynamic result [3,4]. On the contrary to TAVI, clinical and hemodynamic outcomes of BAV were shown to be relatively poor with longer follow-up period, and sometimes the procedure needs to be repeated [4–8]. Due to relatively low access to TAVI, BAV is still a reasonable procedure in developing countries, but such an approach remains rather controversial in light of current ESC guidelines [2]. Thus, we aimed to assess patient flow, procedural complications and clinical outcomes after BAV as rescue or bridge therapy in patients with severe symptomatic AS.

2. Materials and Methods

In current study, the data of all consecutive patients with severe symptomatic AS with an aortic valve area (AVA) < 0.7 cm^2 (indexed AVA < 0.5 cm^2/m^2 body surface area) and/or mean transaortic gradient $\geq$40 mmHg who underwent BAV between December 2008 and May 2021 at two tertiary university centers, were included. Left ventricle ejection fraction (LVEF) was assessed with transthoracic echocardiography (TTE) using the modified Simpson's method of discs, acquiring LV volumes from apical 4- and 2-chamber view. The study was conducted as a two center, retrospective registry. Patients were carefully examined to assess the operative risk, comorbidities and procedural feasibility. Patient screening and selection were performed by a multidisciplinary 'Heart Team'. The institutional ethical board was informed and approved our study. The procedure was preceded by coronary angiography in the vast majority of cases and guided by TTE and fluoroscopy. Femoral access was used, starting with a 6F sheath and the exchanged to destination sheath depending on the balloon size. Anticoagulation was achieved with unfractionated heparin with activated clotting time of 250 to 300 s. Balloons from Osypka Medical Inc. (Berlin, Germany) were used in most cases. Balloon sizes were chosen depending on a minimal annulus diameter measured in TTE or based on CT scans, if available. The exact positioning of the balloon during inflation was obtained with rapid ventricular pacing from either the 0.035" ultra-stiff guidewire inserted into the left ventricle (LV) or the temporary pacemaker inserted into the right ventricle (RV) (via a 6 or 7 Fr venous sheath) [9,10]. The number of balloon inflations was left to the operator's discretion. Successful procedure was described as transaortic gradient drop of more than 30% compared to baseline. Vascular access was closed with manual compression or an Angio-Seal device (Terumo, Tokio, Japan). Baseline clinical, echocardiographic and procedural data, as well as complication rates, were analyzed.

Statistical Analysis

Continuous variables were expressed as a median (interquartile range) and categorical variables were expressed as a number (percentage). Continuous variables were compared by t-test for dependent samples when normally distributed or by Wilcoxon signed-rank test when not normally distributed. Categorical variables were compared by Pearson's v2 test and Fisher's exact test. The Pearson rank correlation coefficient for normally distributed variables or Spearman's rank correlation coefficient for not normally distributed variables were calculated to test the association between two variables. Cox regression models for all-cause mortality were constructed to identify independent predictors of survival. Age, sex, hypertension, coronary artery disease, diabetes, atrial fibrillation, cerebrovascular incident, pulmonary disease, chronic kidney disease, STS score, LVEF < 20% at baseline, LVEF < 30% at 1 month, which were identified a priori as clinically relevant and included in the model. The significance level was set at $p < 0.05$. Statistical analysis was performed using IBM SPSS Statistics for Windows, Version 25.0 (IBM Corporation, Armonk, NY, USA).

3. Results

A total of 382 BAVs in 374 patients was performed. Procedural success was present in 94.6% of patients. Repeat BAV was performed in 8 patients. The main primary indication for BAV was a bridge for TAVI (n = 185, 49.4%). Other indications included a primary bridge for aortic valve implantation (AVR, n = 26, 6.9%) and palliative treatment (n = 139, 37.2%). Twenty-two patients (5.8%) underwent BAV in the course of cardiogenic shock and in 42 (11.2%) patients BAV was performed before urgent non-cardiac surgery. Finally, 183 (48.9%) of patients after BAV underwent TAVI and 52 (13.9%) patients underwent

AVR during follow-up. In some patients who were primarily qualified to TAVI or AVR as described above, the final qualification has changed during the follow-up period (Figure 1). The median follow-up period was 686 days and ranged from 103 to 1245 days.

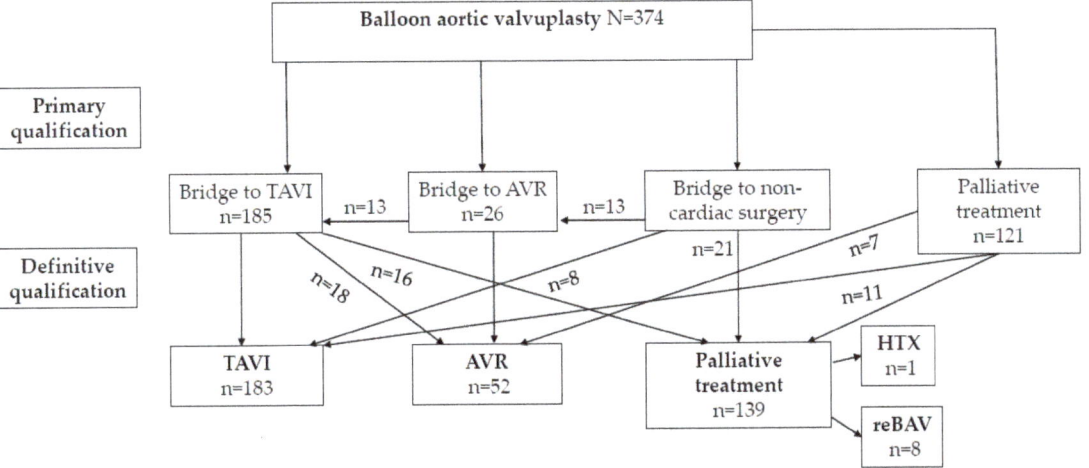

Figure 1. Flowchart of patients undergoing balloon aortic valvuloplasty as a bridge or final therapy. AVR—aortic valve replacement; BAV—balloon aortic valvuloplasty; HTX—heart transplantation; TAVI—transcatheter aortic valve implantation.

3.1. Baseline Characteristics

The median age of the enrolled population was 84 years, with a higher prevalence of females (53%). All patients presented symptoms of NYHA class III or IV. The median STS score was 10.1% and logistic Euroscore II was 7.4. Clinical data are presented in Table 1.

3.2. Procedural Data

Concomitant coronary angiography with BAV was performed in 355 (94.9%) patients and concomitant PCI was performed in 81 (21.6%) patients. Only severe coronary lesions with >70% stenosis were treated in ostial or proximal segments of major epicardial arteries. The median balloon size was 22 mm [IQR 18–24.5 mm]. Wire LV pacing was used in 196 patients (52.4%). Eight patients underwent repeated procedures within a median of 189 days. The remaining procedural data are shown in Table 2.

3.3. Echocardiographic Data

All echocardiographic baseline and follow-up data are showed in Table 3. There were 8 severe aortic regurgitations (AR) after BAV and 4 patients were successfully treated with TAVI, 2 of them underwent successful AVR. The remaining 2 severe ARs resulted in intrahospital death. Echocardiographic examinations performed after BAV and at 30 days, 6 and 12 months showed that AVA was higher up to 6 months, ($p < 0.05$ for all), but the mean transaortic gradient did not show significant differences after 6 months compared to values directly after BAV. Interestingly, in 93 (24.6%) patients with impaired left ventricular function (LVEF <30%) a significant improvement of LVEF (median 18 %) after 30 days ($p = 0.025$) was observed and it was sustained after 6 months ($p = 0.034$). A response to BAV (improvement of LVEF) was observed in 235 patients (63.8%), without any progress of LVEF impairment due to BAV. These circumstances allowed patients to be requalified to definitive therapy, TAVI or AVR. Improvement of LVEF correlated with a change of AVA ($r = 0.6$, $p < 0.0001$) and mean transaortic gradient ($r = 0.72$, $p < 0.0001$).

Table 1. Baseline clinical characteristics.

	All (n = 374)
Age, median (IQR) (years)	84 (81.3–89.5)
Men, n (%)	176 (47.0)
Body mass index, median (IQR) (kg/m^2)	24.7 (22.4–28.4)
Glomerular filtration rate, median (IQR) (mL/min/1.73 m^2)	48 (37.5–75.2)
CCS class, n (%)	
I + II	23 (6.1)
III	289 (77.3)
IV	62 (16.6)
NYHA class, n (%)	
I + II	0
III	228 (60.9)
IV	146 (39.0)
Coronary artery disease, n (%)	324 (79.1)
Arterial hypertension, n (%)	192 (86.6)
Diabetes mellitus, n (%)	158 (42.2)
Atrial fibrillation, n (%)	103 (27.5)
History of myocardial infarction, n (%)	89 (23.8)
History of percutaneous coronary intervention, n (%)	106 (28.3)
History of coronary artery bypass grafting, n (%)	72 (19.2)
Chronic obstructive pulmonary disease, n (%)	79 (21.1)
Peripheral artery disease, n (%)	83 (22.1)
Stroke/transient ischemic attack, n (%)	49 (13.1)
Syncope, n (%)	57 (15.2)
Previous heart failure deterioration, n (%)	226 (60.4)
Cardiogenic shock, n (%)	22 (5.8)
Previous pacemaker, n (%)	43 (11.4)
Neoplasm, n (%)	41 (10.9)
Previous radiotherapy, n (%)	29 (7.7)
Porcelain aorta, n (%)	19 (5.0)
Logistic EuroSCORE II (%), median (IQR)	7.8 (5.6–14.2)
The Society of Thoracic Surgeons score (%), median (IQR)	11.1 (8.1–13.9)

Table 2. Procedural data.

	All (n = 374)
Concomitant coronary angiography, n (%)	355 (94.9)
Concomitant PCI, n (%)	81 (21.6)
Size of femoral arterial sheath, median (IQR) (Fr)	9 (8.0–10.0)
Size of femoral venous sheath if used, median (IQR) (Fr)	6 (6.0–7.0)
Unfractionated heparin dose, median (IQR) (units)	5000 (4000.0–6500.0)
Wire pacing, n (%)	196 (52.4)
Number of inflations, median (IQR)	1 (1–3)
Vascular closure device, n (%)	215 (57.4)
Manual compression after sheath(s) removal, n (%)	159 (42.5)
Balloon size, median (IQR) (mm)	22 (18–24.5)
Radiation dose (BAV alone), median (IQR) (Gy)	0.26 (0.15–0.45)
Contrast media volume (BAV alone), median (IQR) (mL)	10 (5.0–24.0)
Fluoroscopy time (BAV alone), median (IQR) (min)	7.4 (5.2–15.4)
Duration (BAV alone), median (IQR) (min)	26 (17.9–35.5)

BAV—balloon aortic valvuloplasty; PCI—percutaneous coronary intervention.

Table 3. Echocardiografic data.

	Baseline (n = 374)	After BAV (n = 365)	30 Days (n = 335)	6 Months (n = 293)	12 Months (n = 46) ^
Maximal transaortic gradient, median (IQR) (mmHg)	93.8 (81.2–104.82)	64 (47.2–73.5) *	67 (48.4–76.4) *	72.5 (55.3–85.3) *#	86.3 (58.6–97.4) #
Mean transaortic gradient, median (IQR) (mmHg)	41.1 (40.4–55.2)	31.3 (21.4–38.2) *	32.5 (22.4–39.4) *	38.4 (30.3–49.6) *#	40.6 (39.5–54.7) #
Aortic valve area, median (IQR) (cm^2)	0.52 (0.42–0.61)	0.79 (0.65–0.92)	0.77 (0.66–0.90) *	0.71 (0.63–0.88) *#	0.53 (0.44–0.63) #
Left ventricle ejection fraction, median (IQR) (%)	41.2 (33.5–52.0)	44.2 (38.5–54.8)	48.2 (42.6–58.3) *#	46.7 (40.1–55.3)	42.9 (39.1–53.1) #
Right ventricular systolic pressure, median (IQR) (mm Hg)	53 (36.0–68.5)	45.2 (32.2–56.2) *	46.4 (33.2–57.6) *	49.3 (35.2–62.2) #	52 (37.1–65.2) *#
Aortic regurgitation None/trivial, n (%) Mild, n (%) Moderate, n (%) Severe, n (%)	145 (38.7) 157 (41.9) 52 (13.9) 0 (0.0)	93 (24.8) 183 (48.9) 82 (21.9) * 8 (2.1)	86 (22.9) 191 (51.0) * 75 (20.0) * 0 (0.0)	105 (28.0) 206 (55.0) * 67 (17.9) 0 (0.0)	18 (39.1) 12 (26.0) 16 (34.7) 0 (0.0)

* $p < 0.05$ compared with baseline, # $p < 0.05$ compared after BAV. ^ outcomes of the final palliative group not qualified to TAVI or AVR.

3.4. Complications

Detailed data on complications rate are presented in Table 4. Major complications occurred in 97 patients: (1) intraprocedural death (n = 9, 2.4%; 3 fatal tamponades, 1 fatal complete atrioventricular block, 5 cardiogenic shocks due to severe AS), (2) cardiac tamponade (n = 9, 2.4%), (3) severe AR (n = 8, 2.1%), (4) severe cardiac arrhythmias (n = 18, 4.8%), (5) cerebrovascular incident (n = 6, 1.6%), (6) permanent pacemaker implantation (n = 3, 0.8%), (6) need for red blood cells transfusion (n = 31, 8.2%), (7) urgent cardiac surgery (n = 13, 3.5%). Fatal annulus rupture was noted in 1 patient. Of 9 tamponades, 3 resulted in intraprocedural death, 2 with conversion to AVR and 3 were successfully treated with pericardiocentesis. Cardiac tamponade was caused by the temporary electrode placed in the RV in 2 cases confirmed by cardiac surgeons. Two cases were caused by the PM inserted into the RV, based on echo images. One tamponade resulted from annulus rupture. In one case the cause of tamponade remained unclear. Complete atrioventricular block despite stimulation was the cause of one intraprocedural death. Permanent pacemaker implantations were due to complete atrioventricular block occurring directly after BAV. Vascular access site complications occurred in 47 patients (12.5%). Arterial pseudoaneurysms were successfully treated with either manual compression or direct thrombin injection.

3.5. Outcomes

A significant improvement in symptoms (NYHA and CCS) was confirmed after BAV, after 30 days, 6 months and in survivors after 1 year ($p < 0.05$ for all).

In-hospital mortality was 5.1%. In addition to 9 intraprocedural deaths described previously, 4 patients died due to acute respiratory failure despite mechanical ventilation and 6 more had a sudden cardiac arrest (fatal ventricular tachycardia or fibrillation) in the intensive care unit after index procedure.

All-cause mortality rate at 30 days, 6 and 12 months was 10.4%, 21.6%, 28.3%, respectively. However, analyzing the death rate for palliative patients, the rate raised to 66.9% at 12 months (Table 5). Deaths in the palliative group were defined as cardiovascular in 72 (51.8%) cases (recurrent heart failure, sudden cardiac death, major stroke, pulmonary embolism or unknown reason) and non-cardiovascular in 21 (15.1%) cases (cancer, major gastrointestinal bleeding).

Table 4. Complications.

	All (n = 374)
Severe aortic regurgitation after BAV, n (%)	8 (2.1)
Balloon rupture, n (%)	23 (6.1)
Cardiac tamponade, n (%)	9 (2.4)
Severe cardiac arrythmias, n (%)	18 (4.8)
Cerebrovascular incident, n (%)	6 (1.6)
Vascular access site complications, n (%)	47 (12.5)
hematoma, n (%)	18 (4.8)
pseudoaneurysm, n (%)	17 (4.5)
arteriovenous fistula, n (%)	4 (1.0)
retroperitoneal bleeding, n (%)	8 (2.1)
Blood transfusion, n (%)	31 (8.2)
Baseline creatinine level, median (IQR) (g/dL)	107 (87.0–147.6)
Creatinine level after procedures, median (IQR) (g/dL)	104 (91.0–149.2)
Urgent cardiac surgery, n (%)	13 (3.5)
Permanent pacemaker implantation, n (%)	3 (0.8)
Hospital stay duration, median (IQR) (days)	5.5 (4.0–11.5)
Intraprocedural mortality, n (%)	9 (2.4)

BAV—balloon aortic valvuloplasty.

Table 5. Cumulative follow-up mortality data.

	All (n = 374)
In-hospital mortality, n (%)	19 (5.1)
30-day mortality rate, n (%)	39 (10.4)
6-month mortality rate, n (%)	81 (21.6)
12-month morality rate, n (%)	106 (28.3)
12-month mortality in palliative group, n (%)	93 (66.9) *

* n = 139, number of patients undergoing balloon aortic valvuloplasty as destination therapy.

Patients treated with BAV in the course of cardiogenic shock had the worst prognosis with 22.7% intraprocedural mortality and 81.9% in-hospital mortality. 30-day mortality was 100% in this group.

Of 121 palliative patients, one patient was qualified for heart transplantation, 11 have changed qualification for TAVI and subsequently underwent TAVI; 7 were qualified for AVR and subsequently underwent AVR (Figure 1). Eight patients underwent repeat BAV. Among 139 patients in the destination therapy group, we found significant differences in survivors compared to fatal cases in terms of: age (82.2 vs. 86.8 years, $p = 0.001$), logistic EuroSCORE II (7.2% vs. 9.5%, $p = 0.004$), STS score (10.3 vs. 12.8, $p = 0.002$), baseline LVEF (45.3% vs. 31.4%, $p < 0.001$), respectively.

In the subgroup of patients initially bridged for TAVI (Figure 1): 185 successfully underwent TAVI, 24 died before the intended procedure and 16 were excluded due to progressive dementia, mitral stenosis, malignancy, or severe impairment of mobility. Eighteen patients who were to undergo TAVI were switched to AVR because of concomitant severe tricuspid regurgitation, large aortic annulus and improvement of LVEF after BAV. Seven patients were bridged for AVR. All patients bridged to noncardiac surgery successfully underwent their intended procedures, in 13 patients AVR and in 8 - TAVI was performed after noncardiac procedure. The rest of assessed patients remained in the palliative treatment group.

In multivariable logistic regression analysis, we identified following independent predictors of 12-month all-cause mortality (Table 6): baseline STS score [HR (95% CI) 1.25 (1.08 to 1.94), $p = 0.001$], baseline LVEF < 20% [HR (95% CI) 1.65 (1.04–2.67), $p = 0.02$] and LVEF <30% at 1 month [HR (95% CI) 1.87 (1.35–3.43), $p = 0.001$]. Independent predictors of 12-month mortality were baseline STS score [HR (95% CI) 1.42 (1.34 to 2.88), $p < 0.0001$], baseline LVEF < 20% [HR (95% CI) 1.89 (1.55–2.83), $p < 0.0001$] and LVEF < 30% at 1 month [HR (95% CI) 1.97 (1.62–3.67), $p < 0.0001$] adjusted for age/gender.

Table 6. Multivariable Cox model for all-cause mortality.

	HR (95% CI)	p	HR (95% CI) Adjusted for Age/Gender	p
Age	0.87 (0.68–1.15)	0.25	-	-
Sex (female)	0.94 (0.72–2.01)	0.14	-	-
Hypertension	1.12 (0.79–1.79)	0.29	1.05 (0.81–1.63)	0.31
Coronary artery disease	1.06 (0.71–1.56)	0.37	1.03 (0.73–1.43)	0.43
Diabetes	0.82 (0.75–1.34)	0.23	0.83 (0.87–1.29)	0.54
Atrial fibrillation	1.03 (0.86–1.52)	0.30	1.01 (0.90–1.42)	0.47
Cerebrovascular event	1.23 (0.75–2.13)	0.16	1.18 (0.79–2.04)	0.24
Chronic obstructive pulmonary disease	1.19 (0.76–1.99)	0.14	1.14 (0.77–1.87)	0.28
Chronic kidney disease	1.27 (0.80–2.15)	0.19	1.23 (0.78–1.92)	0.32
STS score (per 1%)	1.25 (1.08–2.46)	0.001	1.42 (1.34–2.88)	<0.0001
LVEF < 20% at baseline	1.65 (1.04–2.67)	0.02	1.89 (1.55–2.83)	<0.0001
LVEF < 30% at 1 month	1.87 (1.35–3.43)	0.001	1.97 (1.62–3.67)	<0.0001

LVEF—left ventricle ejection fraction.

4. Discussion

Our study of 374 patients shows that balloon aortic valvuloplasty is a relatively safe and crucial procedure in patients who are at first too sick to be scheduled for TAVI or AVR. Therefore, bridging therapy is necessary to change the primary qualification because of left ventricle function improvement. Moreover, BAV may be an option for extremely comorbid high-risk patients as a palliative intervention for symptom relief, despite very high 12-month all-cause mortality of almost 67%. Left ventricle ejection fraction at baseline and at 1 month as well as baseline STS score were identified as independent predictors of 12-month all-cause mortality. Balloon valvuloplasty may also be important for patients with severe AS who must undergo an urgent non-cardiac surgery.

Hemodynamic results of BAV included an increase of AVA, a decrease of maximal and median transaortic gradient immediately after the procedure what has been presented previously [11–17]. The effect of the procedure was sustained for 1 month and started to diminish gradually at 6 months, however not achieving preprocedural values of AVA, LVEF and transaortic gradients. Nonetheless, at 12 months, the effects of BAV in survivors in the destination therapy group were abated and were similar to baseline values. This highlights the recurrence of AS severity and symptoms with longer time period from BAV. Moreover, a 6-month period following BAV seems to be crucial for bridging to final treatment (TAVI or even AVR) for this subset of patients. Left ventricle ejection fraction recovery after BAV seems to be a turning point for the final treatment pathway, either conservative treatment burdened with high mortality rate or interventional/surgical treatment improving outcomes. Despite favorable acute results, long-term mortality remained high, especially in patients in destination treatment cohort. Also, we noted a relevant rate (ca. 15%) of non-cardiac death for patients after BAV, which may be related to a selection bias wherein those patients are excluded from a more definite treatment due to many comorbidities.

Procedure-related complications rate was similar to that showed in previous studies [3,8,9,13,15,16]. A high rate of vascular complications, up to 12.5%, was reported and mostly related to the use of large arterial sheaths (8–10 F) and peripheral arterial disease. Also, additional venous sheath insertion (in 47.3% of cases) might have contributed to access-site related complications. On the other hand, these rates were lower than reported for TAVI [18]. In the case of peripheral artery disease affecting both iliac arteries, transradial or transbrachial access is possible with the use of one or two balloons [19,20]. Periprocedural deaths were, in fact, limited to patients with hemodynamic instability/cardiogenic shock before the procedure. Once periprocedural death resulted from annulus rupture. In contrast to previous reports, we did not observe myocardial infarction during or after BAV procedure [6,16]. Balloon rupture during BAV may occur due to bulky calcium load from the diseased valve, which was the case in 6.1% of cases in our study. However, none of these resulted in the cerebrovascular incidents. After rupture, removing the balloon with the delivery system is more challenging, especially if a boundary size of the arterial sheath, compatible with the balloon's diameter, was used [21].

Our observations are in line with data shown in other studies showing reprise of BAV in the era of TAVI [3,4,8,9,11–13,15,16,20,22]. When BAV is used as a bridge, it gives some time and opportunity to improve the clinical and hemodynamic response among treated patients with severe AS not being appropriate candidates for final treatment at that time point. The hemodynamic effects of BAV with subsequent LVEF improvement can be a turning point in decision and planning further treatment with TAVI or AVR, especially when serious comorbidities contribute to overall risk profile, extreme frailty or very low ejection fraction affect outcomes seriously [23,24]. In the natural history of conservative course of severe AS during long-term follow-up more significant decrease in AVA and increase of pulmonary artery systolic pressure correlates with a lower reduction of LVEF [25]. This fact may suggest that LV contractility remains proofed longer to unfavorable hemodynamics caused by deteriorating valve disease. On the other hand, a small improvement in AVA after BAV could impact LVEF recovery as presumably, it may be more sensitive to any decrease in afterload. Summing up, current study provides additional evidence for possible improvement of initially depressed LVEF after BAV, what has also been postulated previously [26,27]. Patients become better candidates for TAVI/AVR and this may highlight the actual importance of BAV. However, considering the stepwise and consistent deterioration of valve parameters and the persistent high risk of death, a "watchful waiting strategy" should be preferred over routine follow-up after BAV. Moreover, LVEF >40% at 1 month might be helpful guidance for the decision about final therapy, which should be implemented at the longest of 6 months after BAV [28]. Otherwise, the prognosis would be dramatically worsened, as showed in the palliative group in our study.

Balloon aortic valvuloplasty has also been investigated in patients with severe AS requiring urgent non-cardiac surgery [4,29–33], but no clear evidence has been shown so far, and studies showed disturbing results. In a study by Debry at al., the authors concluded that patients with severe AS managed conservatively before urgent non-cardiac surgery are at high risk of events and a systematic invasive strategy using BAV does not significantly improve clinical outcomes [4]. However, contrary to our results, patients enrolled had higher LVEF (56.6% in the invasive arm and 59.2% in the conservative arm) [4]. Current ESC guidelines for the treatment of valvular heart disease allow BAV to be performed in such patients with class IIb recommendation [2].

The role of cardiac rehabilitation in patients undergoing BAV remains unknown in contrast to the TAVI population [34–36]. Physical exercise conditioning may be, however, limited in these patients due to the profile of comorbidities, frailty and poorer LV function compared to TAVI patients. Nonetheless, close watchful waiting after BAV within an outpatient cardiac rehabilitation program may be beneficial, especially in terms of deterioration of the AS.

Study Limitations

Current study has several limitations which are inherent to the non-randomized design. The study findings were derived from observational analyses, which are subject to well-known limitations. We could not exclude a residual bias related to the age of patients as well as other patient's characteristics.

5. Conclusions

In everyday clinical practice in the TAVI era, there are still clinical indications to BAV a standalone procedure as a bridge to surgery, TAVI or for urgent high risk non-cardiac surgical procedures. Patients may improve clinically after BAV with LV function recovery, allowing to perform final therapy, within a limited time window, for severe AS, which ameliorates long-term outcomes. On the other hand, in patients for whom an isolated BAV becomes a destination therapy, prognosis is extremely poor.

Author Contributions: Conceptualization, P.K., J.L.; methodology, P.K., L.R.; formal analysis, P.K.; investigation, P.K., J.T., L.R.; resources, A.K., P.B., M.S., D.S.; data curation, P.K.; writing—original draft preparation, P.K., A.K.; writing—review and editing, P.K., A.D., S.B., D.D., J.L.; visualization, P.K., A.K.; supervision, P.K. D.D., J.L.; project administration, P.K. All authors have read and agreed to the published version of the manuscript.

Funding: This research received no external funding.

Institutional Review Board Statement: Ethical review and approval were waived for this study, due to retrospective character of the study, yet the institutional board was informed and acknowledged the study.

Informed Consent Statement: Informed consent was obtained from all subjects involved in the study.

Data Availability Statement: The data presented in this study are available on request from the corresponding author.

Conflicts of Interest: The authors declare no conflict of interest.

References

1. Baumgartner, H.; Falk, V.; Bax, J.J.; De Bonis, M.; Hamm, C.; Holm, P.J.; Lansac, E.; Muñoz, D.R.; Rosenhek, R.; Sjögren, J.; et al. 2017 ESC/EACTS Guidelines for the management of valvular heart disease. *Eur. Heart J.* **2017**, *38*, 2739–2791. [CrossRef] [PubMed]
2. Vahanian, A.; Beyersdorf, F.; Praz, F.; Milojevic, M.; Baldus, S.; Bauersachs, J.; Capodanno, D.; Conradi, L.; De Bonis, M.; De Paulis, R.; et al. 2021 ESC/EACTS Guidelines for the management of valvular heart disease: Developed by the Task Force for the management of valvular heart disease of the European Society of Cardiology (ESC) and the European Association for Cardio-Thoracic Surgery (EACTS). *Eur. Heart J.* **2021**, ehab395. [CrossRef]
3. Daniec, M.; Nawrotek, B.; Sorysz, D.; Rakowski, T.; Dziewierz, A.; Rzeszutko, Ł.; Kleczyński, P.; Trębacz, J.; Tomala, M.; Żmudka, K.; et al. Acute and long-term outcomes of percutaneous balloon aortic valvuloplasty for the treatment of severe aortic stenosis. *Catheter. Cardiovasc. Interv.* **2016**, *90*, 303–310. [CrossRef] [PubMed]
4. Debry, N.; Altes, A.; Vincent, F.; Delhaye, C.; Schurtz, G.; Nedjari, F.; Legros, G.; Porouchani, S.; Coisne, A.; Richardson, M.; et al. Balloon Aortic Valvuloplasty for Severe Aortic Stenosis Before Urgent Noncardiac Surgery. *EuroIntervention* **2021**, *17*, e680–e687. [CrossRef] [PubMed]
5. Percutaneous Balloon Aortic Valvuloplasty. Acute and 30-day follow-up results in 674 patients from the NHLBI Balloon Valvuloplasty Registry. *Circulation* **1991**, *84*, 2383–2397. [CrossRef]
6. Lieberman, E.B.; Bashore, T.M.; Hermiller, J.B.; Wilson, J.S.; Pieper, K.S.; Keeler, G.P.; Pierce, C.H.; Kisslo, K.B.; Harrison, J.K.; Davidson, C.J. Balloon aortic valvuloplasty in adults: Failure of procedure to improve long-term survival. *J. Am. Coll. Cardiol.* **1995**, *26*, 1522–1528. [CrossRef]
7. Otto, C.M.; Mickel, M.C.; Kennedy, J.W.; Alderman, E.L.; Bashore, T.M.; Block, P.C.; Brinker, J.A.; Diver, D.; Ferguson, J.; Holmes, D.R. Three-year outcome after balloon aortic valvuloplasty. Insights into prognosis of valvular aortic stenosis. *Circulation* **1994**, *89*, 642–650. [CrossRef]

8. Wacławski, J.; Wilczek, K.; Hudzik, B.; Pres, D.; Hawranek, M.; Milewski, K.; Chodór, P.; Zembala, M.; Gąsior, M. Aortic balloon valvuloplasty as a bridge-to-decision in patients with aortic stenosis. *Adv. Interv. Cardiol.* **2019**, *15*, 195–202. [CrossRef]
9. Kleczynski, P.; Dziewierz, A.; Socha, S.; Rakowski, T.; Daniec, M.; Zawislak, B.; Arif, S.; Wojtasik-Bakalarz, J.; Dudek, D.; Rzeszutko, L. Direct Rapid Left Ventricular Wire Pacing during Balloon Aortic Valvuloplasty. *J. Clin. Med.* **2020**, *9*, 1017. [CrossRef]
10. Stąpór, M.; Trębacz, J.; Wiewiórka, Ł.; Ostrowska-Kaim, E.; Nawara-Skipirzepa, J.; Sobczyński, R.; Konstanty-Kalandyk, J.; Musiał, R.; Trębacz, O.; Kleczyński, P.; et al. Direct left ventricular wire pacing during transcatheter aortic valve implantation. *Kardiol. Pol.* **2020**, *78*, 882–888. [CrossRef]
11. Daniec, M.; Dziewierz, A.; Sorysz, D.; Kleczyński, P.; Rakowski, T.; Rzeszutko, Ł.; Trębacz, J.; Tomala, M.; Nawrotek, B.; Żmudka, K.; et al. Sex-Related Differences in Outcomes After Percutaneous Balloon Aortic Valvuloplasty. *J. Invasive Cardiol.* **2017**, *29*, 188–194. [PubMed]
12. Daniec, M.; Sorysz, D.; Dziewierz, A.; Kleczyński, P.; Rzeszutko, Ł.; Krawczyk-Ożóg, A.; Dudek, D. In-hospital and long-term outcomes of percutaneous balloon aortic valvuloplasty with concomitant percutaneous coronary intervention in patients with severe aortic stenosis. *J. Interv. Cardiol.* **2018**, *31*, 60–67. [CrossRef] [PubMed]
13. Moretti, C.; Chandran, S.; Vervueren, P.; D'Ascenzo, F.; Barbanti, M.; Weerackody, R.; Boccuzzi, G.; Lee, D.-H.; de la Torre Hernandez, J.; Omedè, P.; et al. Outcomes of patients undergoing balloon aortic valvuloplasty in the TAVI Era: A multicenter registry. *J. Invasive Cardiol.* **2015**, *27*, 547–555.
14. McKay, R.G. The Mansfield Scientific aortic valvuloplasty registry: Overview of acute hemodynamic results and procedural complications. *J. Am. Coll. Cardiol.* **1991**, *17*, 485–491. [CrossRef]
15. Malkin, C.J.; Judd, J.; Chew, D.P.; Sinhal, A. Balloon aortic valvuloplasty to bridge and triage patients in the era of trans-catheter aortic valve implantation. *Catheter. Cardiovasc. Interv.* **2013**, *81*, 358–363. [CrossRef]
16. Saia, F.; Marrozzini, C.; Moretti, C.; Ciuca, C.; Taglieri, N.; Bordoni, B.; Dall'ara, G.; Alessi, L.; Lanzillotti, V.; Bacchi-Reggiani, M.L.; et al. The role of percutaneous balloon aortic valvuloplasty as a bridge for transcatheter aortic valve implantation. *EuroIntervention* **2011**, *7*, 723–729. [CrossRef]
17. Doguet, F.; Godin, M.; Lebreton, G.; Eltchaninoff, H.; Cribier, A.; Bessou, J.P.; Litzler, P.Y. Aortic valve replacement after percutaneous valvuloplasty—An approach in otherwise inoperable patients. *Eur. J. Cardiothorac. Surg.* **2010**, *38*, 394–399. [CrossRef]
18. Leon, M.B.; Smith, C.R.; Mack, M.; Miller, D.C.; Moses, J.W.; Svensson, L.G.; Tuzcu, E.M.; Webb, J.G.; Fontana, G.P.; Makkar, R.R.; et al. Transcatheter aortic-valve implantation for aortic stenosis in patients who cannot undergo surgery. *N. Engl. J. Med.* **2010**, *363*, 1597–1607. [CrossRef] [PubMed]
19. Armario, X.; Rosseel, L.; McGrath, B.; Mylotte, D. Balloon aortic valvuloplasty with two simultaneous balloons via ipsilateral transradial and transbrachial access. *EuroIntervention* **2021**, *17*, 88–89. [CrossRef]
20. Tumscitz, C.; Di Cesare, A.; Balducelli, M.; Piva, T.; Santarelli, A.; Saia, F.; Tarantino, F.; Preti, G.; Picchi, A.; Rolfo, C.; et al. Safety, efficacy and impact on frailty of mini-invasive radial balloon aortic valvuloplasty. *Heart* **2021**, *107*, 874–880. [CrossRef]
21. Theodoropoulos, K.C.; Kouparanis, A.; Didagelos, M.; Kassimis, G.; Karvounis, H.; Ziakas, A. Balloon rupture during aortic valvuloplasty: A severe complication or a well-tolerated event? *Kardiol. Pol.* **2021**, *79*, 201–202. [CrossRef]
22. Bularga, A.; Bing, R.; Shah, A.S.; Adamson, P.D.; Behan, M.; Newby, D.E.; Flapan, A.; Uren, N.; Cruden, N. Clinical outcomes following balloon aortic valvuloplasty. *Open Heart* **2020**, *7*, e001330. [CrossRef]
23. Kleczynski, P.; Dziewierz, A.; Bagienski, M.; Rzeszutko, L.; Sorysz, D.; Trebacz, J.; Sobczynski, R.; Tomala, M.; Stapor, M.; Dudek, D. Impact of frailty on mortality after transcatheter aortic valve implantation. *Am. Heart J.* **2017**, *185*, 52–58. [CrossRef] [PubMed]
24. Kleczynski, P.; Tokarek, T.; Dziewierz, A.; Sorysz, D.; Bagienski, M.; Rzeszutko, L.; Dudek, D. Usefulness of Psoas Muscle Area and Volume and Frailty Scoring to Predict Outcomes After Transcatheter Aortic Valve Implantation. *Am. J. Cardiol.* **2018**, *122*, 135–140. [CrossRef] [PubMed]
25. Padmini, V.; Nikhil, K.; Ramesh, C.B.; Ramdas, G.P. Clinical profile and natural history of 453 nonsurgically managed patients with severe aortic stenosis. *Ann. Thorac. Surg.* **2006**, *82*, 2111–2115.
26. Dworakowski, R.; Bhan, A.; Brickham, B.; Monaghan, M.; Maccarthy, P. Effectiveness of balloon aortic valvuloplasty is greater in patients with impaired left ventricular function. *Int. J. Cardiol.* **2011**, *150*, 103–105. [CrossRef]
27. Kefer, J.; Gapira, J.M.; Pierard, S.; De Meester, C.; Gurne, O.; Chenu, P.; Renkin, J. Recovery after balloon aortic valvuloplasty in patients with aortic stenosis and impaired left ventricular function: Predictors and prognostic implications. *J. Invasive Cardiol.* **2013**, *25*, 235–241.
28. Husaini, M.; Soyama, Y.; Kagiyama, N.; Thakker, P.; Thangam, M.; Haque, N.; Deych, E.; Sintek, M.; Lasala, J.; Gorcsan, J., 3rd; et al. Clinical and Echocardiographic Features Associated With Improved Survival in Patients With Severe Aortic Stenosis Undergoing Balloon Aortic Valvuloplasty (BAV). *J. Invasive Cardiol.* **2020**, *32*, E277–E285.
29. Tashiro, T.; Pislaru, S.V.; Blustin, J.M.; Nkomo, V.T.; Abel, M.D.; Scott, C.G.; Pellikka, P.A. Perioperative risk of major non-cardiac surgery in patients with severe aortic stenosis: A reappraisal in contemporary practice. *Eur. Heart J.* **2014**, *35*, 2372–2381. [CrossRef]
30. Leibowitz, D.; Rivkin, G.; Schiffman, J.; Rott, D.; Weiss, A.T.; Mattan, Y.; Kandel, L. Effect of severe aortic stenosis on the outcome in elderly patients undergoing repair of hip fracture. *Gerontology* **2009**, *55*, 303–306. [CrossRef]

31. Calleja, A.M.; Dommaraju, S.; Gaddam, R.; Cha, S.; Khandheria, B.K.; Chaliki, H.P. Cardiac risk in patients aged >75 years with asymptomatic, severe aortic stenosis undergoing noncardiac surgery. *Am. J. Cardiol.* **2010**, *105*, 1159–1163. [CrossRef] [PubMed]
32. Keswani, A.; Lovy, A.; Khalid, M.; Blaufarb, I.; Moucha, C.; Forsh, D.; Chen, D. The effect of aortic stenosis on elderly hip fracture outcomes: A case control study. *Injury* **2016**, *47*, 413–418. [CrossRef] [PubMed]
33. MacIntyre, P.A.; Scott, M.; Seigne, R.; Clark, A.; Deveer, F.; Minchin, I. An observational study of perioperative risk associated with aortic stenosis in non-cardiac surgery. *Anaesth. Intensive Care* **2018**, *46*, 207–214. [CrossRef] [PubMed]
34. Kleczynski, P.; Trebacz, J.; Stapor, M.; Sobczynski, R.; Konstanty-Kalandyk, J.; Kapelak, B.; Zmudka, K.; Legutko, J. Inpatient Cardiac Rehabilitation after Transcatheter Aortic Valve Replacement Is Associated with Improved Clinical Performance and Quality of Life. *J. Clin. Med.* **2021**, *10*, 2125. [CrossRef]
35. Rogers, P.; Al-Aidrous, S.; Banya, W.; Haley, S.R.; Mittal, T.; Kabir, T.; Panoulas, V.; Raja, S.; Bhudia, S.; Probert, H.; et al. Cardiac rehabilitation to improve health-related quality of life following trans-catheter aortic valve implantation: A randomised controlled feasibility study: RECOVER-TAVI Pilot, ORCA 4, For the Optimal Restoration of Cardiac Activity Group. *Pilot Feasibility Stud.* **2018**, *4*, 185. [CrossRef]
36. Tarro Genta, F.; Tidu, M.; Corbo, P.; Bertolin, F.; Salvetti, I.; Bouslenko, Z.; Giordano, A.; Dalla Vecchia, L. Predictors of survival in patients undergoing cardiac rehabilitation after transcatheter aortic valve implantation. *J. Cardiovasc. Med.* **2019**, *20*, 606–615. [CrossRef] [PubMed]

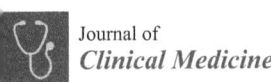

Article

Transcatheter versus Isolated Surgical Aortic Valve Replacement in Young High-Risk Patients: A Propensity Score-Matched Analysis

Markus Mach [1,2,*], Thomas Poschner [1], Waseem Hasan [3], Tillmann Kerbel [1], Philipp Szalkiewicz [1], Ena Hasimbegovic [1,4], Martin Andreas [1], Christoph Gross [1,5], Andreas Strouhal [6], Georg Delle-Karth [6], Martin Grabenwöger [2,7], Christopher Adlbrecht [6,8] and Andreas Schober [6]

1. Department of Cardiac Surgery, Medical University of Vienna, 1090 Vienna, Austria; thomas.poschner@meduniwien.ac.at (T.P.); tillmann.kerbel@meduniwien.ac.at (T.K.); n1405273@students.meduniwien.ac.at (P.S.); ena.hasimbegovic@meduniwien.ac.at (E.H.); martin.andreas@meduniwien.ac.at (M.A.); christoph.gross@meduniwien.ac.at (C.G.)
2. Department of Cardio-Vascular Surgery, Hospital Floridsdorf and Karl Landsteiner Institute for Cardio-Vascular Research, 1210 Vienna, Austria; martin.grabenwoeger@gesundheitsverbund.at
3. Faculty of Medicine, Imperial College London, London SW7 2AZ, UK; waseem.hasan15@imperial.ac.uk
4. Division of Cardiology, Department of Internal Medicine II, Medical University of Vienna, 1090 Vienna, Austria
5. Center of Medical Physics and Biomedical Engineering, Medical University of Vienna, 1090 Vienna, Austria
6. Department of Cardiology, Hospital Floridsdorf and the Karl Landsteiner Institute for Cardiovascular and Critical Care Research Vienna, 1210 Vienna, Austria; andreas.strouhal@gesundheitsverbund.at (A.S.); georg.delle-karth@gesundheitsverbund.at (G.D.-K.); c.adlbrecht@imed19.at (C.A.); andreas.schober@gesundheitsverbund.at (A.S.)
7. Faculty of Medicine, Sigmund Freud University, 1020 Vienna, Austria
8. Imed19, Private Research Center, 1190 Vienna, Austria
* Correspondence: markus.mach@meduniwien.ac.at; Tel.: +43-1-40400-52620

Abstract: Background: Younger patients with severe symptomatic aortic stenosis are a particularly challenging collective with regard to the choice of intervention. High-risk patients younger than 75 years of age are often eligible for both the transcatheter aortic valve replacement (TAVR) and the isolated surgical aortic valve replacement (iSAVR). Data on the outcomes of both interventions in this set of patients are scarce. Methods: One hundred and forty-four propensity score-matched patients aged 75 years or less who underwent TAVR or iSAVR at the Hietzing Heart Center in Vienna, Austria, were included in the study. The mean age was 68.9 years (TAVR 68.7 vs. SAVR 67.6 years; $p = 0.190$) and the average EuroSCORE II was 5.4% (TAVR 4.3 [3.2%] vs. iSAVR 6.4 (4.3%); $p = 0.194$). Results: Postprocedural adverse event data showed higher rates of newly acquired atrial fibrillation (6.9% vs. 19.4%; $p = 0.049$), prolonged ventilation (2.8% vs. 25.0%; $p < 0.001$) and multi-organ failure (0% vs. 6.9%) in the surgical cohort. The in-hospital and 30-day mortality was significantly higher for iSAVR (1.4% vs. 13.9%; $p = 0.012$; 12.5% vs. 2.8%; $p = 0.009$, respectively). The long-term survival (median follow-up 5.0 years (2.2–14.1 years)) of patients treated with the surgical approach was superior to that of patients undergoing TAVR ($p < 0.001$). Conclusion: Although the survival analysis revealed a higher in-hospital and 30-day survival rate for high-risk patients aged ≤75 years who underwent TAVR, iSAVR was associated with a significantly higher long-term survival rate.

Keywords: TAVI; TAVR; SAVR; aortic stenosis; young

1. Introduction

Treating non-geriatric patients with symptomatic aortic stenosis and a high surgical risk profile is challenging in light of the scarcity of data in this patient collective. This collective of patients has not yet been investigated in large randomized trials. Comparing the transcatheter aortic valve replacement (TAVR) to the isolated surgical aortic valve

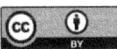

replacement (SAVR), the question of whether young high-risk patients who undergo TAVR share the excellent outcomes of recently published large clinical trials in the field remains unanswered [1,2].

Over the last decade, TAVR has evolved from an initially experimental procedure to a standard therapy option for severe aortic stenosis and is being performed more frequently than SAVR in some countries [2–5]. TAVR is currently indicated for patients suffering from severe symptomatic aortic valve stenosis who are at a high or intermediate surgical risk [6–9]. Furthermore, it has been suggested that TAVR is a safe and suitable option for patients at lower surgical risk levels [10,11]. As the list of possible indications is getting longer, the focus is shifting to concerns regarding prosthesis durability, periinterventional and postinterventional adverse outcomes and patient selection [12–14].

We investigated a cohort of patients under 75 years of age with significant comorbidities and a high surgical risk with symptomatic severe aortic stenosis who underwent either SAVR or TAVR. We performed propensity score matching and investigated the short- and long-term outcomes and procedural differences between TAVR and SAVR.

2. Materials and Methods

2.1. TAVR Cohort

This retrospective analysis was approved by the institutional Ethics Committee of the City of Vienna (EK 20-141—VK). Data from 532 patients enrolled in the Vienna Cardiothoracic Aortic Valve Registry (VICTORY) Registry at the Hietzing Heart Center from June 2009 to December 2016 were reviewed. One hundred and twenty-four patients aged 75 years or less were selected from this collective for further analysis. The 75-year cut-off was chosen according to the treatment allocation recommendations of the 2017 ESC/EACTS guidelines. Although no lower age limit was applied to the analysis, no patients younger than 53 years were included in the study. Patients who exceeded a EuroSCORE II of 4% or a logistic EuroSCORE of 10% were deemed to be at an increased risk for postoperative morbidity or mortality [6]. Each patient was assessed by the institutional Heart Team. The decision to treat these patients with TAVR was based on the risk factors and comorbidities listed in Table 1. Due to existing contraindications to SAVR, 16 patients were excluded from the analysis. Of the remaining 88 patients, 42 were treated via the percutaneous transfemoral and 46 via the transapical access site as previously described [15]. Different generations of transcatheter valves developed by Edwards Lifesciences (Edwards Lifesciences, Irvine, CA, USA), Medtronic (Medtronic, Minneapolis, MN, USA), JenaValve (JenaValve Technology GmbH, Munich, Germany) and Symetis (Symetis SA, a Boston Scientific company, Ecublens, Switzerland) were used.

Table 1. Factors impacting the choice of TAVR over iSAVR.

	TAVR < 75 Years n = 104
Prohibitive surgical risk, n (%) [1]	8 (7.7)
Porcelain aorta, n (%) [1]	9 (8.7)
High-risk reoperation, n (%)	42 (40.4)
Respiratory impairment, n (%)	41 (39.4)
Severely reduced LVEF, n (%)	34 (32.7)
Severe renal insufficiency, n (%)	32 (30.8)
Substance abuse, n (%)	23 (22.1)
Adipositas per magna, n (%)	16 (15.4)
Valve-in-Valve procedure, n (%)	13 (12.5)
Neurological impairment, n (%)	12 (11.5)

Table 1. *Cont.*

	TAVR < 75 Years *n* = 104
Hepatopathy, n (%)	10 (9.6)
History of radiation to the chest, n (%)	9 (8.7)
Severe mental disorder, n (%)	9 (8.7)
Pulmonary hypertension, n (%)	7 (6.7)
Frailty, n (%)	3 (2.9)
Severe rhythm disorder, n (%)	2 (1.9)
History of severe bleeding, n (%)	1 (1.0)
Other, n (%)	17 (16.3)
Patients with 2 or more reasons listed above	74 (71.2)
Patients with 3 or more reasons listed above	35 (33.7)

[1] Excluded from analysis due to absolute SAVR contraindications; LVEF—left ventricular ejection fraction; iSAVR—isolated surgical aortic valve replacement; TAVR—transcatheter aortic valve replacement.

2.2. iSAVR Cohort

Between January 2005 and December 2016, 732 patients younger than 75 years underwent iSAVR without concomitant procedures at the Department of Cardiovascular Surgery, Heart Center Hietzing (Vienna, Austria). iSAVR was performed according to standard surgical practice. A total of 128 patients were excluded from the analysis due to active endocarditis ($n = 54$) or incomplete datasets ($n = 74$). Thus, 604 iSAVR patients were deemed eligible for this study. Patients undergoing aortic valve replacement via a homograft implantation or Ross procedure were excluded from the analysis.

2.3. Study Design and Endpoint Definitions

A propensity score-matched analysis stratified for differences in the patients' baseline characteristics was created to compare the outcome of patients undergoing iSAVR or TAVR. A flowchart depicting patient selection and statistical analysis is shown in Figure 1.

The primary study endpoints were defined as 30-day all-cause mortality and freedom from all-cause mortality after 5 years. The secondary endpoints were the occurrence of adverse events and peri- and postprocedural complications as set out by the updated Valve Academic Research Consortium (VARC)-II criteria including bleeding events, access-related vascular complications, myocardial infarction, acute kidney injury, neurological adverse events, the necessity of pacemaker implantation and reoperations [16].

2.4. Statistical Analysis

Continuous variables were expressed as either the median and interquartile range (IQR) or as mean and standard deviation (±SD), based on their distribution. Categorical variables were expressed as absolute numbers and percentages and compared with the chi^2 test or Fisher's exact test.

2.5. Propensity Score Matching

Propensity score matching was performed according to the recommendations proposed by McMurry et al. [17]. A non-parsimonious multivariable logistic regression model was used to calculate the propensity score. Rigorous adjustment for significant differences in the patients' baseline characteristics relevant for the treatment assignment and potential outcomes was performed with 1-to-1 matching using the following algorithm: nearest neighbor matching with a caliper width of 0.1 standard deviation of the propensity score and no replacement. The propensity score model was adjusted for differences in the following baseline characteristics: sex, age at time of procedure, body mass index (BMI), preprocedural serum creatinine level, chronic obstructive lung disease, peripheral vascular disease, arterial hypertension, previous cardiac surgery, insulin-dependent diabetes mellitus and left ventricular ejection fraction. The average absolute standardized difference was 1.5 and 0.04 after matching (Figure 2).

Differences in categorical variables between the matched cohorts were analyzed with McNemar's test, and continuous variables were compared using the Wilcoxon signed-rank test or paired samples t-test based on variable distribution. A Kaplan–Meier estimate of long-term survival was performed, and survival curves were compared by the test described by Klein and Moeschberger [18]. Baseline, procedural and outcome characteristics of patients excluded from the analysis after propensity score matching are summarized in Supplementary Tables S1–S3.

All reported p-values were two-sided, and the results were categorized as statistically significant with an alpha level set at <0.05; due to the exploratory nature of the analyses, p-values may be interpreted as descriptive rather than confirmatory. All analyses were performed using SPSS, version 24.0 (IBM Corp, Armonk, NY, USA).

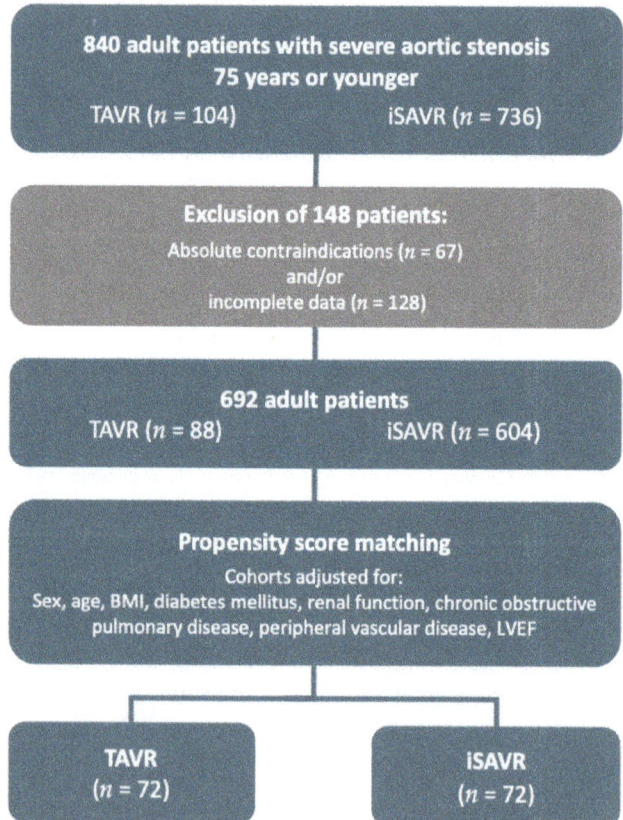

Figure 1. Patient selection and propensity score matching flow-chart (BMI—body mass index, LVEF—left ventricular ejection fraction).

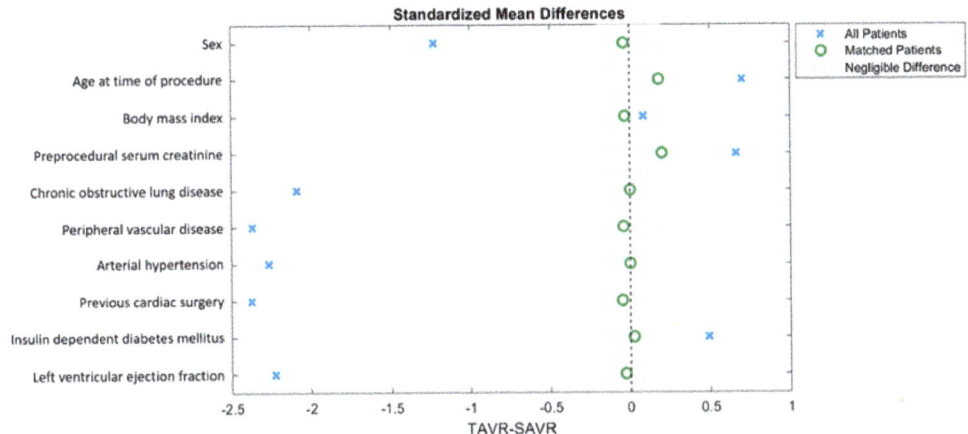

Figure 2. Standardized mean differences in matching variables before and after propensity score matching.

3. Results

3.1. Baseline Characteristics

Baseline characteristics, procedural characteristics and adverse events for the unmatched and matched population are presented in Tables 2–4, respectively. Eighty-eight TAVR patients and 604 iSAVR patients were included in the retrospective analysis (64.1 ± 9.5 years, 287 (41.5%) female, median follow-up 5.5 years (2.2–14.1 years)). After propensity score matching, 72 matched pairs were compared. The cohorts did not differ regarding baseline characteristics used for adjustment in the analysis model (Figure 2). No differences were observed in the EuroSCORE II (4.3 ± 3.2% vs. 6.4 ± 4.3%; $p = 0.194$). However, patients undergoing TAVR had more often been treated with a percutaneous coronary intervention (PCI) prior to the procedure (TAVR: 19.4% vs. iSAVR: 5.6%; $p = 0.021$).

Table 2. Baseline clinical characteristics of the unmatched and matched cohorts.

	Overall $n = 692$	Unmatched-Population ($n = 692$)		PS-Matched-Population ($n = 144$)		p-Value
		iSAVR < 75 Years $n = 604$	TAVR < 75 Years $n = 88$	iSAVR < 75 Years $n = 72$	TAVR < 75 Years $n = 72$	
Demographics						
Age, mean (±SD)	64.1 (9.5)	63.4 (9.8)	68.9 (5.2)	67.6 (7)	68.7 (5.5)	0.190
Female, n (%)	287 (41.5)	237 (39.2)	50 (56.8)	33 (45.8)	39 (54.2)	0.418
Body mass index kg/m^2, median (IQR)	28.7 (5.5)	28.6 (5.4)	29.2 (6.5)	29.3 (4.8)	29.1 (6.7)	0.854
Risk profile						
EuroSCORE II, median (IQR)	2.7 (3.7)	1.7 (2.2)	5.9 (5.3)	6.4 (4.3)	4.3 (3.2)	0.194
Chronic Health Conditions and Risk Factors						
Hypertension, n (%)	538 (77.7)	464 (92.2)	74 (84.1)	53 (73.6)	62 (86.1)	0.089
Dyslipidaemia, n (%)	433 (62.6)	380 (82.3)	53 (60.2)	42 (36.2)	41 (35.3)	0.999
Diabetes mellitus, n (%)	200 (28.9)	164 (27.2)	36 (40.9)	9 (12.5)	8 (11.1)	0.371
Active smoker, n (%)	126 (18.2)	106 (17.5)	20 (22.7)	9 (12.5)	18 (25.0)	0.121
Serum creatinine mg/dL, mean (±SD)	1.1 (0.6)	1.0 (0.4)	1.5 (1.2)	1.4 (0.7)	1.3 (0.6)	0.894
Preoperative dialysis, n (%)	6 (0.9)	2 (0.3)	4 (4.5)	2 (2.8)	1 (1.4)	0.999
Chronic obstructive pulmonary disease, n (%)	217 (31.4)	168 (24.3)	49 (7.1)	41 (56.9)	37 (51.4)	0.608
Peripheral vascular disease, n (%)	67 (9.7)	43 (6.2)	24 (27.3)	14 (19.4)	14 (19.4)	0.999
Cerebrovascular disease, n (%)	111 (16.0)	87 (14.4)	24 (3.5)	9 (12.5)	19 (26.4)	0.031
Previous cerebrovascular accident, n (%)	17 (2.5)	7 (1.2)	10 (11.4)	4 (5.6)	9 (12.5)	0.227
Atrial fibrillation, n (%)	119 (17.2)	101 (16.7)	18 (20.5)	14 (19.4)	13 (18.1)	0.999

Table 2. Cont.

		Unmatched-Population (n = 692)		PS-Matched-Population (n = 144)		
	Overall n = 692	iSAVR < 75 Years n = 604	TAVR < 75 Years n = 88	iSAVR < 75 Years n = 72	TAVR < 75 Years n = 72	p-Value
Previous myocardial infarction, n (%)	54 (7.8)	37 (6.1)	17 (19.3)	10 (13.9)	13 (18.1)	0.629
New York Heart Association class III/IV, n (%)	367 (53.1)	288 (47.7)	79 (90)	51 (70.8)	63 (87.5)	0.072
Preprocedural PCI, n (%)	43 (6.2)	26 (4.3)	17 (19.3)	4 (5.6)	14 (19.4)	0.021
Previous pacemaker implantation, n (%)	32 (4.6)	17 (2.8)	15 (17)	5 (6.9)	11 (15.3)	0.210
Previous cardiac surgery, n (%)	64 (9.2)	26 (4.3)	38 (43.2)	16 (22.2)	26 (36.1)	0.064
Previous CABG, n (%)	34 (4.9)	11 (1.8)	23 (26.1)	9 (12.5)	17 (23.6)	
Previous valve surgery, n (%)	34 (4.9)	16 (2.6)	18 (20.5)	10 (13.9)	10 (13.9)	
aortic, n (%)	25 (3.6)	12 (2.0)	13 (14.8)	9 (12.5)	10 (13.9)	
mitral, n (%)	9 (1.5)	4 (0.7)	5 (5.7)	1 (1.4)	0 (0)	
tricuspid, n (%)	3 (0.4)	2 (0.3)	1 (1.0)	0 (0)	0 (0)	
Previous other cardiac surgery, n (%)	17 (2.5)	2 (0.3)	15 (17)	0 (0)	10 (13.9)	
Preoperative Echocardiographic Data						
Mean pressure gradient, mean (±SD)	48 (17.3)	48.6 (17.6)	46.3 (18.3)	48.3 (17.9)	46.7 (18.6)	0.266
Left ventricular ejection fraction %, mean (±IQR) [1]	52.7 (9.9)	53.4 (9.2)	46.5 (11.9)	51.7 (12.8)	47.7 (11.3)	0.061

[1] McNemar (for binary variables) and Wilcoxon signed-rank test or paired samples t-test (for continuous variables); PS—propensity score; CABG—coronary artery bypass graft; EuroSCORE—European System for Cardiac Operative Risk Evaluation; IQR—interquartile range; PCI—percutaneous coronary intervention; PS—propensity score SD—standard deviation.

Table 3. Procedural characteristics of the unmatched and matched cohorts.

		Unmatched-Population (n = 692)		PS-Matched-Population (n = 144)		
	Overall n = 692	iSAVR < 75 Years n = 604	TAVR < 75 Years n = 88	iSAVR < 75 Years n = 72	TAVR < 75 Years n = 72	p-Value
Procedural Characteristics						
Biological valve prosthesis, n (%)	595 (86.0)	507 (83.9)	88 (100)	62 (86.1)	72 (100)	n/a ‡
Balloon-expandable THV, n (%)			56 (63.6)		43 (59.7)	n/a ‡
Prosthesis size in mm, mean (±SD)	23.2 (3.2)	22.8 (3.1)	26.3 (2.2)	22.7 (2.2)	26.5 (2.1)	<0.001
Full sternotomy, n (%)		494 (81.2)		66 (91.7)		n/a ‡
Cross-clamp time, mean (±SD)	58.3 (31)	58.3 (31)	0 (0)	62.8 (21.5)	0 (0)	n/a ‡
Perfusion time, mean (±SD)	87.8 (52.1)	87.8 (52.1)	0 (0)	111.2 (40.2)	0 (0)	n/a ‡
Transfemoral access, n (%)			42 (47.7)		29 (40.3)	n/a ‡
Predilatation, n (%)			43 (48.9)		38 (52.8)	n/a ‡
Postdilatation, n (%)			9 (10.2)		5 (6.9)	n/a ‡
Paravalvular leak > mild, n (%)	1 (0.1)	0 (0)	1 (1.1)	0 (0)	1 (1.4)	0.999
Postoperative circulatory support, n (%)	8 (1.2)	7 (1.2)	1 (1.1)	4 (5.6)	0 (0)	n/a ‡
Extubated in the operating room, n (%)	10 (1.4)	0 (0)	10 (12)	0 (0)	6 (8.3)	n/a ‡
Total hours ventilated, median (±IQR)	8 (8)	8.0 (8)	4 (7)	12 (27)	4 (7)	<0.001
Re-intubated during hospital stay, n (%)	22 (3.2)	19 (3.1)	3 (3.6)	4 (5.6)	3 (4.5)	0.999
Number of administered red blood cell units, mean (±SD)	0.6 (1.6)	0.6 (1.6)	0.6 (1.2)	1.0 (3.0)	0.6 (1.2)	0.242
Length of stay, median (±IQR)	11.0 (5)	11 (5)	9 (7)	11.5 (6)	9.0 (7)	0.188

n/a ‡—not calculated if a variable is constant in one cohort; PS—propensity score; IQR—Interquartile range; SD—standard deviation; THV—transcatheter heart valve.

Table 4. Adverse events in the unmatched and matched cohorts.

	Unmatched-Population (n = 692)			PS-Matched-Population (n = 144)		
	Overall n = 692	iSAVR < 75 Years n = 604	TAVR < 75 Years n = 88	iSAVR < 75 Years n = 72	TAVR < 75 Years n = 72	p-Value
	VARC-2 Adverse Events					
Myocardial infarction, n (%)	2 (0.3)	1 (0.2)	1 (1.1)	0 (0)	1 (1.4)	n/a ‡
Neurological adverse event, n (%)	9 (1.3)	7 (1.2)	2 (2.3)	2 (2.8)	2 (2.8)	0.999
Major vascular access complication, n (%)	5 (0.7)	0 (0)	5 (5.7)	0 (0)	4 (5.6)	n/a ‡
Major bleeding complication, n (%)	28 (4.0)	24 (4.0)	4 (4.6)	6 (8.3)	3 (4.2)	0.508
Postoperative dialysis, n (%)	10 (1.4)	8 (1.3)	2 (2.3)	2 (2.8)	2 (2.8)	0.999
New-onset atrial fibrillation, n (%)	84 (12.1)	79 (13.1)	5 (5.7)	14 (19.4)	5 (6.9)	0.049
AV-Block III, n (%)	16 (2.3)	11 (1.8)	5 (5.7)	0 (0)	2 (2.8)	n/a ‡
Pacemaker implantation, n (%)	18 (2.6)	13 (2.2)	5 (5.7)	0 (0)	2 (2.8)	n/a ‡
Reoperation for valvular dysfunction, n (%)	2 (0.3)	2 (0.3)	0 (0)	1 (1.4)	0 (0)	n/a ‡
Reoperation for bleeding/tamponade, n (%)	16 (2.3)	15 (2.5)	1 (1.1)	4 (5.6)	1 (1.4)	0.375
Reoperation for other cardiac problem, n (%)	5 (0.7)	2 (0.3)	3 (0.4)	1 (1.4)	2 (2.8)	0.999
Reoperation for non-cardiac problem, n (%)	15 (2.2)	10 (1.7)	5 (5.7)	0 (0)	5 (6.9)	n/a ‡
Postoperative sepsis, n (%)	4 (0.6)	4 (0.7)	0 (0)	2 (2.8)	0 (0)	n/a ‡
Pronounced wound infection, n (%)	9 (1.3)	9 (1.5)	0 (0)	5 (5.6)	0 (0)	n/a ‡
Prolonged ventilation > 6 h, n (%)	64 (9.2)	61 (10.1)	3 (0.4)	18 (25.0)	2 (2.8)	<0.001
Multi-organ dysfunction syndrome, n (%)	10 (1.4)	10 (1.7)	0 (0)	5 (6.9)	0 (0)	n/a ‡
In-hospital death, n (%)	17 (2.5)	16 (2.3)	1 (1.1)	10 (13.9)	1 (1.4)	0.012
30-day all-cause mortality, n (%)	19 (2.7)	16 (2.7)	3 (3.4)	9 (12.5)	2 (2.8)	0.022

n/a ‡—not calculated if the variable is constant in one cohort; AV—atrioventricular.

3.2. Survival and Safety Outcome

After propensity score matching, a significant difference in ventilation times (TAVR: 4 ± 7 h vs. iSAVR: 12 ± 27 h; $p < 0.001$) was observed. Patients undergoing iSAVR demonstrated higher rates of new-onset atrial fibrillation (TAVR: 6.9% vs. iSAVR: 19.4%; $p = 0.049$), sepsis (TAVR: 0% vs. iSAVR: 2.8%, $p = n/a$) and pronounced wound infection (TAVR: 0% vs. iSAVR: 5.6%, $p = n/a$). Of the 43 patients (59.7%) receiving transapical TAVR only 6 patients (8.3%) were extubated in the operating theatre. Prolonged ventilation times of longer than 6 h were more frequent in the iSAVR cohort (TAVR: 2.8% vs. iSAVR: 25%; $p < 0.001$). Conduction disorders and pacemaker implantation only occurred in the TAVR cohort, and the overall incidence was exceptionally low (TAVR: 0% vs. iSAVR 2.8%, $p = n/a$). Major vascular access complications occurred only in patients treated with TAVR (TAVR: 5.6% vs. iSAVR 0.0%, $p = n/a$), resulting in a higher re-operation rate for non-cardiac causes (TAVR 6.9% vs. iSAVR 0%, $p = n/a$). Multi organ dysfunction syndrome, in hospital death and 30-day all-cause mortality were significantly higher in the iSAVR cohort ([iSAVR: 0% vs. TAVR: 6.9%, $p = n/a$]; [1.4% vs. 13.9%; $p = 0.012$]; [2.8% vs. 12.5%; $p = 0.022$]).

The 5-year Kaplan–Meier curve is depicted in Figure 3. Although TAVR was associated with an improved 30-day survival, iSAVR patients had higher long-term survival rates ($p < 0.001$).

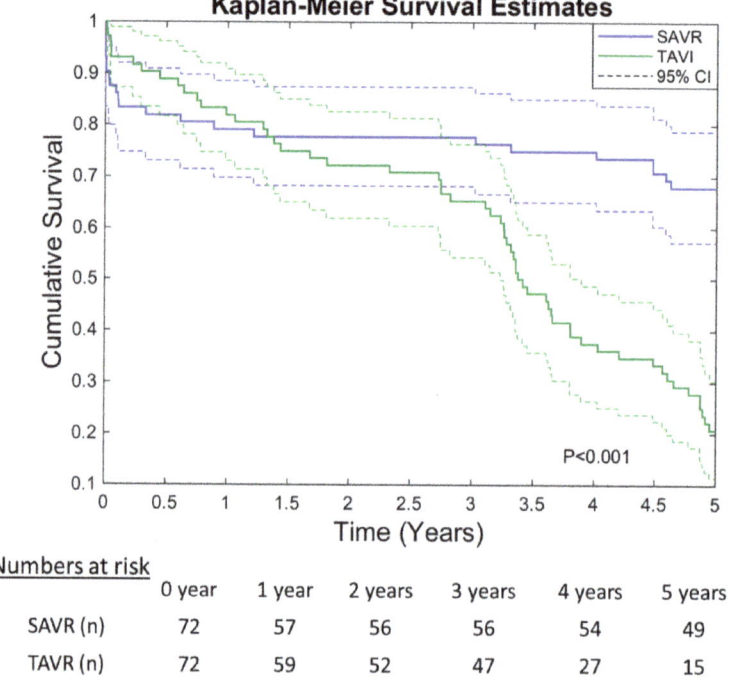

Figure 3. Five-year Kaplan–Meier survival curves (CI—Confidence Interval).

4. Discussion

This study is the first propensity-matched comparison of TAVR and iSAVR in non-geriatric high-risk patients. Although the 30-day survival is higher after TAVR, iSAVR is linked to a higher long-term survival rate. This study confirms the known strengths and weaknesses of the respective therapy options: on the one hand, iSAVR was associated with a higher incidence of new-onset atrial fibrillation and prolonged ventilation times, and on the other hand, TAVR patients had a higher incidence of associated vascular access complications. This led to the conclusion that, while for non-geriatric patients who are at a high risk of suffering significant adverse events or dying during or immediately following surgery, prohibitive risk of morbidity or mortality can be treated effectively with TAVR, those likely to recover from surgery benefit from iSAVR in the long run.

The observed mortality differences in young high-risk patients provide new insights compared to isolated reports from either high-risk or non-geriatric populations. The PARTNER 1A trial investigated outcomes in TAVR and SAVR in a high-risk cohort and found no differences in the 30-day and 5-year mortality [19,20]. The intermediate risk PARTNER 2 trial similarly showed no differences in 30-day mortality between the procedures [21]. The difference between these reported survival rates between the interventions and the results observed in our patients suggest a different pattern in the younger subgroup of the high-risk population. A higher rate of recovery from adverse events as well as the lower prevalence of frailty among non-geriatric patients may account for the higher long-term survival rate after SAVR, whereas the higher 30-day survival rates following TAVR are likely the result of the minimally invasive nature of the procedure.

Potential TAVR-related survival benefits in low-risk septuagenarians and octogenarians (average age 79 years) were studied in the Nordic NOTION trial and the GARY registry. Both studies found no differences in the 1-year mortality between TAVR and SAVR. Additionally, the NOTION trial showed no significant difference in the mortality between TAVR and SAVR at five years [14,22,23]. On the other hand, the most recent real-world analysis of the GARY registry, published by Beyersdorf et al., in 2021, showed a difference in the 5-year outcomes. The study, conducted on a propensity score-matched collective chosen from a total of 18010 patients (1820 TAVR vs. 1820 iSAVR), showed a significantly reduced long-term survival (hazard ratio 1.51, 95% confidence interval 1.35–1.68; $p < 0.0001$) after an implantation of early generation TAVI valves compared with SAVR [24].

Device improvements made between subsequent valve generations mainly aimed to reduce the paravalvular leakage rate by redesigning perivalvular skirts and reducing the size of delivery systems, and to improve access to the coronary ostia by increasing the cell size in the stent frame. Therefore, in light of the minimal changes made to the method of leaflet suspension and the anticalcification methods, and the consequently similar expected rates of structural valve deterioration, it is likely that similar survival curves might be seen after analysis of data with most recent valve designs. However, the PVL rate after TAVR has decreased significantly over the years and can have a substantial impact on long-term survival [25]. Among younger low-risk TAVR patients, whose mean age was closer to 74, the PARTNER 3 trial reported significantly lower rates of 30-day mortality or stroke for TAVR compared to SAVR, and the EVOLUT trial found that TAVR was noninferior with regard to death or disabling stroke at 24 months [10,11]. While our analysis seems to indicate a short-term survival benefit of TAVI in young high-risk patients, iSAVR is linked to a higher long-term survival rate, in contrast to the findings of the abovementioned trials. Although high-risk patients appear to share a few similarities with previously investigated populations, they require an individually tailored approach.

The differences in procedural outcomes between TAVR and iSAVR found in our analysis corroborate results from previous studies. iSAVR patients experienced significantly longer ventilating times and more instances where the ventilation time exceeded six hours. Prolonged ventilation times have been linked to delirium after cardiac surgery, which in turn has been shown to reduce the 30-day survival rate for both TAVR and SAVR [26,27]. New onset atrial fibrillation has consistently been found to occur more commonly after SAVR, which is in line with our findings [10,11,19,21]. Our TAVR cohort had a higher incidence of AV block and correspondingly higher rates of pacemaker implantation, both of which are in accordance with previous findings [10,22,28].

Certain differences in procedural outcomes between our cohorts are due to inherent differences between TAVR and iSAVR. Pronounced wound infections only occurred in the iSAVR cohort. The higher rates of major vascular access complications in the TAVR population are a consequence of the sheath size and manipulation during TAVR [19,21]. A higher incidence of major vascular access complications was not found in the NOTION, PARTNER 3 or EVOLUT trials [10,11,22]. The difference likely stems from the use of early-generation TAVR devices—the newer-generation valves used in these trials have low-profile sheaths.

This study has several limitations, most of them inherent to retrospective analysis. The single-center study with limited patient numbers may impede generalization of events yet emphasizes the necessity of larger randomized trials in this unusual, young high-risk population. The possibility of the presence of unidentified confounding variables cannot be excluded as the patients were not randomized. Propensity score matching cannot replace a prospective randomized analysis. The higher rate of certain comorbidities and potential other unidentified confounders including frailty may have played a role in the divergence of the survival curves after 1.5 years. Furthermore, individual patient preferences and the interdisciplinary decision-making process in the Heart Team may result in individual deviations from guideline recommendations.

Discrepancies between the results of our study and other trials may result from propensity score matching. For example, the 30-day mortality in our matched iSAVR cohort deviates from previously reported values (VICTORY: 12.5%, PARTNER 1A: 6.5%, PARTNER 2: 4.1%, PARTNER 3: 1.1%, EVOLUT: 1.3%, NOTION: 3.7%, GARY: 2.9%, Schaefer et al.: 1.1%) [10,11,14,19,21,26]. However, examining non-geriatric high-risk TAVR patients using propensity score matching inevitably resulted in an iSAVR cohort with an unusually high mortality rate compared to our overall iSAVR population and previous studies. The EuroSCORE II of the iSAVR population increased almost fourfold after propensity score matching (unmatched iSAVR: 1.7 vs. propensity score-matched iSAVR: 6.4) and the 30-day mortality increased almost five times (unmatched iSAVR 2.7% vs. propensity score-matched iSAVR 12.5%). Our results are more susceptible to biases caused by propensity score matching due to the small cohort size. However, the propensity score matching may have eliminated TAVR patients with numerous comorbidities and extremely high risk levels, as evidenced by the reduced EuroSCORE II (unmatched TAVR: 5.9 vs. matched TAVR: 4.3) and mortality (unmatched TAVR 3.4% vs. matched TAVR: 2.8%).

The use of risk scores to compare TAVR and iSAVR patients is problematic. TAVR patients often have substantially different risk profiles compared to iSAVR patients. Furthermore, not all relevant parameters are represented in existing surgical risk scores. As a result, despite analyzing a high-risk TAVR cohort, its EuroSCORE II was lower than that of the iSAVR cohort. Although frailty typically appears to be a minor contributing factor to postprocedural outcome in younger low-risk patients, the patients compared in our analysis were often significantly advanced in their biological age as a result of the higher number of comorbidities and the consecutively increased risk profile. Therefore, effectively comparing iSAVR and TAVR patients requires an appropriate scoring system that includes both the well-established traditional risk factors as well as frailty assessment tools.

5. Conclusions

Among younger high-risk patients, 30-day mortality rates are lower after TAVR, but the long-term survival is decidedly higher iSAVR. Other postprocedural outcomes were similar to patterns observed in other TAVR/SAVR studies. The only notable differences most likely stem from the use of first-generation TAVR devices and propensity score matching. Further research is required to determine when interventional procedures are futile and patients too frail for either procedure. Decisions regarding the method of aortic valve replacement should be led by the likelihood of surviving surgery and the immediate postoperative period in order for the patient to reap the long-term benefits of a surgical valve replacement.

Supplementary Materials: The following are available online at https://www.mdpi.com/article/10.3390/jcm10153447/s1, Supplementary Table S1: Baseline clinical characteristics of the excluded cohorts; Supplementary Table S2: Procedural characteristics of the excluded cohorts; Supplementary Table S3: Adverse events of the excluded cohorts.

Author Contributions: Conceptualization and methodology, M.M., A.S. (Andreas Schober), M.A., C.A., M.G. and G.D.-K.; software, C.G.; validation, M.M., W.H., E.H. and P.S.; formal analysis, M.M. and C.G.; investigation and data curation, T.P., W.H., T.K., P.S.; resources, M.G. and G.D.-K.; writing—original draft preparation, M.M., E.H., W.H., A.S. (Andreas Strouhal); writing—review and editing, T.P., W.H., T.K., P.S., M.A., C.G., A.S. (Andreas Schober), A.S. (Andreas Strouhal), G.D.-K., M.G., C.A.; visualization, M.M., T.P. and C.G.; supervision, M.M., M.G. and G.D.-K.; project administration, M.M. All authors have read and agreed to the published version of the manuscript.

Funding: This research received no external funding.

Institutional Review Board Statement: The study was conducted according to the guidelines of the Declaration of Helsinki, and approved by the Institutional Ethics Committee of the City of Vienna (EK 20-141—VK; 9 July 2020).

Informed Consent Statement: Patient consent was waived due to the retrospective nature of the analysis.

Data Availability Statement: The datasets for this study will be made available from the corresponding author upon reasonable request.

Acknowledgments: The authors would like to express their special gratitude to Francesco Maisano, Maurizio Taramasso, Carlos Mestres, Barbara Jenny, and the extended CAS—cardiac structural interventions faculty for creating an immensely inspiring environment that supports the clinical, academic, and scientific pillars of our field of work, and helped us to transcend traditional boundaries into a new, modern, and pioneering era of structural heart interventions.

Conflicts of Interest: M. Mach has received a research grant from Edwards Lifesciences, JenaValve and Symetis. M. Andreas is a proctor for Edwards Lifesciences and Abbott Laboratories and an adviser to Medtronic. All other authors have reported that they have no relationships relevant to the content.

References

1. De Backer, O.; Sondergaard, L. Challenges When Expanding Transcatheter Aortic Valve Implantation to Younger Patients. *Front. Cardiovasc. Med.* **2018**, *5*, 45. [CrossRef] [PubMed]
2. De Backer, O.; Luk, N.H.; Olsen, N.T.; Olsen, P.S.; Sondergaard, L. Choice of Treatment for Aortic Valve Stenosis in the Era of Transcatheter Aortic Valve Replacement in Eastern Denmark (2005 to 2015). *JACC Cardiovasc. Interv.* **2016**, *9*, 1152–1158. [CrossRef] [PubMed]
3. Popma, J.J.; Adams, D.H.; Reardon, M.J.; Yakubov, S.J.; Kleiman, N.S.; Heimansohn, D.; Hermiller, J., Jr.; Hughes, G.C.; Harrison, J.K.; Coselli, J.; et al. Transcatheter aortic valve replacement using a self-expanding bioprosthesis in patients with severe aortic stenosis at extreme risk for surgery. *J. Am. Coll. Cardiol.* **2014**, *63*, 1972–1981. [CrossRef]
4. Luscher, T.F. TAVI: From an experimental procedure to standard of care. *Eur. Heart J.* **2018**, *39*, 2605–2608. [CrossRef]
5. De Sciscio, P.; Brubert, J.; De Sciscio, M.; Serrani, M.; Stasiak, J.; Moggridge, G.D. Quantifying the Shift Toward Transcatheter Aortic Valve Replacement in Low-Risk Patients: A Meta-Analysis. *Circ. Cardiovasc. Qual. Outcomes* **2017**, *10*, e003287. [CrossRef] [PubMed]
6. Baumgartner, H.; Falk, V.; Bax, J.J.; De Bonis, M.; Hamm, C.; Holm, P.J.; Lung, B.; Lancellotti, P.; Lansac, E.; Muñoz, D.R.; et al. 2017 ESC/EACTS Guidelines for the Management of Valvular Heart Disease. *Rev. Esp. Cardiol. (Engl. Ed.)* **2018**, *71*, 110.
7. Gleason, T.G.; Reardon, M.J.; Popma, J.J.; Deeb, G.M.; Yakubov, S.J.; Lee, J.S.; Kleiman, N.S.; Chetcuti, S.; Hermiller, J.B.; Heiser, J.; et al. 5-Year Outcomes of Self-Expanding Transcatheter Versus Surgical Aortic Valve Replacement in High-Risk Patients. *J. Am. Coll. Cardiol.* **2018**, *72*, 2687–2696. [CrossRef] [PubMed]
8. Nishimura, R.A.; Otto, C.M.; Bonow, R.O.; Carabello, B.A.; Erwin, J.P.; Guyton, R.A., 3rd; O'Gara, P.T.; Ruiz, C.E.; Skubas, N.J.; Sorajja, P.; et al. 2014 AHA/ACC guideline for the management of patients with valvular heart disease: Executive summary: A report of the American College of Cardiology/American Heart Association Task Force on Practice Guidelines. *J. Am. Coll. Cardiol.* **2014**, *63*, 2438–2488. [CrossRef]
9. Webb, J.G.; Doshi, D.; Mack, M.J.; Makkar, R.; Smith, C.R.; Pichard, A.D.; Kodali, S.; Kapadia, S.; Miller, D.C.; Babaliaros, V.; et al. A Randomized Evaluation of the SAPIEN XT Transcatheter Heart Valve System in Patients With Aortic Stenosis Who Are Not Candidates for Surgery. *JACC Cardiovasc. Interv.* **2015**, *8*, 1797–1806. [CrossRef]
10. Popma, J.J.; Deeb, G.M.; Yakubov, S.J.; Mumtaz, M.; Gada, H.; O'Hair, D.; Bajwa, T.; Heiser, J.C.; Merhi, W.; Kleiman, N.S.; et al. Transcatheter Aortic-Valve Replacement with a Self-Expanding Valve in Low-Risk Patients. *N. Engl. J. Med.* **2019**, *380*, 1706–1715. [CrossRef]
11. Mack, M.J.; Leon, M.B.; Thourani, V.H.; Makkar, R.; Kodali, S.K.; Russo, M.; Kapadia, S.R.; Malaisrie, S.C.; Cohen, D.J.; Pibarot, P.; et al. Transcatheter Aortic-Valve Replacement with a Balloon-Expandable Valve in Low-Risk Patients. *N. Engl. J. Med.* **2019**, *380*, 1695–1705. [CrossRef] [PubMed]
12. Del Trigo, M.; Munoz-Garcia, A.J.; Wijeysundera, H.C.; Nombela-Franco, L.; Cheema, A.N.; Gutierrez, E.; Serra, V.; Kefer, J.; Amat-Santos, I.J.; Benitez, L.M.; et al. Incidence, Timing, and Predictors of Valve Hemodynamic Deterioration After Transcatheter Aortic Valve Replacement: Multicenter Registry. *J. Am. Coll. Cardiol.* **2016**, *67*, 644–655. [CrossRef] [PubMed]
13. Cerrato, E.; Nombela-Franco, L.; Nazif, T.M.; Eltchaninoff, H.; Sondergaard, L.; Ribeiro, H.B.; Barbanti, M.; Nietlispach, F.; De Jaegere, P.; Agostoni, P.; et al. Evaluation of current practices in transcatheter aortic valve implantation: The WRITTEN (WoRldwIde TAVI ExperieNce) survey. *Int. J. Cardiol.* **2017**, *228*, 640–647. [CrossRef] [PubMed]
14. Bekeredjian, R.; Szabo, G.; Balaban, U.; Bleiziffer, S.; Bauer, T.; Ensminger, S.; Frerker, C.; Herrmann, E.; Beyersdorf, F.; Hamm, C.; et al. Patients at low surgical risk as defined by the Society of Thoracic Surgeons Score undergoing isolated interventional or surgical aortic valve implantation: In-hospital data and 1-year results from the German Aortic Valve Registry (GARY). *Eur. Heart J.* **2019**, *40*, 1323–1330. [CrossRef] [PubMed]
15. Mach, M.; Koschutnik, M.; Wilbring, M.; Winkler, B.; Reinweber, M.; Alexiou, K.; Kappert, U.; Adlbrecht, C.; Delle-Karth, G.; Grabenwöger, M.; et al. Impact of COPD on Outcome in Patients Undergoing Transfemoral versus Transapical TAVI. *Thorac. Cardiovasc. Surg.* **2019**, *67*, 251–256. [CrossRef]
16. Kappetein, A.P.; Head, S.J.; Genereux, P.; Piazza, N.; van Mieghem, N.M.; Blackstone, E.H.; Brott, T.G.; Cohen, D.J.; Cutlip, D.E.; Van Es, G.-A.; et al. Updated standardized endpoint definitions for transcatheter aortic valve implantation: The Valve Academic Research Consortium-2 consensus document. *Eur. Heart J.* **2012**, *33*, 2403–2418. [CrossRef]
17. McMurry, T.L.; Hu, Y.; Blackstone, E.H.; Kozower, B.D. Propensity scores: Methods, considerations, and applications in the Journal of Thoracic and Cardiovascular Surgery. *J. Thorac. Cardiovasc. Surg.* **2015**, *150*, 14–19. [CrossRef]
18. Klein, J.P.; Moeschberger, M.L. *Survival Analysis: Techniques for Censored and Truncated Data*, 2nd ed.; Springer: New York, NY, USA, 1997.

19. Smith, C.R.; Leon, M.B.; Mack, M.J.; Miller, D.C.; Moses, J.W.; Svensson, L.G.; Tuzcu, E.M.; Webb, J.G.; Fontana, G.P.; Makkar, R.R.; et al. Transcatheter versus surgical aortic-valve replacement in high-risk patients. *N. Engl. J. Med.* **2011**, *364*, 2187–2198. [CrossRef]
20. Mack, M.J.; Leon, M.B.; Smith, C.R.; Miller, D.C.; Moses, J.W.; Tuzcu, E.M.; Webb, J.G.; Douglas, P.S.; Anderson, W.N.; Blackstone, E.H.; et al. 5-year outcomes of transcatheter aortic valve replacement or surgical aortic valve replacement for high surgical risk patients with aortic stenosis (PARTNER 1): A randomised controlled trial. *Lancet* **2015**, *385*, 2477–2484. [CrossRef]
21. Leon, M.B.; Smith, C.R.; Mack, M.J.; Makkar, R.R.; Svensson, L.G.; Kodali, S.K.; Thourani, V.H.; Tuzcu, E.M.; Miller, D.C.; Herrmann, H.C.; et al. Transcatheter or Surgical Aortic-Valve Replacement in Intermediate-Risk Patients. *N. Engl. J. Med.* **2016**, *374*, 1609–1620. [CrossRef]
22. Thyregod, H.G.; Steinbruchel, D.A.; Ihlemann, N.; Nissen, H.; Kjeldsen, B.J.; Petursson, P.; Chang, Y.; Franzen, O.W.; Engstrøm, T.; Clemmensen, P.; et al. Transcatheter Versus Surgical Aortic Valve Replacement in Patients With Severe Aortic Valve Stenosis: 1-Year Results From the All-Comers NOTION Randomized Clinical Trial. *J. Am. Coll. Cardiol.* **2015**, *65*, 2184–2194. [CrossRef] [PubMed]
23. Thyregod, H.G.H.; Ihlemann, N.; Jorgensen, T.H.; Nissen, H.; Kjeldsen, B.J.; Petursson, P.; Chang, Y.; Franzen, O.W.; Engstrøm, T.; Clemmensen, P.; et al. Five-Year Clinical and Echocardiographic Outcomes from the Nordic Aortic Valve Intervention (NOTION) Randomized Clinical Trial in Lower Surgical Risk Patients. *Circulation* **2019**, *139*, 2714–2723. [CrossRef] [PubMed]
24. Beyersdorf, F.; Bauer, T.; Freemantle, N.; Walther, T.; Frerker, C.; Herrmann, E.; Bleiziffer, S.; Möllmann, H.; Landwehr, S.; Ensminger, S.; et al. Five-year outcome in 18 010 patients from the German Aortic Valve Registry. *Eur. J. Cardiothorac. Surg.* **2021**, ezab216. [CrossRef] [PubMed]
25. Maisano, F.; Taramasso, M.; Nietlispach, F. Prognostic influence of paravalvular leak following TAVI: Is aortic regurgitation an active incremental risk factor or just a mere indicator? *Eur. Heart J.* **2015**, *36*, 413–415. [CrossRef] [PubMed]
26. Burkhart, C.S.; Dell-Kuster, S.; Gamberini, M.; Moeckli, A.; Grapow, M.; Filipovic, M.; Seeberger, M.; Monsch, A.U.; Strebel, S.P.; Steiner, L.A. Modifiable and nonmodifiable risk factors for postoperative delirium after cardiac surgery with cardiopulmonary bypass. *J. Cardiothorac. Vasc. Anesth.* **2010**, *24*, 555–559. [CrossRef]
27. Maniar, H.S.; Lindman, B.R.; Escallier, K.; Avidan, M.; Novak, E.; Melby, S.J.; Damiano, M.S.; Lasala, J.; Quader, N.; Rao, R.S.; et al. Delirium after surgical and transcatheter aortic valve replacement is associated with increased mortality. *J. Thorac. Cardiovasc. Surg.* **2016**, *151*, 815–823.e2. [CrossRef]
28. Schaefer, A.; Schofer, N.; Gossling, A.; Seiffert, M.; Schirmer, J.; Deuschl, F.; Schneeberger, Y.; Voigtländer, L.; Detter, C.; Schaefer, U.; et al. Transcatheter aortic valve implantation versus surgical aortic valve replacement in low-risk patients: A propensity score-matched analysis. *Eur. J. Cardiothorac. Surg.* **2019**, *56*, 1131–1139. [CrossRef]

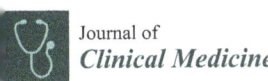

Article

Calculated Plasma Volume Status Is Associated with Adverse Outcomes in Patients Undergoing Transcatheter Aortic Valve Implantation

Hatim Seoudy [1,2,†], Mohammed Saad [1,†], Mostafa Salem [1], Kassem Allouch [1], Johanne Frank [1,2], Thomas Puehler [2,3], Mohamed Salem [2], Georg Lutter [2,3], Christian Kuhn [1] and Derk Frank [1,2,*]

1. Department of Internal Medicine III, Cardiology and Angiology, Campus Kiel, University Hospital Schleswig-Holstein, D-24105 Kiel, Germany; hatim.seoudy@uksh.de (H.S.); mohammed.saad@uksh.de (M.S.); mostafa.salem@uksh.de (M.S.); kassem.allouch@gmx.de (K.A.); johanne.frank@uksh.de (J.F.); chris_kuhn@gmx.de (C.K.)
2. DZHK (German Centre for Cardiovascular Research), Partner Site Hamburg/Kiel/Lübeck, D-24105 Kiel, Germany; thomas.puehler@uksh.de (T.P.); mohamed.salem@uksh.de (M.S.); georg.lutter@uksh.de (G.L.)
3. Department of Cardiac and Vascular Surgery, Campus Kiel, University Hospital Schleswig-Holstein, D-24105 Kiel, Germany
* Correspondence: derk.frank@uksh.de; Tel.: +49-(0)4-31500-22801
† These authors have contributed equally to this work and share first authorship.

Abstract: Background: Calculated plasma volume status (PVS) reflects volume overload based on the deviation of the estimated plasma volume (ePV) from the ideal plasma volume (iPV). Calculated PVS is associated with prognosis in the context of heart failure. This single-center study investigated the prognostic impact of PVS in patients undergoing transcatheter aortic valve implantation (TAVI). Methods: A total of 859 TAVI patients had been prospectively enrolled in an observational study and were included in the analysis. An optimal cutoff for PVS of -5.4% was determined by receiver operating characteristic curve analysis. The primary endpoint was a composite of all-cause mortality or heart failure hospitalization within 1 year after TAVI. Results: A total of 324 patients had a PVS $< -5.4\%$ (no congestion), while 535 patients showed a PVS $\geq -5.4\%$ (congestion). The primary endpoint occurred more frequently in patients with a PVS $\geq -5.4\%$ compared to patients with PVS $< -5.4\%$ (22.6% vs. 13.0%, $p < 0.001$). After multivariable adjustment, PVS was confirmed as a significant predictor of the primary endpoint (HR 1.53, 95% CI 1.05–2.22, $p = 0.026$). Conclusions: Elevated PVS, as a marker of subclinical congestion, is significantly associated with all-cause mortality and heart failure hospitalization within 1 year after TAVI.

Keywords: aortic stenosis; transcatheter aortic valve implantation; valvular heart disease; congestion; plasma volume; risk stratification

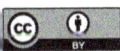

1. Introduction

Transcatheter aortic valve implantation (TAVI) has become an essential treatment option for severe aortic stenosis (AS) across the whole spectrum of surgical risk [1,2]. In patients undergoing TAVI, subclinical congestion is associated with worse clinical outcomes. However, it is often not detected by routine clinical assessment [3]. While right heart catheterization is considered the gold standard to quantify fluid status in patients with volume overload, its use is limited by its invasive nature [4]. Radiotracer indicator-dilution methods using labeled albumin or red blood cells were previously proposed as alternative techniques to accurately quantify plasma volume (PV), but are not applicable in daily clinical practice [5,6]. In contrast, non-invasive PV calculations based on weight and hematocrit have been shown to correlate well with quantitative measurements using gold-standard radioisotope assays [7]. Plasma volume status (PVS) reflects the degree of deviation of the estimated plasma volume (ePV) from the ideal plasma volume (iPV) and has been shown to be associated with prognosis in patients with heart failure [8].

The aim of this study was to determine the incidence and prognostic impact of subclinical volume overload, detected by elevated calculated PVS, in patients undergoing TAVI. We hypothesized that PVS is significantly associated with adverse outcomes after TAVI.

2. Materials and Methods

Between February 2014 and February 2020, a total of 979 patients undergoing transfemoral TAVI were prospectively enrolled in an observational study at the University Hospital Schleswig-Holstein, Kiel, Germany. Patients with incomplete clinical or follow-up data as well as those with intraprocedural conversion to open-heart surgery were excluded from the analysis. The final study population comprised 859 patients.

An optimal PVS cutoff value of −5.4% (AUC 0.601, 95% confidence interval 0.55–0.65, $p < 0.001$) was determined using receiver operating characteristic (ROC) curve analysis. According to calculated PVS, patients were divided into two groups: PVS < −5.4% (no congestion) versus PVS ≥ −5.4% (congestion). The primary endpoint was a composite of all-cause mortality or heart failure hospitalization. The secondary study endpoints were both individual components of the primary endpoint.

The decision to perform TAVI was based on careful evaluation by the multidisciplinary heart team. All procedures were performed using third-generation SAPIEN devices (Edwards Lifesciences, Irvine, CA, USA) or CoreValve devices (Medtronic, Minneapolis, MN, USA). Type and size of the transcatheter heart valve were determined using pre-procedural multidetector computed tomography measurements and evaluation with the 3 mensio Structural Heart software (3 mensio Medical Imaging BV, Bilthoven, the Netherlands). Procedures were done by experienced implanters and pre- and post-dilatation were left to the physician's discretion. During TAVI, unfractionated heparin was administered to achieve an activated clotting time of 250–300 s. Closure of the vascular access was conducted using two Perclose ProGlide™ vascular closure systems (Abbott Laboratories, Chicago, IL, USA).

PVS was calculated after obtaining ePV and iPV using two well-established equations which have been previously reported in detail elsewhere [9,10]:

$$ePV = ((1 - \text{hematocrit}) \times (a + (b \times \text{weight (kg)}))),$$

with a = 864 in females and 1530 in males, and b = 47.9 in females and 41 in males.

$$iPV = k \times \text{weight [kg]}, \text{ with } k = 40 \text{ in females and } 39 \text{ in males}.$$

PVS is an index of deviation of ePV from iPV and was subsequently calculated as follows:

$$PVS = ((ePV - iPV) \times 100\%)/iPV$$

Written informed consent was obtained from each patient. The study was approved by the Ethics Committee of the University of Kiel and conformed to the ethical guidelines of the Declaration of Helsinki. Patient data and blood samples were collected 1–3 days prior to TAVI. Patients were followed up through clinical visits, communication with ambulatory physicians, or telephone consultations after the procedure. Patient outcomes were reported according to the incidence of life-threatening bleeding, myocardial infarction, stroke with disability, acute kidney injury stage 3/4, and new permanent pacemaker implantation in accordance with the definitions of the Valve Academic Research Consortium-3 (VARC-3) consensus document [11]. Hospitalization for heart failure was defined as hospitalization due to typical symptoms and objective signs of worsening heart failure. The Society of Thoracic Surgeons (STS) risk score was calculated using the updated model released in 2018 [12,13].

All continuous data showed a skewed distribution and were thus expressed as median with interquartile range (IQR). Categorical variables were summarized as counts and percentages. Differences between both groups were assessed using the Mann-Whitney U test, χ^2-test, and Fisher's exact test, as appropriate. Outcome data were evaluated using

Kaplan-Meier curves and the log-rank test. For the Cox regression model, all factors linked to mortality in univariable (p-value < 0.25) were considered as candidate variables. The backward selection was based on the likelihood ratio criteria. Continuous variables were dichotomized to keep the Cox model simple. Cox regression results were presented as adjusted hazard ratios (HR) with 95% confidence intervals (CI). The proportional hazard assumption was confirmed using weighted residuals. In order to minimize collinearity, covariables directly related to PVS including hemoglobin, hematocrit, and anemia were not included in the regression model. Statistical analyses were performed using R software, version 4.0.4 (URL: https://www.R-project.org/ (accessed on 27 July 2021)), and GraphPad PRISM, version 8 (GraphPad Software, San Diego, CA, USA). All tests were two-tailed, and a p-value < 0.05 was considered statistically significant.

3. Results

3.1. Baseline Characteristics

A total of 859 TAVI patients were available for analysis. Based on the calculated PVS cutoff, 324 patients (37.7%) had a PVS < −5.4% (no congestion), while 535 patients (62.3%) had a PVS ≥ −5.4% (congestion). Compared to patients with PVS < −5.4%, the PVS ≥ −5.4% group was significantly older, had a higher proportion of female patients as well as higher STS Scores, higher levels of NT-proBNP, higher rates of impaired left ventricular ejection fraction (LVEF), higher prevalence of anemia, lower eGFR, lower hematocrit and hemoglobin, lower BMI and lower prevalence of dyslipidemia. Diuretics were more frequently prescribed in patients with a PVS ≥ −5.4% compared to the PVS < −5.4% group (Table 1).

Table 1. Baseline characteristics and heart failure medication.

	Total (n = 859)	PVS < −5.4% (n = 324)	PVS ≥ −5.4% (n = 535)	p-Value
Age (years)	81.9 (78.7–85.8)	81.0 (77.6–84.1)	82.8 (79.5–86.9)	<0.001
Female, n (%)	452 (52.6)	152 (46.9)	300 (56.1)	0.009
BMI (kg/m^2)	26.2 (23.9–29.6)	28.9 (25.9–32.0)	25.0 (22.7–27.7)	<0.001
Atrial fibrillation, n (%)	373 (43.4)	134 (41.4)	239 (44.7)	0.342
CAD, n (%)	550 (64.0)	199 (61.4)	351 (65.6)	0.215
COPD, n (%)	94 (10.9)	31 (9.6)	63 (11.8)	0.315
CVD, n (%)	150 (17.5)	56 (17.3)	94 (17.6)	0.915
Diabetes mellitus, n (%)	258 (30.0)	96 (29.6)	162 (30.3)	0.840
Dyslipidemia, n (%)	431 (50.2)	177 (54.6)	254 (47.5)	0.042
Hypertension, n (%)	759 (88.4)	286 (88.3)	473 (88.4)	0.951
NYHA class III or IV, n (%)	612 (71.2)	219 (67.6)	393 (73.5)	0.067
PAD, n (%)	72 (8.4)	26 (8.0)	46 (8.6)	0.769
PAH, n (%)	115 (13.4)	46 (14.2)	69 (12.9)	0.588
Prev. cardiac surgery, n (%)	126 (14.7)	54 (16.7)	72 (13.5)	0.198
STS-Score (%)	3.7 (2.4–5.5)	2.9 (2.1–4.6)	4.2 (2.6–6.3)	<0.001
Hematocrit (%)	0.36 (0.32–0.39)	0.40 (0.38–0.42)	0.34 (0.31–0.36)	<0.001
Hemoglobin (g/dL)	12.4 (11.1–13.4)	13.6 (12.8–14.4)	11.5 (10.4–12.4)	<0.001
Anemia				
Mild	253 (29.5)	52 (16.0)	201 (37.6)	<0.001
Moderate	173 (20.1)	5 (1.5)	168 (31.4)	<0.001
Severe	5 (0.6)	0 (0)	5 (0.9)	0.081
Non-Anemia	428 (49.8)	267 (82.4)	161 (30.1)	<0.001
eGFR (mL/min/1.73 m^2)	54 (40–67)	59 (48–70)	51 (37–63)	<0.001
NT-proBNP (pg/mL)	1461 (573–3462)	986 (445–2287)	2102 (704–4529)	<0.001
LVEF				
≥55%, n (%)	555 (64.6)	226 (69.8)	329 (61.5)	0.014
45–54%, n (%)	162 (18.9)	52 (16.0)	110 (20.6)	0.101
35–44%, n (%)	72 (8.4)	19 (5.9)	53 (9.9)	0.038
<35%, n (%)	70 (8.1)	27 (8.3)	43 (8.0)	0.878

Table 1. Cont.

	Total (n = 859)	PVS < −5.4% (n = 324)	PVS ≥ −5.4% (n = 535)	p-Value
AVA (cm^2)	0.8 (0.6–0.9)	0.8 (0.6–0.9)	0.8 (0.6–0.9)	0.075
MPG (mmHg)	38 (29–50)	38 (30–49)	38 (29–50)	0.838
MR III-IV, n (%)	72 (8.4)	26 (8.0)	46 (8.6)	0.769
TR III-IV, n (%)	36 (4.2)	14 (4.3)	22 (4.1)	0.882
Calculated actual PV (mL)	2907 (2621–3264)	2951 (2693–3321)	2883 (2566–3235)	0.003
Calculated ideal PV (mL)	3000 (2613–3393)	3315 (3000–3783)	2800 (2457–3120)	<0.001
PVS (%)	−2.6 (−8.6–4.1)	−10.4 (−14.0–−7.5)	1.8 (−2.0–7.2)	<0.001
Heart failure medication				
ACE-I/ARB	714 (83.1)	275 (84.9)	439 (82.1)	0.285
Betablocker	639 (74.4)	235 (72.5)	404 (75.5)	0.332
MRA	108 (12.6)	35 (10.8)	73 (13.6)	0.223
Diuretics	598 (69.6)	211 (65.1)	387 (72.3)	0.026

Legend: ACE-I, angiotensin-converting enzyme inhibitor; ARB, angiotensin receptor blocker; AVA, aortic valve area; BMI, body mass index; CAD, coronary artery disease; COPD, chronic obstructive pulmonary disease; CVD, cerebrovascular disease; eGFR, estimated glomerular filtration rate; LVEF, left ventricular ejection fraction; MPG, mean pressure gradient; MR, mitral regurgitation; MRA, mineralocorticoid receptor antagonist; NT-proBNP, N-terminal Pro-B-Type Natriuretic Peptide; NYHA, New York Heart Association; PAD, peripheral artery disease; PAH, pulmonary arterial hypertension; Prev., previous; PV, plasma volume; PVS, plasma volume status; STS, Society of Thoracic Surgeons; TR, tricuspid regurgitation. Values are presented as median (interquartile range) or counts (percentages).

3.2. Periprocedural Complications

There was no statistically significant difference regarding the type of transcatheter heart valve used for the procedure. Periprocedural complications defined as individual endpoints of type 3 (life-threatening) bleeding, myocardial infarction, stroke with disability, acute kidney injury stage 3/4, and new pacemaker implantation after TAVI did also not differ between both groups (Table 2).

Table 2. Procedural variables and outcomes.

	Total (n = 859)	PVS < −5.4% (n = 324)	PVS ≥ −5.4% (n = 535)	p-Value
Valve type				0.146
Self-expanding, n (%)	433 (50.4)	153 (47.2)	280 (52.3)	
Balloon-expandable, n (%)	426 (49.6)	171 (52.8)	255 (47.7)	
Procedural duration (min)	50 (40–63)	49 (40–61)	49 (40–65)	0.302
Contrast medium (mL)	84 (70–105)	85 (70–107)	80 (68–103)	0.219
VARC-3				
New permanent pacemaker, n (%)	101 (11.8)	43 (13.3)	58 (10.8)	0.284
Myocardial infarction, n (%)	3 (0.3)	1 (0.3)	2 (0.4)	>0.999
AKIN stage 3/4, n (%)	9 (1.0)	2 (0.6)	7 (1.3)	0.496
Type 3 (life-threatening) bleeding, n (%)	21 (2.4)	4 (1.2)	17 (3.2)	0.108
Stroke with disability, n (%)	3 (0.3)	1 (0.3)	2 (0.4)	>0.999
Primary composite outcome, n (%)	163 (19.0)	42 (13.0)	121 (22.6)	<0.001
All-cause mortality, n (%)	110 (12.8)	22 (6.8)	88 (16.4)	<0.001
Heart failure hospitalization, n (%)	77 (9.0)	21 (6.5)	56 (10.5)	0.048

Legend: AKIN, Acute Kidney Injury Network; PVS, plasma volume status; VARC-3, Valve Academic Research Consortium-3. Values are presented as median (interquartile range) or counts (percentages).

3.3. Clinical Outcome during Long-Term Follow-Up

The primary composite outcome (all-cause mortality or heart failure hospitalization) occurred in 121/535 patients (22.6%) in the PVS ≥ −5.4% group compared to 42/324 patients (13.0%) with a PVS < −5.4% (Table 1, Figure 1). Furthermore, the PVS ≥ −5.4% group had higher rates of both secondary endpoints of all-cause mortality (16.4% vs. 6.8%, $p < 0.001$) and heart failure hospitalization (10.5% vs. 6.5%, $p = 0.031$; Table 1, Figure 2A,B). In univariable Cox regression analysis, PVS was significantly associated with the primary endpoint (HR 1.99, 95%, CI 1.39–2.84, $p < 0.001$). After multivariable adjustment for other variables, PVS remained a significant predictor of the composite of all-cause mortality or heart failure hospitalization (HR 1.53, 95% CI 1.05–2.22, p = 0.026; Table 3).

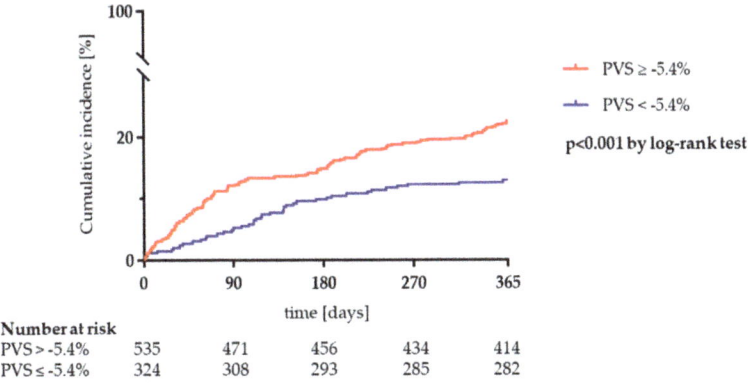

Figure 1. Elevated plasma volume status (PVS) is associated with the primary composite endpoint of all-cause mortality or heart failure hospitalization after transcatheter aortic valve implantation. Legend: Kaplan-Meier survival curves for the primary endpoint comparing patients with a PVS ≥ −5.4% (congestion) to patients with a PVS < −5.4% (no congestion).

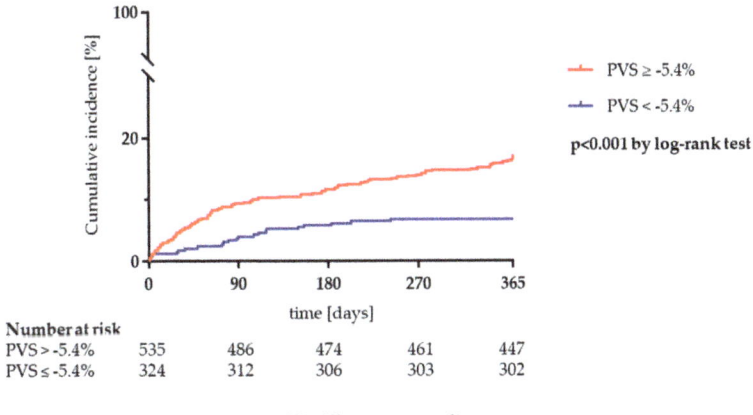

(**A**) All-cause mortality

Figure 2. *Cont.*

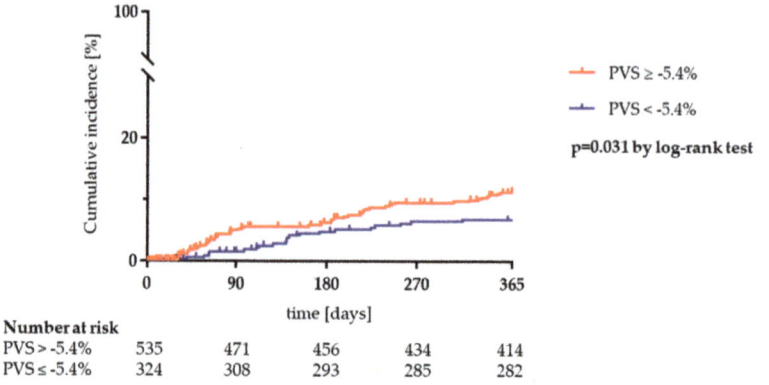

(B) Heart failure hospitalization

Figure 2. Elevated plasma volume status (PVS) is associated with adverse outcomes after transcatheter aortic valve implantation. (A) All-cause mortality. (B) Heart failure hospitalization. Legend: Kaplan-Meier survival curves for the secondary endpoints of all-cause mortality and heart failure hospitalization comparing patients with a PVS $\geq -5.4\%$ (congestion) to patients with a PVS $< -5.4\%$ (no congestion).

Table 3. Cox regression analysis for the primary composite endpoint of all-cause mortality or heart failure hospitalization.

Variable	HR (95% CI)	p-Value	HR (95% CI)	p-Value
PVS $\geq -5.4\%$	1.99 (1.39–2.84)	<0.001	1.53 (1.05–2.22)	0.026
Atrial fibrillation	1.70 (1.25–2.31)	<0.001		
Age > median (81.9 years)	1.27 (0.93–1.73)	0.132		
BMI > median (26.2 kg/m^2)	0.66 (0.48–0.90)	0.008		
STS score > median (3.7%)	2.23 (1.61–3.08)	<0.001	1.67 (1.17–2.38)	0.005
COPD	1.58 (1.03–2.42)	0.036	1.54 (0.99–2.39)	0.056
NT-proBNP > median (1461 pg/mL)	1.94 (1.41–2.67)	<0.001	1.48 (1.06–2.09)	0.023
eGFR < 60 mL/min/1.73 cm^2	1.85 (1.29–2.65)	<0.001		
LVEF < 55%	1.73 (1.27–2.35)	<0.001		
TR III-IV	3.37 (2.04–5.57)	<0.001	2.87 (1.72–4.80)	<0.001
MR III-IV	2.36 (1.55–3.59)	<0.001		
PAH	1.55 (1.04–2.30)	0.030		
AKIN stage 3/4	10.10 (4.72–21.70)	<0.001	8.50 (3.91–18.51)	<0.001
Myocardial infarction	5.11 (1.27–20.60)	0.022	6.12 (1.47–25.40)	0.013
Stroke with disability	7.73 (1.92–31.20)	0.004		
Type 3 (life-threatening) bleeding	4.60 (2.55–8.28)	<0.001	6.34 (3.50–11.49)	<0.001

Legend: AKIN, Acute Kidney Injury Network; BMI, body mass index; COPD, chronic obstructive pulmonary disease; eGFR, estimated glomerular filtration rate; LVEF, left ventricular ejection fraction; MR, mitral regurgitation; NT-proBNP, N-terminal Pro-B-Type Natriuretic Peptide; PAH, pulmonary arterial hypertension; PVS, plasma volume status; STS, Society of Thoracic Surgeons; TR, tricuspid regurgitation. Results are presented as adjusted hazard ratios (HR) with 95% confidence intervals (CI).

4. Discussion

This study found that calculated PVS as a marker of hypervolemia was significantly associated with all-cause mortality and heart failure hospitalization in patients undergoing TAVI.

In our study, 62.3% of patients had a preprocedural PVS $\geq -5.4\%$ reflecting relevant (subclinical) congestion. This relatively high incidence of hypervolemia as well as the ROC-derived cutoff for PVS of -5.4% in TAVI patients is consistent with previously published reports [14]. In another study using a PVS cut-off value of -4%, an elevated

PVS was present in 59.6% of patients admitted for TAVI [15]. Compared to patients with PVS < −5.4%, patients with a PVS ≥ −5.4% in our study were older and had multiple co-morbidities. Again, this was consistent with previously published investigations, where elevated PVS was associated with increased comorbidities in patients undergoing TAVI [14–17]. The lower BMI in patients with a PVS ≥ −5.4% was most probably a result of malnutrition and frailty, which are associated with an increased risk of all-cause mortality in patients undergoing TAVI [16,18]. In our study, the median calculated PVS was −2.6% (−8.6–4.1%) which is in line with previously reported PVS in the context of TAVI [14]. Notably, PVS values in TAVI patients seem to be higher than in patients with chronic heart failure [8]. This finding indicates that patients with severe symptomatic AS may suffer from unrecognized hypervolemia and subclinical congestion to a greater extent compared to patients with chronic heart failure. This may be explained by the typical clinical profile of the TAVI population including advanced age, high prevalence of comorbidities, and suboptimal heart failure medication in elderly patients [19]. In our study, patients with a PVS ≥ −5.4% showed higher rates of diuretic therapy, while there was no significant difference in prognostic heart failure medication. This finding highlights the potential role of PVS as a tool to optimize medical treatment.

During follow-up, both mortality and heart failure hospitalization were significantly higher in patients with PVS ≥ −5.4% compared to patients with PVS < −5.4% ($p < 0.001$ and $p = 0.031$, respectively; Figure 2A,B). Consistently, other studies showed adverse outcomes in TAVI patients with elevated PVS. Maznyczka et al. reported that a PVS > 0% was linked to a two-fold risk for mortality as well as prolonged ICU and hospital stay [14]. Shimura et al. reported a significantly higher all-cause mortality and heart failure hospitalization rate in the high-PVS group than in the low-PVS group [17]. In addition, patients with high PVS and NYHA I/II had a worse prognosis than those with low PVS and NYHA III/IV. Adlbrecht et al. reported that patients with a high PVS did not only demonstrate a substantially impaired long-term survival during follow-up but were also at increased risk for a 30-day composite of all-cause mortality, stroke, life-threatening bleeding, acute kidney injury, coronary artery obstruction requiring intervention, major vascular complication and valve-related dysfunction requiring repeat procedure [15]. The prognostic significance of PVS was also previously reported in patients with heart failure. In an analysis of 3414 patients with heart failure with preserved ejection fraction, higher calculated estimates of PVS were independently associated with an elevated risk of long-term clinical outcomes, and particularly, heart failure hospitalization [20]. In an analysis of 186 patients who received a continuous-flow left ventricular assist device, high PVS was associated with higher mortality during follow-up [21].

Importantly, previous studies investigating calculated PVS have not reported the prevalence of anemia [14,15,17]. Based on WHO definitions, anemia (<12.0 g/dL in women; <13.0 g/dLs in men) was prevalent in 50.2% of the total population in our study (69.9% in the PVS ≥ −5.4% groups compared to 17.6% the PVS < −5.4% group, $p < 0.001$). This was mostly attributed to mild and moderate forms of anemia [22]. While anemia is known to be multifactorial in patients with severe AS, hemodilution due to congestion is likely to have had a significant impact on the high prevalence of anemia in patients with PVS ≥ −5.4% [23–25]. As was the case in previous studies, our analysis is unable to differentiate between "true" anemia and anemia due to hemodilution in patients with congestion. Thus, future studies should focus on the close relationship between anemia and PVS in order to correct for confounding effects.

It has been previously suggested that volume overload associated with elevated PVS might add to the pressure overload on the stiff, non-compliant ventricle in severe AS, leading to a higher risk of pulmonary and systemic edema, global hypoperfusion, and adverse outcomes after TAVI [14]. Thus, calculated PVS could be a simple tool to guide fluid management and medical treatment including diuretic therapy in patients with heart failure. Similarly, NT-proBNP has been previously proposed as a simple marker to guide therapy in the context of heart failure and TAVI [26,27]. Additionally, a number of cardiovascular biomarkers, such as high-sensitivity Troponin T, soluble ST2, and GDF-15 have also been studied in the context of TAVI and are associated with outcomes in patients undergoing TAVI [28]. Using PVS in patients with severe AS and optimizing heart failure treatment in addition to TAVI may result in more favorable outcomes in this vulnerable patient group. Prospective randomized trials are needed to study the utility of PVS as part of an integrated approach for improved risk stratification and management of TAVI patients.

There are several study limitations that have to be acknowledged. First, this is a single-center study which may limit the conclusions that can be drawn from the analysis. Second, in line with previous studies, hemoglobin/hematocrit and anemia were not included in the Cox regression model in order to minimize collinearity. However, comorbidities such as frailty, heart failure, and chronic kidney disease are known to be closely associated with hemoglobin concentrations, which may have significantly influenced PVS [29]. Third, as anemia and PVS are closely intertwined, this study is unable to differentiate between true anemia and anemia caused by hemodilution. Thus, anemia potentially remains a major confounding factor. Fourth, the relative low HR for PVS in the Cox regression analysis indicates that PVS should only be used as part of an integrative approach. Fifth, additional endpoints such as heart failure symptoms and physical capacity were not accounted for. Sixth, factors affecting PVS, such as blood transfusions and extensive heart failure therapy during a hospital stay, were not taken into consideration during the calculation of PVS. Finally, ePV in this study was not validated by the measured PV. However, ePV has been shown to correlate well with PV levels measured using gold-standard radioisotope assays [8,26].

5. Conclusions

Elevated PVS was an independent predictor of all-cause mortality and heart failure hospitalization within 1 year after TAVI. Future trials are necessary to determine the potential role of PVS as part of an integrative strategy towards improved risk stratification and therapeutic management of patients undergoing TAVI.

Author Contributions: Conceptualization, H.S., M.S. (Mohammed Saad), J.F., C.K., D.F.; methodology, H.S., M.S. (Mostafa Salem), K.A.; software, H.S., M.S. (Mohammed Saad), G.L., D.F.; validation, J.F., T.P., C.K.; formal analysis, H.S., M.S. (Mohammed Saad), K.A., D.F.; investigation, H.S., M.S. (Mohammed Saad), K.A., T.P., G.L., C.K.; resources, H.S., M.S. (Mohammed Saad), J.F., T.P.; data curation, H.S., M.S. (Mohammed Saad), M.S. (Mohamed Salem), G.L.; writing—original draft preparation, H.S., M.S. (Mohammed Saad), K.A.; writing—review and editing, M.S. (Mostafa Salem), J.F., T.P., G.L., C.K., D.F.; visualization, H.S., K.A.; supervision, C.K., D.F.; project administration, H.S., M.S. (Mohammed Saad), D.F. All authors have read and agreed to the published version of the manuscript.

Funding: This research received no external funding.

Institutional Review Board Statement: The study was conducted according to the guidelines of the Declaration of Helsinki, and approved by the Ethics Committee of the University of Kiel (protocol code D 529/16).

Informed Consent Statement: Informed consent was obtained from all subjects involved in the study.

Data Availability Statement: The datasets for this study will not be made available to other researchers due to data protection reasons. However, calculation of PVS is simple and easily reproducible, and we encourage scientists to validate our findings in other TAVI cohorts.

Conflicts of Interest: G.L. is a consultant for Edwards Lifesciences, Medtronic, Boston Scientific and Abbott. C.K. received speaker's honoraria from Medtronic. D.F. is a consultant for Edwards Lifesciences and Medtronic and has received research funding from Edwards Lifesciences. All other authors have no commercial or financial relationships that could be construed as a potential conflict of interest.

References

1. Carroll, J.D.; Mack, M.J.; Vemulapalli, S.; Herrmann, H.C.; Gleason, T.G.; Hanzel, G.; Deeb, G.M.; Thourani, V.H.; Cohen, D.J.; Desai, N.; et al. STS-ACC TVT Registry of Transcatheter Aortic Valve Replacement. *J. Am. Coll. Cardiol.* **2020**, *76*, 2492–2516. [CrossRef]
2. Writing Committee Members; Otto, C.M.; Nishimura, R.A.; Bonow, R.O.; Carabello, B.A.; Erwin, J.P., III; Gentile, F.; Jneid, H.; Krieger, E.V.; Mack, M.; et al. 2020 ACC/AHA Guideline for the Management of Patients With Valvular Heart Disease: A Report of the American College of Cardiology/American Heart Association Joint Committee on Clinical Practice Guidelines. *J. Am. Coll. Cardiol.* **2021**, *77*, e25–e197. [CrossRef] [PubMed]
3. Nitsche, C.; Kammerlander, A.A.; Koschutnik, M.; Sinnhuber, L.; Forutan, N.; Eidenberger, A.; Donà, C.; Schartmueller, F.; Dannenberg, V.; Winter, M.; et al. Fluid overload in patients undergoing TAVR: What we can learn from the nephrologists. *ESC Heart Fail.* **2021**, *8*, 1408–1416. [CrossRef]
4. Binanay, C.; Califf, R.M.; Hasselblad, V.; O'Connor, C.M.; Shah, M.R.; Sopko, G.; Stevenson, L.W.; Francis, G.S.; Leier, C.V.; Miller, L.W.; et al. Evaluation Study of Congestive Heart Failure and Pulmonary Artery Catheterization Effectiveness. *JAMA* **2005**, *294*, 1625–1633. [CrossRef]
5. Miller, W.L.; Mullan, B.P. Volume Overload Profiles in Patients with Preserved and Reduced Ejection Fraction Chronic Heart Failure. *JACC Heart Fail.* **2016**, *4*, 453–459. [CrossRef]
6. Gibson, J.G.; Seligman, A.M.; Peacock, W.C.; Aub, J.C.; Fine, J.; Evans, R.D. The distribution of red cells and plasma in large and minute vessels of the normal dog, determined by radioactive isotopes of iron and iodine 1. *J. Clin. Investig.* **1946**, *25*, 848–857. [CrossRef]
7. Martens, P.; Nijst, P.; Dupont, M.; Mullens, W. The Optimal Plasma Volume Status in Heart Failure in Relation to Clinical Outcome. *J. Card. Fail.* **2019**, *25*, 240–248. [CrossRef]
8. Ling, H.Z.; Flint, J.; Damgaard, M.; Bonfils, P.K.; Cheng, A.; Aggarwal, S.; Velmurugan, S.; Mendonca, M.; Rashid, M.; Kang, S.; et al. Calculated plasma volume status and prognosis in chronic heart failure. *Eur. J. Heart Fail.* **2015**, *17*, 35–43. [CrossRef]
9. Hakim, R.M. Plasmapheresis. In *Handbook of Dialysis*, 3rd ed.; Daugirdas, J.T., Blake, P.G., Ing, T.S., Eds.; Lippincott, Williams and Wilkins: Philadelphia, PA, USA, 2001; p. 236.
10. Longo, D. Table 218: Body fluids and other mass data. In *Harrison's Principles of Internal Medicine*, 18th ed.; Longo, D.L., Fauci, A.S., Kasper, D.L., Hauser, S.L., Jameson, J.L., Loscalzo, J., Eds.; McGraw-Hill: New York, NY, USA, 2011; p. A-1.
11. VARC-3 Writing Committee; Généreux, P.; Piazza, N.; Alu, M.C.; Nazif, T.; Hahn, R.T.; Pibarot, P.; Bax, J.J.; A Leipsic, J.; Blanke, P.; et al. Valve Academic Research Consortium 3: Updated endpoint definitions for aortic valve clinical research. *Eur. Heart J.* **2021**, *42*, 1825–1857. [CrossRef]
12. Shahian, D.M.; Jacobs, J.P.; Badhwar, V.; Kurlansky, P.A.; Furnary, A.P.; Cleveland, J.C.; Lobdell, K.W.; Vassileva, C.; von Ballmoos, M.C.W.; Thourani, V.H.; et al. The Society of Thoracic Surgeons 2018 Adult Cardiac Surgery Risk Models: Part 1—Background, Design Considerations, and Model Development. *Ann. Thorac. Surg.* **2018**, *105*, 1411–1418. [CrossRef] [PubMed]
13. O'Brien, S.M.; Feng, L.; He, X.; Xian, Y.; Jacobs, J.P.; Badhwar, V.; Kurlansky, P.A.; Furnary, A.P.; Cleveland, J.C.; Lobdell, K.W.; et al. The Society of Thoracic Surgeons 2018 Adult Cardiac Surgery Risk Models: Part 2—Statistical Methods and Results. *Ann. Thorac. Surg.* **2018**, *105*, 1419–1428. [CrossRef] [PubMed]
14. Maznyczka, A.M.; Barakat, M.; Aldalati, O.; Eskandari, M.; Wollaston, A.; Tzalamouras, V.; Dworakowski, R.; Deshpande, R.; Monaghan, M.; Byrne, J.; et al. Calculated plasma volume status predicts outcomes after transcatheter aortic valve implantation. *Open Heart* **2020**, *7*, e001477. [CrossRef]
15. Adlbrecht, C.; Piringer, F.; Resar, J.; Watzal, V.; Andreas, M.; Strouhal, A.; Hasan, W.; Geisler, D.; Weiss, G.; Grabenwöger, M.; et al. The impact of subclinical congestion on the outcome of patients undergoing transcatheter aortic valve implantation. *Eur. J. Clin. Investig.* **2020**, *50*, e13251. [CrossRef] [PubMed]
16. Afilalo, J.; Lauck, S.; Kim, D.H.; Lefèvre, T.; Piazza, N.; Lachapelle, K.; Martucci, G.; Lamy, A.; Labinaz, M.; Peterson, M.D.; et al. Frailty in Older Adults Undergoing Aortic Valve Replacement. *J. Am. Coll. Cardiol.* **2017**, *70*, 689–700. [CrossRef]
17. Shimura, T.; Yamamoto, M.; Yamaguchi, R.; Adachi, Y.; Sago, M.; Tsunaki, T.; Kagase, A.; Koyama, Y.; Otsuka, T.; Yashima, F.; et al. Calculated plasma volume status and outcomes in patients undergoing transcatheter aortic valve replacement. *ESC Heart Fail.* **2021**, *8*, 1990–2001. [CrossRef]
18. Seoudy, H.; Al-Kassou, B.; Shamekhi, J.; Sugiura, A.; Frank, J.; Saad, M.; Bramlage, P.; Seoudy, A.K.; Puehler, T.; Lutter, G.; et al. Frailty in patients undergoing transcatheter aortic valve replacement: Prognostic value of the Geriatric Nutritional Risk Index. *J. Cachex Sarcopenia Muscle* **2021**, *12*, 577–585. [CrossRef] [PubMed]
19. Komajda, M.; Hanon, O.; Hochadel, M.; Lopez-Sendon, J.L.; Follath, F.; Ponikowski, P.; Harjola, V.-P.; Drexler, H.; Dickstein, K.; Tavazzi, L.; et al. Contemporary management of octogenarians hospitalized for heart failure in Europe: Euro Heart Failure Survey II. *Eur. Heart J.* **2008**, *30*, 478–486. [CrossRef]
20. Grodin, J.L.; Philips, S.; Mullens, W.; Nijst, P.; Martens, P.; Fang, J.C.; Drazner, M.H.; Tang, W.W.; Pandey, A. Prognostic implications of plasma volume status estimates in heart failure with preserved ejection fraction: Insights from TOPCAT. *Eur. J. Heart Fail.* **2019**, *21*, 634–642. [CrossRef]
21. Imamura, T.; Narang, N.; Combs, P.; Siddiqi, U.; Mirzai, S.; Stonebraker, C.; Bullard, H.; Simone, P.; Jeevanandam, V. Impact of plasma volume status on mortality following left ventricular assist device implantation. *Artif. Organs* **2021**, *45*, 587–592. [CrossRef] [PubMed]

22. *Haemoglobin Concentrations for the Diagnosis of Anaemia and Assessment of Severity. Vitamin and Mineral Nutrition Information System*; WHO/NMH/NHD/MNM/11.1; World Health Organization: Geneva, Switzerland, 2011; Available online: http://www.who.int/vmnis/indicators/haemoglobin.pdf (accessed on 18 July 2021).
23. Nagao, K.; CURRENT AS Registry Investigators; Taniguchi, T.; Morimoto, T.; Shiomi, H.; Ando, K.; Kanamori, N.; Murata, K.; Kitai, T.; Kawase, Y.; et al. Anemia in Patients with Severe Aortic Stenosis. *Sci. Rep.* **2019**, *9*, 1924. [CrossRef]
24. Androne, A.-S.; Katz, S.D.; Lund, L.; LaManca, J.; Hudaihed, A.; Hryniewicz, K.; Mancini, D.M. Hemodilution Is Common in Patients with Advanced Heart Failure. *Circulation* **2003**, *107*, 226–229. [CrossRef]
25. Otto, J.; Plumb, J.; Clissold, E.; Kumar, S.B.; Wakeham, D.J.; Schmidt, W.; Grocott, M.; Richards, T.; Montgomery, H.E. Hemoglobin concentration, total hemoglobin mass and plasma volume in patients: Implications for anemia. *Haematologica* **2017**, *102*, 1477–1485. [CrossRef]
26. Felker, G.M.; Anstrom, K.J.; Adams, K.F.; Ezekowitz, J.A.; Fiuzat, M.; Houston-Miller, N.; Januzzi, J.L.; Mark, D.B.; Piña, I.L.; Passmore, G.; et al. Effect of Natriuretic Peptide-Guided Therapy on Hospitalization or Cardiovascular Mortality in High-Risk Patients With Heart Failure and Reduced Ejection Fraction. *JAMA* **2017**, *318*, 713–720. [CrossRef]
27. Seoudy, H.; Frank, J.; Neu, M.; Güßefeld, N.; Klaus, Y.; Freitag-Wolf, S.; Lambers, M.; Lutter, G.; Dempfle, A.; Rangrez, A.Y.; et al. Periprocedural Changes of NT-proBNP Are Associated with Survival After Transcatheter Aortic Valve Implantation. *J. Am. Heart Assoc.* **2019**, *8*, e010876. [CrossRef]
28. Oury, C.; Nchimi, A.; Lancellotti, P.; Bergler-Klein, J. Can Blood Biomarkers Help Predicting Outcome in Transcatheter Aortic Valve Implantation? *Front. Cardiovasc. Med.* **2018**, *5*, 31. [CrossRef] [PubMed]
29. Wu, P.Y.; Chao, C.-T.; Chan, D.-C.; Huang, J.-W.; Hung, K.-Y. Contributors, risk associates, and complications of frailty in patients with chronic kidney disease: A scoping review. *Ther. Adv. Chronic Dis.* **2019**, *10*. [CrossRef] [PubMed]

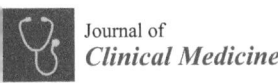

Article

Proper Selection Does Make the Difference: A Propensity-Matched Analysis of Percutaneous and Surgical Cut-Down Transfemoral TAVR

Marco Gennari [1,*], Marta Rigoni [2,3], Giorgio Mastroiacovo [1], Piero Trabattoni [1], Maurizio Roberto [1], Antonio L. Bartorelli [4], Franco Fabbiocchi [5], Gloria Tamborini [6], Manuela Muratori [6], Laura Fusini [6], Mauro Pepi [7], Paola Muti [3,8], Gianluca Polvani [8,9] and Marco Agrifoglio [1,8]

1 Department of Cardiovascular Surgery, IRCCS Centro Cardiologico Monzino, 20100 Milan, Italy; gio.mastroiacovo@hotmail.it (G.M.); piero.trabattoni@ccfm.it (P.T.); maurizio.roberto@ccfm.it (M.R.); marco.agrifoglio@ccfm.it (M.A.)
2 Department of Industrial Engineering, University of Trento, 38100 Trento, Italy; marta.rigoni@unitnt.it
3 Department of Oncology and Health, Evidence, and Impact, McMaster University, Hamilton, ON L8S 4L8, Canada; Paola.Muti@unimi.it
4 Department of Biomedical and Clinical Sciences "Luigi Sacco", University of Milan, 20100 Milan, Italy; antonio.bartorelli@ccfm.it
5 Department of Invasive Cardiology, IRCCS Centro Cardiologico Monzino, 20100 Milan, Italy; franco.fabbiocchi@ccfm.it
6 Department of Cardiovascular Imaging, IRCCS Centro Cardiologico Monzino, 20100 Milan, Italy; gloria.tamborini@ccfm.it (G.T.); manuela.muratori@ccfm.it (M.M.); laura.fusini@ccfm.it (L.F.)
7 Clinical Area Director, IRCCS Centro Cardiologico Monzino, 20100 Milan, Italy; mauro.pepi@ccfm.it
8 Department of Biomedical, Surgical and Dental Sciences, University of Milan, 20100 Milan, Italy; gianluca.polvani@ccfm.it
9 Chief of Cardiovascular Surgery Department, IRCCS Centro Cardiologico Monzino, 20100 Milan, Italy
* Correspondence: marcogennari.md@gmail.com; Tel.: +39-02-58-0022-96

Abstract: Background. Transcatheter aortic valve replacement (TAVR) is an established technique to treat severe symptomatic aortic stenosis patients with a wide range of surgical risk. Currently, the common femoral artery is the first choice as the main access route for the procedure. The objective of this observational study is to report our experience on percutaneous and surgical cut-down transfemoral TAVRs comparing the two approaches. Methods. From January 2014 to January 2019, five hundred eleven consecutive patients underwent TAVR for severe symptomatic aortic stenosis. We analyzed only elective transfemoral procedures. After propensity score-matching based on age, sex, EuroSCORE II, mean aortic gradient, and left ventricular ejection fraction, we obtained two homogeneous populations: surgical cut-down (n = 119) and percutaneous (n = 225), which were labeled Group 1 and Group 2, respectively. Results. The main findings were that there were no significant procedural outcome differences between the two groups, but Group 2 patients had a shorter length of hospital stay and were more frequently discharged home. At follow-up, Group 1 patients had lower survival rates. Conclusions. An accurate preoperative assessment of the femoral access is mandatory to achieve satisfactory outcomes with transfemoral TAVRs. Nevertheless, the percutaneous approach allows shorter in-hospital stay and the need for rehabilitation, thus potentially decreasing the costs of the procedure.

Keywords: TAVR; percutaneous access; vascular complications; surgical cut-down; transfemoral approach

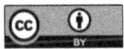

1. Background

Transcatheter aortic valve replacement (TAVR) is an established procedure to treat patients with severe symptomatic aortic stenosis (AS) at high and intermediate surgical risk. After PARTNER 3 and Evolut R low-risk trials [1,2] showing non-inferiority to surgical aortic valve replacement (SAVR) of the latest generation balloon-expandable and self-expanding valves, it is expected for there to be an increase of the number of transcatheter-based replacements of the aortic valve.

Currently, the transfemoral route is the preferred main access for the procedure [3] gained by either surgical cut-down or the percutaneous approach (Figure 1), the latter being the first choice whenever feasible. Despite the lower profile of the delivery catheters of the latest generation of transcatheter aortic valves (TAVs) and that the improvements of the performance of large-bore vascular closure devices (VCDs) had turned into an overall reduction in bleedings or major vascular complications, troubles at the vascular access site still have an impact on the outcome [4].

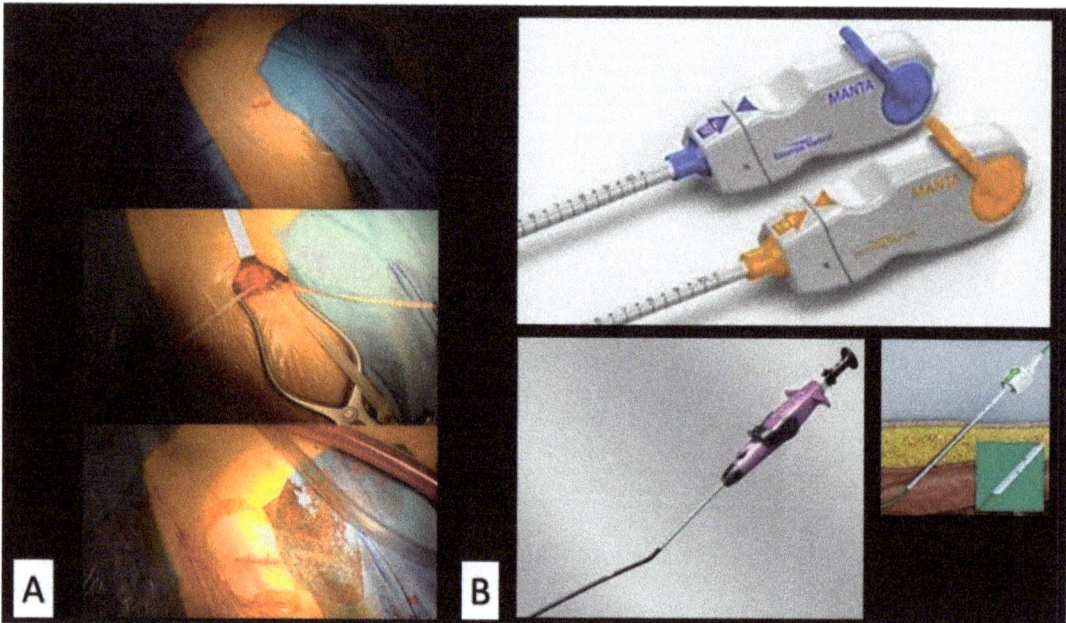

Figure 1. (**A**) Minimal surgical incision at the groin for the isolation of the common femoral artery. (**B**) Currently the most widely used vascular closure devices for large-bore arterial holes.

Surgical cut-down of the common femoral artery may allow better control and repair in case of complications, but it is burdened by all the classical surgical access-related problems [5] such as invasiveness, longer recovery, infection risk, lymphatic or neurological issues, and currently, a fully percutaneous approach with VCDs use is the preferred choice [6].

The aim of this observational study is to report our experience, outcomes, and follow-up of the transfemoral TAVRs with the currently available devices performed by either a surgical cut-down or a percutaneous approach.

2. Methods

This is an observational study of the perioperative and follow-up outcomes of both surgical cut-down and percutaneous transfemoral TAVRs, compared by a propensity score-matching of the two populations. Figure 2 depicts the patients' selection process flow chart.

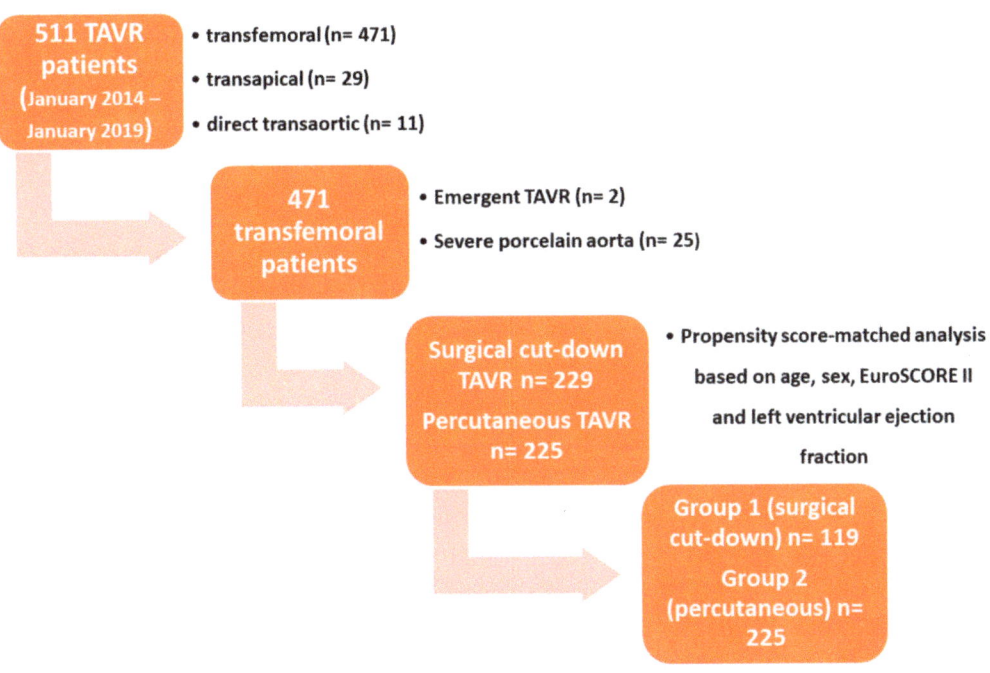

Figure 2. Flow chart of the study. Legend. TAVR = trancatheter aortic valve replacement.

2.1. Patients

From January 2014 to January 2019, five hundred-eleven patients with severe symptomatic aortic stenosis were treated at our institution with both transfemoral balloon-expandable and self-expanding TAVR by the same surgical group. The decision to perform the transcatheter procedure was made by the local Heart Team according to established criteria [7]. The routes of delivery of the transcatheter heart valves (THVs) were femoral (n = 471), left ventricular apex (n = 29), and direct aortic (n = 11). Only elective transfemoral TAVRs have been analyzed in this work. Emergency procedures (n = 2) and patients with challenging porcelain aorta (n = 25) were excluded from the analysis.

We divided the remaining 444 patients into two groups—according to the surgical (n = 219) or percutaneous access (n = 225) to the femoral artery. Since these raw populations presented a relevant mismatch of the baseline characteristics (Table 1), we performed a propensity score-matched analysis based on age, sex, EuroSCORE II, body mass index (BMI), hypertension, diabetes, mean aortic gradient, and left ventricular rejection fraction, obtaining two homogeneous populations of 119 and 225 patients for the surgical and percutaneous group that we labeled Group 1 and Group 2, respectively. The majority of the patients were at intermediate surgical risk (Group 1 presenting a median EuroSCORE II of 4.09 and Group 2 presenting a score 3.77). The frailty burden was considered comparable for both populations after Heart Team evaluation. The decision to perform a surgical or a percutaneous approach was made in the Heart Team context after careful analysis of a contrast-enhanced non-electrocardiogram-guided multi-slice computed tomography (MSCT) of the abdominal aorta and femoral vessels. Briefly, in case of moderate, non-anterior wall calcifications and in the presence of adequate arterial diameters, the percutaneous approach was preferred. In case of borderline diameter with a sheath-to-femoral artery ratio (STFR) > 1.05 [8] or severe concentric calcifications and tortuosity, a direct surgical cut-down of the vessel was favored. Anyway, a final decision on the type of the femoral access was left to the discretion of the operator.

Table 1. Baseline characteristics of the unmatched groups (surgical cut-down versus percutaneous) transcatheter aortic valve replacement (TAVR).

Variables	Unmatched		
	Surgical Cut-Down	Percutaneous	p-Value
Total Population (n)	219	225	
Age, Median (q1–q3)	81 (77–85)	83 (79–86)	<0.01
Male, n (%)	105 (47.9)	130 (57.8)	0.04
Female, n (%)	114 (52.1)	95 (42.2)	
BMI, Median (q1–q3), kg/m^2	25.1 (22.2–28.7)	25.1 (23.4–28.0)	0.37
Hypertension, n (%)	166 (76.2)	180 (80.0)	0.36
Diabetes, n (%)	55 (25.2)	52 (23.1)	0.66
COPD	13 (6)	11 (5)	0.33
Peripheral Vascular Disease, n (%)	82 (37.6)	55 (24.4)	<0.01
Creatinin, Median (q1–q3), mg/dL	1.00 (0.81–1.26)	1.02 (0.81–1.29)	0.35
Hb, Mean (SD), (g/dL)	12.4 (1.7)	12.6 (1.6)	0.34
EuroSCORE II log, Median (q1–q3)	4.13 (2.52–6.75)	3.77 (2.33–5.22)	0.21
Atrial Fibrillation, n (%)	36 (16.7)	34 (15.3)	0.70
Mean Aortic Gradient, Median (q1–q3), mmHg	46 (39–55)	43 (35–52)	0.02
EF, Median (q1–q3)	61 (53–67)	59 (50–66)	0.05
PAPs, median (q1–q3), mmHg	35 (31–42)	35 (31–42)	0.22

Legend: BMI = body mass index; COPD = chronic obstructive pulmonary disease; Hb = hemoglobin; EF = ejection fraction; PAPs = pulmonary artery pressures; q1 = first quartile; q3 = third quartile.

2.2. Ethical Committee

This work is based on a retrospective review of data prospectively collected with follow-up information retrieved by telephone calls and hospital records. This research has been approved by the Institutional Review Board (IRB), in accordance with the principles of the Declaration of Helsinki. The local ethical committee waived the requirement for individual consent for the study due to the retrospective nature of our analysis.

2.3. Surgical Cut-Down Technique

A 3-cm long transversal incision is made ≈1 cm above the inguinal fold. After that, the subcutaneous tissue is longitudinally dissected, and the common femoral artery is approached laterally to decrease the hazard of lymphatic injury. Once the proximal and distal segments of the artery are encircled with a vascular lace, the anterior wall is manually palpated to find the best area for the access. Hereby, a non-calcific area is chosen, a double (180° degrees apart) 5–0 purse-string proline stitch is placed, and a tourniquet snaring system is applied. Afterwards, the artery is directly punctured under vision and tactile feedback. At the end of the procedure, the sutures are tight and the pulse is evaluated; if a relevant stenosis is suspected, the artery is temporary clamped, the purse-string sutures are removed, and the arterial wall is repaired.

2.4. Percutaneous Access Technique

For all the percutaneous procedures, we utilize the double pre-closing technique with two 6Fr Proglide (Abbott, Chicago, IL, USA) deployed at the 10 and 2 o'clock positions. After removing the procedural sheath and tightening the sutures, a bleeding check is performed; if satisfactory hemostasis is achieved, the sutures are further bounded and then cut. If bleeding is still an issue, manual compression or contralateral crossover management is performed (with peripheral balloon occlusion and stent-graft placement when indicated). A similar management is adopted in case of significant femoral stenosis.

2.5. Outcomes and Follow-Up

Most of the patients were followed up in our outpatient clinic, and the follow-up was completed in 100% of them. About 85% were clinical follow-ups, while the remaining were made by phone calls. The outcomes analyzed were procedural results according to VARC-2 (Valve Academic Research Consortium-2) definitions [9], median length of hospital stay, discharge destination, mortality at follow-up, New York Heart Association (NYHA) class, and rehospitalizations. Major adverse cardiovascular and cerebrovascular events (MACCE) as well as survival data were collected.

2.6. Statistical Analysis

Descriptive variables were expressed by mean ± standard deviation (SD) in case of normal distribution, or by median and first and third quartiles (q1, q3 respectively) in case of non-normal distribution. The normality of the variables was tested with the Shapiro–Wilk test. The dichotomous variables or scores were expressed as frequencies and occurrence percentages.

Variables and outcomes were compared between the two groups using the most appropriate test according to the type and nature of the data among the t-test for independent samples, nonparametric Mann–Whitney U-test, Pearson's chi-squared test, or Fisher's exact test.

The Cox proportional hazard model was used to estimate the hazard ratio (HR) and 95% confidence Interval (95% CI) for all-cause mortality for the percutaneous group in respect to the surgical cut-down group. Moreover, Kaplan–Meier estimates analysis was used to generate a time-to-event curve for all-cause mortality, and all event mortality was stratified by access type (surgical cut-down or percutaneous).

All tests were 2-tailed, and a p-value < 0.05 was set for statistical significance.

Statistical analyses were performed using the Stata software (StataCorp LLC 1996-2021, 4905 Lakeway Drive, College Station, TX, USA).

3. Results

3.1. Baseline Characteristics

The baseline characteristics of the two matched groups are listed in Table 2. After the propensity-score matching, only the body mass index (BMI) differed between the two populations, being higher in Group 2 (p = 0.05). No differences were found in the incidence of previous coronary interventions (Table 3), either coronary artery bypass or percutaneous coronary interventions, while Group 1 presented a higher incidence of previous surgical aortic valve replacements (SAVRs) (n = 8, p < 0.01).

Table 2. Baseline characteristics of the matched groups (surgical cut-down versus percutaneous) TAVR.

	Unmatched		
Variables	Group 1 Surgical Cut-Down	Group 2 Percutaneous	p-Value
Total Population (n)	119	225	
Age, Median (q1–q3)	83 (78–85)	83 (79–86)	0.45
Male, n (%)	67 (56.3)	130 (57.8)	0.79
Female, n (%)	52 (43.7)	95 (42.2)	
BMI, Median (q1–q3), kg/m2	24.7 (22.3–27.5)	25.1 (23.4–28.0)	0.05
Hypertension, n (%)	89 (74.8)	180 (80.0)	0.27
Diabetes, n (%)	27 (22.7)	52 (23.1)	0.93
COPD	7 (6)	11 (5)	0.21
Peripheral Vascular Disease, n (%)	37 (31.1)	55 (24.4)	0.19
Creatinin, Median (q1–q3), mg/dL	1.00 (0.82–1.32)	1.02 (0.81–1.29)	0.81
Hb, Mean (SD), (g/dL)	12.5 (1.6)	12.6 (1.6)	0.57
EuroSCORE II log, Median (q1–q3)	4.09 (2.61–7.29)	3.77 (2.33–5.22)	0.22
Atrial Fibrillation, n (%)	22 (18.6)	34 (15.3)	0.44
Mean Aortic Gradient, Median (q1–q3), mmHg	45 (38–54)	43 (35–52)	0.30
EF, Median (q1–q3)	61 (48–67)	59 (50–66)	0.35
PAPs, Median (q1–q3), mmHg	35 (31–42)	35 (31–42)	0.37

Legend: BMI = body mass index; COPD = chronic obstructive pulmonary disease; Hb = hemoglobin; EF = ejection fraction; PAPs = pulmonary artery pressures; q1 = first quartile; q3 = third quartile.

Table 3. Cardiovascular baseline characteristics of the matched populations.

	Matched Populations		
Variables	Group 1	Group 2	p-Value
History of Coronaropathy, n (%)	45 (37.8)	92 (40.9)	0.58
Previous CABG o PCI, n (%)	19 (16.0)	50 (22.2)	0.17
Previous Cardiac Surgery (%)	31 (26.1)	39 (17.3)	0.07
Previous SAVR, n (%)	8 (7.0)	0 (0.0)	<0.01
Severe Peripheral Vascular Disease, n (%)	37 (31.1)	55 (24.4)	0.19
EF, Median (q1–q3)	61 (48–67)	59 (50–66)	0.35

Legend: CABG = coronary artery bypass grafting; PCI = percutaneous coronary interventions; SAVR = surgical aortic valve replacement; EF = ejection fraction.

All the procedures (except one) were performed in deep sedation and oro-tracheal intubation. We analyzed only third-generation devices (Sapien 3, Edwards Lifesciences, Irvine, USA and Evolut R, Medtronic, Minneapolis, USA). Most of the procedures were accomplished using the balloon-expandable platform. No differences between the two groups were recorded on the diameter of the TAVs (Table 4).

Similarly, we did not observe any statistical differences in the femoral sheath diameter (14Fr and 16Fr Edwards eSheath or 14Fr EnVeo R InLine Medtronic sheath).

3.2. In-Hospital Outcomes

No relevant intraprocedural or periprocedural differences were found between the surgical and percutaneous groups in terms of MACCE, major bleedings, major vascular complications, or neurological complications according to VARC-2 criteria (Table 5).

Table 4. Procedural features of the matched populations.

Variable	Group 1	Group 2	p-Value
Type of Anesthesia			
Deep Sedation, n (%)	119 (100.0)	224 (99.5)	1.0
Local Anesthesia + Mild Sedation, n (%)	0 (0.0)	1 (0.5)	
Type of TAV			
Self-Expanding TAV, n (%)	5 (4.2)	12 (5.3)	0.80
Balloon-Expandable TAV, n (%)	114 (95.8)	213 (94.7)	
TAV's Diameter			
20 mm, n (%)	3 (2.5)	1 (0.5)	
23 mm, n (%)	52 (43.7)	87 (38.7)	0.17
26 mm, n (%)	47 (39.5)	109 (48.4)	
29 mm, n (%)	17 (14.3)	28 (12.4)	
Femoral Sheaths			
14F eSheath n (%)	100 (84)	191 (84.9)	
14F EnVeo R InLine Sheath n (%)	5 (4.2)	12 (5.3)	0.35
16F eSheath n (%)	14 (11.8)	22 (9.8)	

Legend: TAV = transcatheter aortic valve.

3.3. Clinical Outcome at Follow-Up

The median follow-up for Group 1 was 949 days (interquartile range 624–1434) and for Group 2, it was 1039 days (interquartile range 703–1553, $p = 0.27$). The main differences are listed in Table 6.

The percutaneous group had a significantly shorter length of hospital stay and was more frequently discharged home, while the surgical group frequently needed a postoperative rehabilitation. We generally offer postoperative rehabilitation to the surgical patients because we want to follow the correct healing of the surgical access, while the percutaneous patients are candidates to rehabilitation only in case of specific situations, such as post procedural rhythm disturbances.

Kaplan–Meier survival estimates (Figure 3) showed a survival rate higher for Group 2, with a crude HR = 0.61; 95% CI = 0.40–0.94; $p = 0.03$. This means that in our analysis, the percutaneous approach was associated with a reduction in the morality hazard of 39% compared with the surgical counterpart.

Table 5. Procedural results (Valve Academic Research Consortium-2 definitions) of the matched populations.

Outcome	Group 1	Group 2	p-Value
Intraprocedural Death, n (%)	1 (0.8)	5 (2.2)	0.67
Cardiac Arrest, n (%)	1 (0.8)	4 (1.8)	0.66
Cardiovascular Mortality, n (%)	1 (0.8)	4 (1.8)	0.66
More than Mild PVL, n (%)	7 (6.0)	19 (8.7)	0.09
Device Embolization, n (%)	0 (0)	0 (0)	0.00
Need for CPB/ECMO, n (%)	1 (0.8)	1 (0.4)	1.00
Conversion to Sternotomy, n (%)	1 (0.8)	1 (0.4)	1.00
Device Success, n (%)	116 (98.3)	219 (97.3)	0.72
Minor Vascular Complications, n (%)	6 (5.1)	10 (4.5)	0.97
Major Vascular Complications, n (%)	3 (2.6)	6 (2.7)	1.00
Coronary Occlusion, n (%)	0 (0)	1 (0.4)	1.00
New Onset AF, n (%)	6 (5.1)	13 (5.8)	0.79
AMI, n (%)	1 (0.8)	0 (0)	0.34
Minor Neurological Events, n (%)	1 (0.85)	2 (0.9)	0.48
Major Neurological Events, n (%)	0 (0.0)	5 (2.2)	0.38
Major Bleedings, n (%)	9 (7.7)	22 (9.9)	0.78
Minor Bleedings, n (%)	3 (2.6)	3 (1.3)	0.44
PPI, n (%)	3 (5.6)	12 (5.4)	0.28
Temporary Postoperative CVVH, n (%)	1 (0.8)	2 (0.9)	1.00

Legend: PVL = paravalvular leak; CPB = cardio-pulmonary bypass; ECMO = extracorporeal membrane oxygenation; AF = atrial fibrillation; AMI = acute myocardial infarction; PPI = permanent pacemaker implantation; CVVH = continuous veno-venous hemofiltration.

Table 6. Outcomes and follow-up of the matched populations.

Outcomes	Group 1	Group 2	p-Value
Length of Stay, Median (q1–q3), days	7 (5–9)	5 (4–7)	<0.01
Discharged Home, n (%)	18 (15.5)	194 (88.2)	<0.01
Rehabilitation, n (%)	98 (84.5)	26 (11.8)	<0.01
Follow-Up Mortality, n (%)	37 (31.6)	48 (21.8)	0.05
Follow-Up Cardiovascular Mortality al, n (%)	11 (9.4)	22 (10.1)	0.85
Median Follow-Up (q1–q3), Days	949 (624–1434)	1039 (703–1553)	0.27
NYHA 1 at Follow-Up, n (%)	94 (83.9)	184 (86.4)	0.83
NYHA 2 at Follow-Up, n (%)	16 (14.3)	26 (12.2)	
NYHA 3 at Follow-Up, n (%)	2 (1.8)	3 (1.4)	
Cardiovascular Rehospitalization, n (%)	7 (6.3)	22 (10.3)	0.22

Legend: NYHA = New York Heart Association; q1 = first quartile; q3 = third quartile.

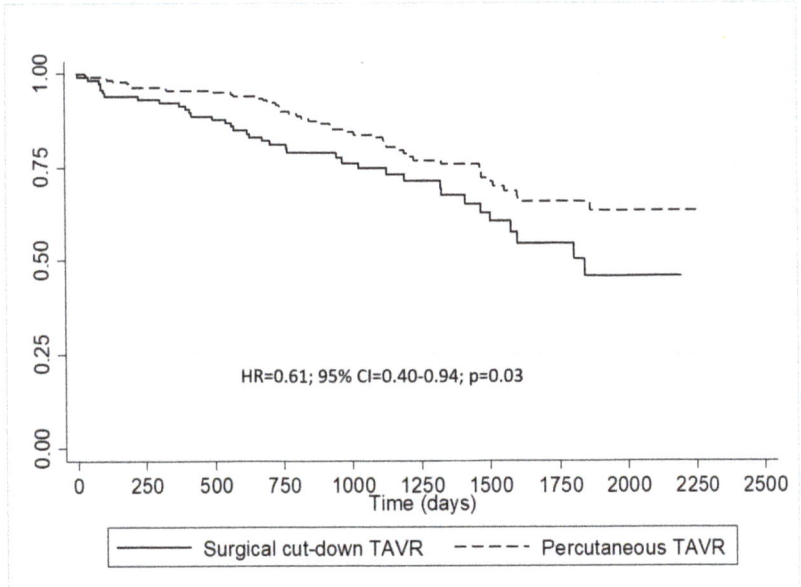

Figure 3. Kaplan–Meier survival estimates. Legend. CI= confidential interval; HR= hazard ratio; TAVR= transcatheter aortic valve replacement.

4. Discussion

The main findings of this report are as follows: (i) an accurate preoperative assessment of the femoral vasculature is mandatory to achieve a low rate of major access-related complications; (ii) even though the operative results were similar for the two groups, patients underwent percutaneous access had a significantly lower length of hospital stay and were more frequently discharged home, potentially reducing the overall costs of the procedure; (iii) and finally, the percutaneous group presented higher survival rates at follow-up.

The latest generation of TAVs are deployed with a lower profile regarding their delivery catheters compared to the early generation devices [10,11]; this has led to a progressive shift toward a less invasive totally percutaneous approach to the femoral artery [12]. Although technical and expertise improvements in the last years have yielded to better outcomes, the incidence of vascular complications after TAVR is still reported to be between 8% and 30% [12].

Whatever the way of access, vascular complications after TAVR are linked to an excess mortality.

Accurate pre-procedural planning of the access is crucial for a safe vascular outcome. The MSCT is currently the main stem of the pre-TAVR assessment [13]; in particular, minimum diameters of the ilio-femoral axes, calcifications burden, and degrees of tortuosity are well-established features that may affect the risk of vascular injury. Although a profile reduction of the delivery systems and an ultrasound-guided approach to the femoral vessels [14] can reduce the hazard of vascular troubles, the choice of the right way of access still play a role. We report our Heart Team experience depicting comparable operative outcomes of both surgical and percutaneous approach, given a deep pre-procedural assessment of the clinical and anatomical characteristics (Figure 4).

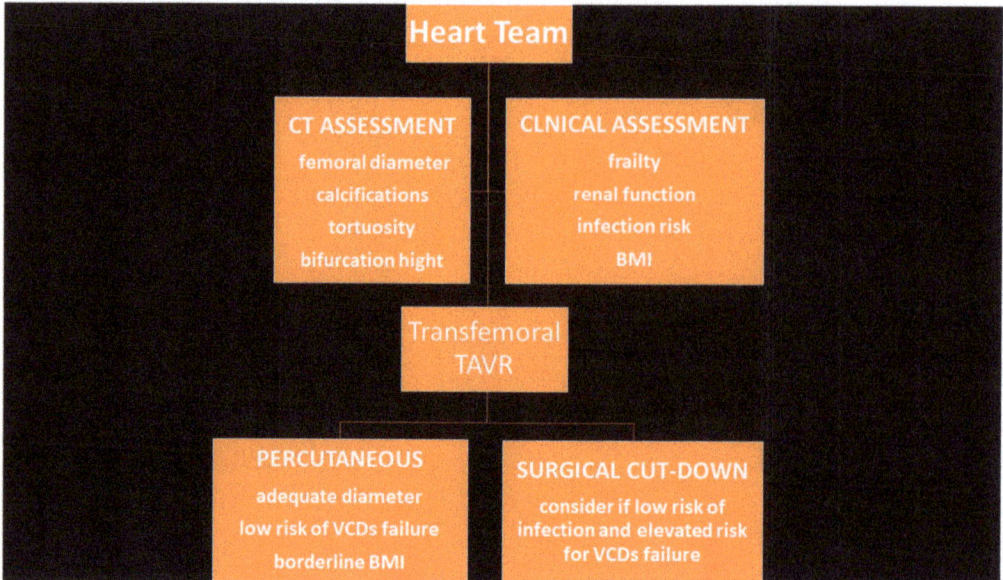

Figure 4. Flow chart of the decision-making to perform surgical cut-down versus percutaneous femoral access.

Despite the favorable results, the greater invasiveness of the surgical cut-down of the femoral artery has led to an overall prolonged in-hospital stay and the need for postoperative rehabilitation.

This may affect the outcome in two ways. The slower recovery of the surgical group may predispose to prolonged immobilization and increased infections rates [15,16], which are all known concerns in these frail surgical candidates. Indeed, lymphoceles and paresthesia complications are quite more common when a surgical femoral isolation is performed [17]. We do not insert an inguinal drain on a regular basis, but only in selected populations such as obese patients or if an extensive arterial dissection is performed; in these cases, the drain can help reduce the common local post-procedural complications (such as infections, lymphoceles) at the expense of a prolonged in-hospital stay.

Secondly, the prolonged hospitalization may affect the costs of the procedure [18], despite the intrinsic costs of the percutaneous toolbox including the vascular closure devices (VCDs).

Most of the available data on the outcome of surgical or percutaneous transfemoral TAVR are derived from registries, case series, and observational studies, whose results are in line with our report [19].

Only a small, randomized clinical trial [20] has prospectively evaluated the outcomes between the two groups, determining that high-volume experienced centers may perform a total percutaneous approach with a low rate of vascular problems.

Finally, we report a higher mortality rate for the surgical group. Although definitive conclusions could not be driven from this evidence, a possible explanation is that the surgical group could have presented a higher global atherosclerotic cardiovascular burden (witnessed by eight valve-in-valve procedures), determining an increased mortality at follow-up. In fact, we speculated that even though the matched baseline characteristics were similar between the two groups, the impact of the cardiovascular risk factors might have a more deep impact on patients who have previously undergone open-heart surgery.

Limitations

This report is affected by several limitations. First, it is a single-center observational analysis. Secondly, the preoperative decision to perform a surgical or percutaneous approach may resent several inter-operator biases. Another limitation is related to our practice in the management of the discharge of the surgical or percutaneous transfemoral TAVR patient; as it is an internal routine and there is currently a lack of evidence-based guidelines, a final conclusion on the benefit of either the rehabilitation or home discharge can not be reached. Finally, most of the experience was along the balloon-expandable platform, making it hard to drive comparison with other platform sheaths.

5. Conclusions

The preoperative selection of the patients based on MSCT is mandatory to improve the vascular and general outcome of the TAVR procedures. The percutaneous approach in the selected population drives a fast in-hospital length of stay and home-based recovery. In our series, it is also linked to better survival rates. In the new parading of tailoring the management of the structural heart disease patient, we believe that handling both techniques (i.e., surgical and percutaneous) could be of worth in the best-option treatment, given their feasibility and good results when properly chosen.

Author Contributions: Conceptualization, M.G. and M.A.; methodology, M.G.; software, M.R. (Marta Rigoni); validation, M.A., G.P. and M.P.; formal analysis, M.R. (Marta Rigoni), P.M.; investigation, M.G.; resources, M.G., M.A., A.L.B.; data curation, G.M., P.T., M.R. (Maurizio Roberto), F.F., G.T., L.F., M.M.; writing—original draft preparation, M.G.; writing—review and editing, M.G.; visualization, M.A.; supervision, M.A.; project administration, M.P.; funding acquisition, N/A. All authors have read and agreed to the published version of the manuscript.

Funding: This research received no external funding.

Institutional Review Board Statement: The study was conducted according to the guidelines of the Declaration of Helsinki, and approved by the Institutional Review Board (or Ethics Committee) of IRCCS Centro Cardiologico Monzino (protocol code CCM 1459 10.02.2021).

Informed Consent Statement: Informed consent was obtained from all subjects involved in the study.

Data Availability Statement: All the data concerning this work are available from the corresponding author upon reasonable request.

Conflicts of Interest: The authors declare no conflict of interest for this work.

References

1. Mack, M.J.; Leon, M.B.; Thourani, V.H.; Makkar, R.; Kodali, S.K.; Russo, M.; Kapadia, S.R.; Malaisrie, S.C.; Cohen, D.J.; Pibarot, P. Transcatheter Aortic-Valve Replacement with a Balloon-Expandable Valve in Low-Risk Patients. *N. Engl. J. Med.* **2019**, *380*, 1695–1705. [CrossRef] [PubMed]
2. Popma, J.J.; Deeb, G.M.; Yakubov, S.J.; Mumtaz, M.; Gada, H.; O'Hair, D.; Bajwa, T.; Heiser, J.C.; Merhi, W.; Kleiman, N.S.; et al. Transcatheter Aortic-Valve Replacement with a Self-Expanding Valve in Low-Risk Patients. *N. Engl. J. Med.* **2019**, *380*, 1706–1715. [CrossRef] [PubMed]
3. Ates, I.; Cilingiroglu, M. Percutaneous access versus surgical cut down for TAVR: Where do we go from here? *Catheter Cardiovasc. Interv.* **2018**, *91*, 1363–1364. [CrossRef] [PubMed]
4. Généreux, P.; Webb, J.G.; Svensson, L.G.; Kodali, S.K.; Satler, L.F.; Fearon, W.F.; Davidson, C.J.; Eisenhauer, A.C.; Makkar, R.R.; Bergman, G.W.; et al. Vascular complications after transcatheter aortic valve replacement: Insights from the PARTNER (Placement of AoRTic TraNscathetER Valve) trial. *J. Am. Coll. Cardiol.* **2012**, *60*, 1043–1052. [CrossRef] [PubMed]
5. Ando, T.; Briasoulis, A.; Holmes, A.A.; Takagi, H.; Slovut, D.P. Percutaneous versus surgical cut-down access in transfemoral transcatheter aortic valve replacement: A meta-analysis. *J. Card. Surg.* **2016**, *31*, 710–717. [CrossRef] [PubMed]
6. Drafts, B.C.; Choi, C.H.; Sangal, K.; Cammarata, M.W.; Applegate, R.J.; Gandhi, S.K.; Kincaid, E.H.; Kon, N.; Zhao, D.X. Comparison of outcomes with surgical cut-down versus percutaneous transfemoral transcatheter aortic valve replacement: TAVR transfemoral access comparisons between surgical cut-down and percutaneous approach. *Catheter Cardiovasc. Interv.* **2018**, *91*, 1354–1362. [CrossRef] [PubMed]

7. Hayashida, K.; Lefèvre, T.; Chevalier, B.; Hovasse, T.; Romano, M.; Garot, P.; Mylotte, D.; Uribe, J.; Farge, A.; Donzeau-Gouge, P.; et al. Transfemoral aortic valve implantation new criteria to predict vascular complications. *JACC Cardiovasc. Interv.* **2011**, *4*, 851–858. [CrossRef] [PubMed]
8. Baumgartner, H.; Falk, V.; Bax, J.J.; De Bonis, M.; Hamm, C.; Holm, P.J.; Lung, B.; Lancellotti, P.; Lanac, E.; Muñoz, D.R.; et al. 2017 ESC/EACTS Guidelines for the management of valvular heart disease. *Eur. Heart J.* **2017**, *38*, 2739–2791. [CrossRef] [PubMed]
9. Kappetein, A.P.; Head, S.J.; Généreux, P.; Piazza, N.; van Mieghem, N.M.; Blackstone, E.H.; Brott, T.G.; Cohen, D.J.; Cutlip, D.E.; van Es, G.A.; et al. Valve Academic Research Consortium (VARC)-2. Updated standardized endpoint definitions for transcatheter aortic valve implantation: The Valve Academic Research Consortium-2 consensus document (VARC-2). *Eur. J. Cardiothorac. Surg.* **2012**, *42*, 45–60. [CrossRef] [PubMed]
10. Van Mieghem, N.M.; Nuis, R.J.; Piazza, N.; Apostolos, T.; Ligthart, J.; Schultz, C.; de Jaegere, P.P.; Serruys, P.W. Vascular complications with transcatheter aortic valve implantation using the 18 Fr Medtronic CoreValve System: The Rotterdam experience. *EuroIntervention* **2010**, *5*, 673–679. [CrossRef] [PubMed]
11. Ducrocq, G.; Francis, F.; Serfaty, J.M.; Himbert, D.; Maury, J.M.; Pasi, N.; Marouene, S.; Provenchère, S.; Iung, B.; Castier, Y.; et al. Vascular complications of transfemoral aortic valve implantation with the Edwards SAPIEN prosthesis: Incidence and impact on outcome. *EuroIntervention* **2010**, *5*, 666–672. [CrossRef] [PubMed]
12. Toggweiler, S.; Gurvitch, R.; Leipsic, J.; Wood, D.A.; Willson, A.B.; Binder, R.K.; Cheung, A.; Ye, J.; Webb, J.G. Percutaneous aortic valve replacement: Vascular outcomes with a fully percutaneous procedure. *J. Am. Coll. Cardiol.* **2012**, *59*, 113–118. [CrossRef] [PubMed]
13. Okuyama, K.; Jilaihawi, H.; Kashif, M.; Takahashi, N.; Chakravarty, T.; Pokhrel, H.; Patel, J.; Forrester, J.S.; Nakamura, M.; Cheng, W.; et al. Transfemoral access assessment for transcatheter aortic valve replacement: Evidence-based application of computed tomography over invasive angiography. *Circ. Cardiovasc. Imaging* **2014**, *8*, e001995. [CrossRef] [PubMed]
14. Vincent, F.; Spillemaeker, H.; Kyheng, M.; Belin-Vincent, C.; Delhaye, C.; Piérache, A.; Denimal, T.; Verdier, B.; Debry, N.; Moussa, M. Ultrasound Guidance to Reduce Vascular and Bleeding Complications of Percutaneous Transfemoral Transcatheter Aortic Valve Replacement: A Propensity Score-Matched Comparison. *J. Am. Heart Assoc.* **2020**, *9*, e014916. [CrossRef] [PubMed]
15. Yanagawa, B.; Graham, M.M.; Afilalo, J.; Hassan, A.; Arora, R.C. Frailty as a risk predictor in cardiac surgery: Beyond the eyeball test. *J. Thorac. Cardiovasc. Surg.* **2019**, *157*, 1905–1909. [CrossRef] [PubMed]
16. Baekke, P.S.; Jørgensen, T.H.; Søndergaard, L. Impact of early hospital discharge on clinical outcomes after transcatheter aortic valve implantation. *Catheter Cardiovasc. Interv.* **2020**. [CrossRef] [PubMed]
17. Torsello, G.B.; Kasprzak, B.; Klenk, E.; Tessarek, J.; Osada, N.; Torsello, G.F. Endovascular suture versus cutdown for endovascular aneurysm repair: A prospective randomized pilot study. *J. Vasc. Surg.* **2003**, *38*, 78–82. [CrossRef]
18. Goldsweig, A.M.; Tak, H.J.; Chen, L.W.; Aronow, H.D.; Shah, B.; Kolte, D.; Desai, N.R.; Szerlip, M.; Velagapudi, P.; Abbott, J.D. Relative Costs of Surgical and Transcatheter Aortic Valve Replacement and Medical Therapy. *Circ. Cardiovasc. Interv.* **2020**, *13*, e008681. [CrossRef] [PubMed]
19. Nakamura, M.; Chakravarty, T.; Jilaihawi, H.; Doctor, N.; Dohad, S.; Fontana, G.; Cheng, W.; Makkar, R.R. Complete percutaneous approach for arterial access in transfemoral transcatheter aortic valve replacement: A comparison with surgical cut-down and closure. *Catheter Cardiovasc. Interv.* **2014**, *84*, 293–300. [CrossRef] [PubMed]
20. Holper, E.M.; Kim, R.J.; Mack, M.; Brown, D.; Brinkman, W.; Herbert, M.; Stewart, W.; Vance, K.; Bowers, B.; Dewey, T. Randomized trial of surgical cutdown versus percutaneous access in transfemoral TAVR. *Catheter Cardiovasc. Interv.* **2014**, *83*, 457–464. [CrossRef] [PubMed]

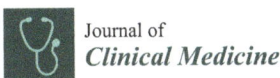

Article

Feasibility and Safety of Cerebral Embolic Protection Device Insertion in Bovine Aortic Arch Anatomy

Ana Paula Tagliari [1,2,*], Enrico Ferrari [1,3], Philipp K. Haager [1,4], Martin Oliver Schmiady [1], Luca Vicentini [1], Mara Gavazzoni [1], Marco Gennari [1,5], Lucas Jörg [1,4], Ahmed Aziz Khattab [6,7], Stefan Blöchlinger [8], Francesco Maisano [1] and Maurizio Taramasso [1]

1. Cardiac Surgery Department, University Hospital of Zurich, University of Zurich, 8091 Zurich, Switzerland; enrico.ferrari@cardiocentro.org (E.F.); philipp.haager@kssg.ch (P.K.H.); martinoliver.schmiady@usz.ch (M.O.S.); luca.vicentini@usz.ch (L.V.); mara.gavazzoni@usz.ch (M.G.); marco.gennari@usz.ch (M.G.); lucas.joerg@kssg.ch (L.J.); francesco.maisano@usz.ch (F.M.); m.taramasso@gmail.com (M.T.)
2. Postgraduate Program in Health Sciences: Cardiology and Cardiovascular Sciences—Faculdade de Medicina, Universidade Federal do Rio Grande do Sul, Porto Alegre 90035003, Brazil
3. Cardiac Surgery Department, Cardiocentro Ticino, 6900 Lugano, Switzerland
4. Cardiology Department, Kantonsspital St. Gallen, 9007 St. Gallen, Switzerland
5. Cardiac Surgery Department, IRCCS Centro Cardiologico Monzino, 20138 Milan, Italy
6. Cardiology Department, University Hospital of Zurich, University of Zurich, 8091 Zurich, Switzerland; ahmedaziz.khattab@usz.ch
7. Cardiology Department, Cardiance Clinic, 8808 Pfäffikon, Switzerland
8. Cardiology Department, Kantonsspital Winterthur KSW, 8400 Winterthur, Switzerland; stefan.bloechlinger@ksw.ch
* Correspondence: anapaulatagliari@gmail.com; Tel.: +41-(44)-255-3728

Received: 19 November 2020; Accepted: 16 December 2020; Published: 20 December 2020

Abstract: Background: Cerebral embolic protection devices (CEPDs) have emerged as a mechanical barrier to prevent debris from reaching the cerebral vasculature, potentially reducing stroke incidence. Bovine aortic arch (BAA) is the most common arch variant and represents challenge anatomy for CEPD insertion during transcatheter aortic valve replacement (TAVR). Methods: Cohort study reporting the Sentinel^{TM} Cerebral Protection System insertion's feasibility and safety in 165 adult patients submitted to a transfemoral TAVR procedure from April 2019 to April 2020. Patients were divided into 2 groups: (1) BAA; (2) non-BAA. Results: Median age, EuroScore II, and STS score were 79 years (74–84), 2.9% (1.7–6.2), and 2.2% (1.6–3.2), respectively. BAA was present in 12% of cases. Successful two-filter insertion was 86.6% (89% non-BAA vs. 65% BAA; $p = 0.002$), and debris was captured in 95% (94% non-BAA vs. 95% BAA; $p = 0.594$). No procedural or vascular complications associated with Sentinel insertion and no intraprocedural strokes were reported. There were two postprocedural non-disabling strokes, both in non-BAA. Conclusion: This study demonstrated Sentinel insertion feasibility and safety in BAA. No procedural and access complications related to Sentinel deployment were reported. Being aware of the bovine arch prevalence and having the techniques to navigate through it allows operators to successfully use CEPDs in this anatomy.

Keywords: cerebral protection device; transcatheter aortic valve replacement; stroke; cerebrovascular events; bovine aortic arch

1. Introduction

Although newer-generation transcatheter heart valve devices and increased operator experience have reduced the incidence of cerebrovascular events during transcatheter aortic valve replacement (TAVR) [1,2], stroke remains one of the most feared procedural complications. This concern is especially relevant since TAVR is moving to low-risk and younger patients, a population in which a cerebrovascular event has even more impact on survival and quality of life [3–6].

Cerebral embolic protection devices (CEPDs) have been developed to work as a mechanical barrier to prevent embolic debris from reaching the cerebral vasculature, potentially reducing neurological events during TAVR procedures. The dual-filter-based Sentinel™ Cerebral Protection System (Sentinel) (Boston Scientific, Marlborough, MA, USA) received CE Mark approval in 2013 and Food and Drug Administration (FDA) approval in 2017, and it is now the most widely used CEPD system [7,8].

Although no single study had demonstrated Sentinel benefits in terms of hard outcomes, two recently published propensity scoring match analyses have suggested that Sentinel use was associated with reduced post-procedural stroke and mortality rates. In the Society of Thoracic Surgeons/American College of Cardiology Transcatheter Valve Therapy (STS/ACC TVT) Registry, after propensity-weighted analysis, significant reduction in in-hospital stroke [relative risk (RR) 0.82; 95% confidence interval (CI) 0.69-0.97], in-hospital death or stroke (RR 0.84; 95% CI 0.73-0.98), 30-day stroke (RR 0.85; 95% CI 0.73-0.99), and 30-day mortality rate (RR 0.78; 95% CI 0.64-0.95) was observed in patients submitted to a protected TAVR [9]. Corroborating these findings, another propensity-weighted analysis from the National Inpatient Sample showed that Sentinel use was associated with lower risk of in-hospital ischemic stroke [odds ratio (OR) 0.24; 95% CI 0.09-0.62] and in-hospital death (0 vs. 1%; $p = 0.036$) [10].

Bovine aortic arch is the most common aortic arch variant and occurs when the brachiocephalic artery (or innominate artery) shares a common origin with the left common carotid artery. The bovine aortic arch prevalence is around 15% (range from 8% to 25%) [11], and its presence carries important implications for preprocedural planning and open or endovascular interventions involving the aortic arch. Indeed, the bovine arch has been associated with consistent geometric hostile features for endovascular procedures, namely angulation, tortuosity, and elongation [12]. Bovine arch is also a recognized anatomic risk factor for carotid stenting, increasing the procedural difficulty level [13], and thoracic aortic disease development [14]. In this respect, in younger patients with this anatomical configuration, TAVR may represent a valid option considering that they could, in time, require an open aortic valve repair.

Regarding CEPD insertion in bovine aortic arches, though there is no formal contraindication to apply the Sentinel system in this scenario, the angulation and tortuosity features related to this anatomical variant are frequent reasons to preclude Sentinel use in real-life procedures. Therefore, many patients who could benefit from cerebral protection are deprived of this strategy.

Herein, we report the feasibility and safety of Sentinel insertion in bovine aortic arch anatomy and bovine arch prevalence in patients undergoing a TAVR procedure. This is the first study evaluating a cohort of patients with bovine aortic arch anatomy submitted to TAVR under cerebral protection.

2. Material and Methods

Single-center cohort study. Patients who underwent a transfemoral-protected TAVR from April 2019 to April 2020 were analyzed and divided into two groups according to the aortic arch anatomy: Group 1: Non-bovine aortic arch anatomy; Group 2: Bovine aortic arch anatomy.

All procedures involving human participants followed the institutional research committee ethical standards in accordance with the 1964 Helsinki declaration and its later amendments. TAVR indication decisions were driven by the institutional heart team, and patients provided written informed consent before the procedure. Patients undergoing TAVR procedures in our institution are included in the nationwide Swiss TAVI Registry (NCT01368250; 2016-00587), a prospective multi-center and observational national registry collecting clinical characteristics of patients undergoing TAVR in Switzerland, which had been previously approved by local ethics committees [15,16].

Clinical, echocardiographic, and tomographic data were collected at baseline, discharge, and 30 days after the procedure. Clinical events were adjudicated according to the updated Valve Academic Research Consortium (VARC-2) criteria [17]. Combined procedures were defined as simultaneous elective interventions, such as coronary artery angiogram, percutaneous coronary artery intervention, left atrial appendage occlusion, intravascular lithotripsy, bioprosthetic or native aortic scallop intentional laceration to prevent coronary artery obstruction (BASILICA), or pacemaker generator change. Significant tortuosity was defined, based on subjective operator judgment, as a brachiocephalic or left common carotid artery S- or C-shaped elongation or undulation, evaluated in the preoperative computed tomography (CT) scan.

The cerebral embolic protection device used was the dual-filter-based Sentinel™ Cerebral Protection System (Sentinel) (Boston Scientific, Marlborough, MA, USA), which consists of a 6-Fr-compatible steerable catheter (100 cm long) carrying two cone-shaped, biocompatible polyurethane filters equipped with 140 µm pores to capture and retrieve debris during TAVR procedures. The sheath is inserted through the right radial artery, and the filters are targeted to the brachiocephalic artery (proximal target vessel) and the left common carotid artery (distal target vessel). Using an articulating sheath, the device's curve can be adjusted to accommodate anatomic variations of the aortic arch (Figure 1, Movie 1). In patients in whom the insertion of both filters was not possible, only the proximal filter was deployed. At the end of the procedure, both filters were checked for the presence of captured material. Successful Sentinel insertion was defined as a successful positioning and deployment of both filters in the correct anatomical position.

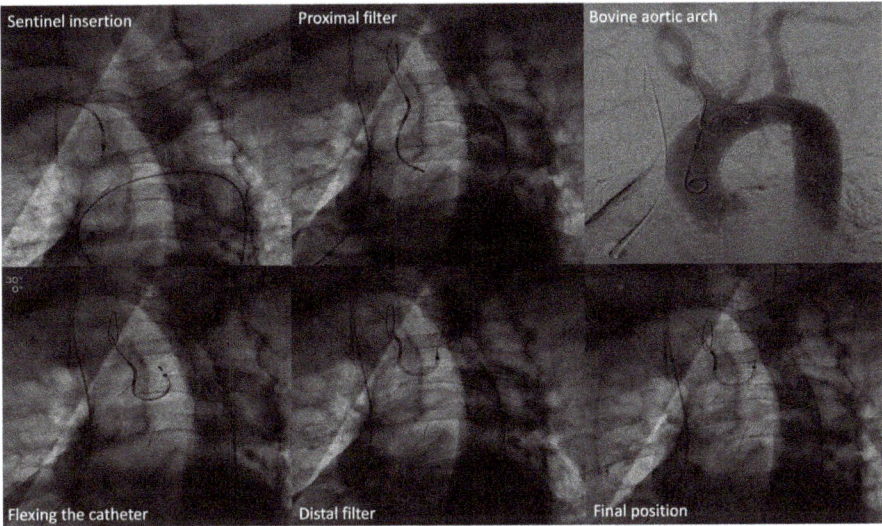

Figure 1. Sentinel insertion in a bovine aortic arch anatomy.

3. Statistical Analysis

Quantitative data were expressed as mean ± standard deviation (SD) or median and interquartile range (IQR). Qualitative variables were expressed as frequency and percentage. Analyses were performed using the statistical package SPSS 19.0 software (Chicago, IL, USA). Categorical variables were analyzed using the chi-square test, continuous variables were analyzed using the Student's T-test or the Mann–Whitney U test. A two-sided p-value lower than 0.05 was considered significant for all tests.

4. Results

From April 2019 to April 2020, 231 patients were submitted to a transfemoral TAVR procedure, 165 (71.5%) of them under cerebral embolic protection. The most common reasons to preclude Sentinel use were significant aortic arch branch tortuosity (22.3%, $n = 15$); emergency procedure or procedure performed under hemodynamic instability (10.4%, $n = 7$); no right radial artery suitable for Sentinel insertion (9%, $n = 6$) or no Sentinel progression (3%, $n = 2$); aberrant right subclavian artery (3%, $n = 2$); and previous left carotid endarterectomy (3%, $n = 2$).

Overall, bovine aortic arch (Figure 2) was identified in 37 patients (16%, $n = 37/231$) and in 20 (12.12%; $n = 20/165$) of those submitted to a protected TAVR procedure. Type I (common origin of the brachiocephalic and left common carotid artery) bovine arch anatomy was presented in 97.3% (*n* = 36) of the cases, and type II (left common carotid artery originating directly from the brachiocephalic artery, rather than as a common trunk) in 2.7% (*n* = 1). Comparison between patients who received a Sentinel device with those who did not are presented in the Supplementary Material (Table S1). There was no difference in procedural time (55 min (46–67) vs. 51.5 min (41.7–62.7); $p = 0.492$) or injected contrast volume (87 mL (69–133) vs. 102 (77–120); $p = 0.071$) between protected and unprotected TAVR.

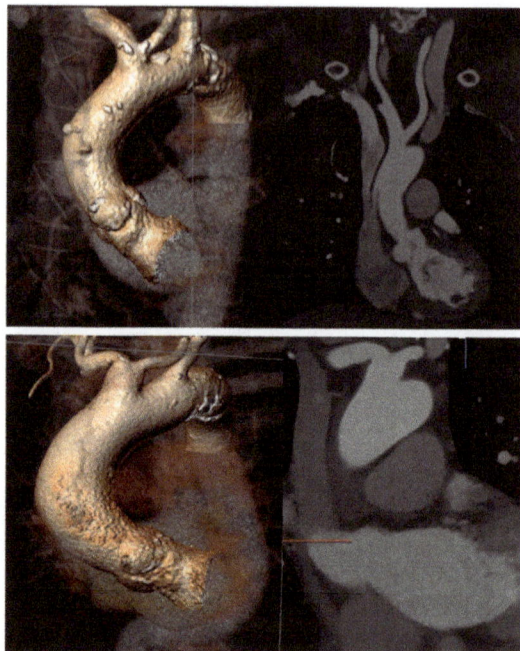

Figure 2. Two examples of bovine aortic arch anatomy suitable for Sentinel insertion.

Among the 165 patients who underwent a transfemoral TAVR under cerebral protection, baseline clinical and aortic valve characteristics were similar between the bovine and non-bovine anatomy groups and are presented in Table 1. Significant aortic arch branch tortuosity was present in 27 patients (16.3%; 17.2% in non-bovine vs. 2% in bovine; $p = 0.412$). Successful insertion of two Sentinel filters was achieved in 143 (86.6%; 89.7% in non-bovine vs. 65% in bovine; $p = 0.002$). Debris was captured in the filters of 158 patients (95.7%; 94.5% in non-bovine vs. 95% in bovine; $p = 0.594$).

Procedure characteristics and outcomes are presented in Tables 2 and 3, respectively. There were no procedural or vascular complications associated with Sentinel insertion, nor intraprocedural strokes. Two non-disabling ischemic strokes (1.21%) were reported in the non-bovine group: the first case showed-up as aphasia on the first postoperative day, which completely regressed one day after; the second case presented hemiplegia on the third postoperative day, which also totally regressed at the hospital discharge. No new cerebrovascular events were reported between hospital discharge and 30-day outpatient evaluation. Total procedure time (55 min vs. 55 min; $p = 0.654$) and volume of contrast used (87mL vs. 89mL; $p = 0.727$) were similar in bovine and non-bovine aortic arches, respectively.

Table 1. Baseline clinical and aortic valve characteristics in patients undergoing transcatheter aortic valve replacement (TAVR) with concomitant cerebral protection.

Variable	Non-Bovine n = 145	Bovine n = 20	p-Value
Age, years median (IQR)	79 (74–83)	80 (77–84)	0.318
Male gender	86 (59.3)	14 (70)	0.359
EuroScore II, % median (IQR)	2.8 (1.6–6.2)	3.2 (2.2–6.3)	0.328
STS score, % median (IQR)	2.1 (1.6–3.2)	2.8 (1.6–3.7)	0.732
Weight, Kg mean ± SD	77.2 ± 14	75.9 ± 16	0.717
Height, cm mean ± SD	166.4 ± 8	170 ± 10	0.051
Severe aortic valve stenosis	142 (97.9)	20 (100)	0.516
Aortic valve regurgitation ≥ moderate	11 (6.6)	1 (5)	0.561
NYHA functional class III/IV	77 (53)	11 (55)	0.982
Arterial hypertension	103 (71)	13 (65)	0.580
Diabetes mellitus	41 (28.3)	2 (10)	0.081
Dyslipidemia	84 (57.9)	12 (60)	0.182
Coronary artery disease	64 (44.1)	12 (60)	0.191
Previous myocardial infarction	17 (12.4)	4 (20)	0.349
Previous stroke	11 (7.6)	3 (15)	0.265
Atrial fibrillation	50 (34.5)	11 (55)	0.075
Chronic obstructive pulmonary disease	17 (11.7)	3 (15)	0.674
Chronic kidney disease	44 (30.3)	6 (30)	0.975
Anemia	16 (11)	0	0.118
Peripheral artery disease	12 (8.3)	1 (5)	0.610
Active smoker	46 (31.7)	8 (40)	0.460
Previous PCI	37 (25.5)	9 (45)	0.069
Previous CABG	8 (5.5)	3 (15)	0.111
Previous aortic valve surgery	9 (6.2)	1 (5)	0.832
Previous permanent pacemaker	11 (7.6)	2 (10)	0.707
Bicuspid aortic valve	14 (9.7)	1 (5)	0.497
Aortic valve area, cm^2 median (IQR)	0.75 (0.6–0.9)	0.85 (0.7–0.97)	0.099
Aortic valve mean gradient, mmHg median (IQR)	42 (35–51)	45 (37–52)	0.703
LVEF, % median (IQR)	58 (45–65)	55 (47–60)	0.301

Values expressed as numbers (%) unless otherwise indicated. IQR = interquartile range; SD = standard deviation; CABG = coronary artery bypass graft; LVEF = left ventricular ejection fraction; NYHA = New York Heart Association; PCI = percutaneous coronary intervention; STS = The Society of Thoracic Surgeons.

Table 2. Procedural characteristics.

Variable	Non-Bovine n = 145	Bovine n = 20	p-Value
Sedation	136 (94.4)	19 (95)	0.959
Combined procedure	9 (6.2)	0	0.252
Two Sentinel filters inserted	130 (89.7)	13 (65)	0.002
Type of bioprosthesis			0.908
Portico	49 (33.8)	9 (45)	
Edwards Sapien 3/Ultra	43 (29.6)	5 (25)	
Medtronic Evolut R/Pro	36 (24.8)	3 (15)	
Acurate Neo	12 (8.3)	2 (10)	
Allegra	3 (2.1)	1 (5)	
Lotus	2 (1.4)	0	
Procedure time, min median (IQR)	55 (45–67)	55 (48–61)	0.654
Contrast injection, mL median (IQR)	87 (68–130)	89 (72–145)	0.727

Values expressed as numbers (%) unless otherwise indicated. IQR = interquartile range.

Table 3. In-hospital outcomes.

Variable	Non-Bovine n = 145	Bovine n = 20	p-Value
All-cause mortality	1 (0.7)	0	0.710
Permanent pacemaker implantation	20 (13.8)	5 (25)	0.190
Non-disabling stroke	2 (1.3)	0	0.516
New onset of atrial fibrillation	6 (4.1)	0	0.354
Delirium	3 (2.1)	0	0.516
Aortic valve mean gradient, mmHg median (IQR)	8.8 (5–11)	7.7 (5–9)	0.309
Aortic valve regurgitation ≤ mild	135 (93.1)	18 (90)	0.909
LVEF, % median (IQR)	57 (49–63)	54 (49–57)	0.214
Hospital length of stay, days median (IQR)	5 (4–7)	6 (4–7)	0.554

Values expressed as numbers (%) unless otherwise indicated. IQR = interquartile range; LVEF = left ventricular ejection fraction.

5. Discussion

Cerebrovascular events are one of the most devastating TAVR complications, not only in terms of mortality but also regarding the potential sequelae and impaired quality of life [3–6]. Clinical strokes are related to an up-to-nine-fold increase in postprocedural mortality [4,18,19], non-return to working life in 50% of the cases [20,21], and an increase in index hospitalization cost of approximately 25,000 USD [22].

Almost 50% of all early post-TAVR strokes are directly procedure-related and occur within the first 24 h [3,19,23]. This post-TAVR stroke incidence peak is consistent with what has been observed in carotid stenting procedures, suggesting that stroke occurrence is related to hostile aortic arch and anatomical features of supra-aortic vessels [24].

CEPDs were developed with the purpose of offering a safer procedure, mitigating cerebrovascular event risk, and improving TAVR-related outcomes [25–29]. Despite the worldwide spread of CEPD use, evidence about anatomical features associated with its unsuccessful implantation remains scarce [29]. As bovine aortic arch is the most common aortic arch branching variant in humans, the present study aimed to report the feasibility and safety of performing a Sentinel device insertion in this anatomy, as well as the prevalence of bovine aortic arch anatomy in patients who underwent a protected TAVR.

Previous studies have indicated that bovine left common carotid artery configuration occurs in 8–25% of patients [11], a prevalence similar to that observed in our cohort (12%; $n = 20/165$). The presence of this type of anatomical configuration is associated with an increased endovascular device navigation complexity [30,31]. Comparing patients with or without aortic arch anomalies who underwent a carotid artery stent, Faggioli et al. observed that bovine arch was associated with increased neurologic events (20% vs. 5.3%; $p = 0.039$) and technical failure (89.6% vs. 76.4%; $p = 0.1$) due to the greater difficulty in navigating devices through tortuous vessels [30]. In addition, the presence of increased aortic arch angulation also reflects a hostile take-off angle of the supra-aortic branches [12]. In this scenario, Rozado et al. advocated that an extreme device tip flexure could help to advance a wire into the left carotid artery, allowing proper Sentinel advancement and positioning [32].

In our study, despite bovine aortic arch anatomy being associated with reduced two-filter insertion (89.7% vs. 65%; $p = 0.002$), this feature did not reflect an increase in procedural complication rate or postprocedural neurological events. Total procedure time (55 min vs. 55 min; $p = 0.654$) and volume of contrast used (87 mL vs. 89 mL; $p = 0.727$) were also similar in bovine and non-bovine aortic arches. Higher tortuosity degree and challenging device navigation were probably factors related to a lower rate of two-filter insertion in bovine group. However, since in bovine aortic arches, both common carotid arteries have the same origin and are in a close position, one filter properly positioned beyond their origins is probably enough to provide adequate cerebral protection. Furthermore, even if bi-carotid protection is not feasible, a single-filter insertion is possibly better than no cerebral protection at all. Indeed, further computational fluid dynamics studies may shed some light on stroke risk related to debris distribution along the arch and supra-aortic branches according to the aortic arch anatomy.

In our study, the Sentinel was not used in 28.5% ($n = 66$) of patients, a rate similar to that recently reported by Voss et al. (38.5%; $n = 122$). In this study, the authors reported that Sentinel ineligibility reasons, based on MSCT criteria, were as follows: inappropriate diameter within the target landing zone ($n = 116$); significant subclavian artery stenosis ($n = 4$) or an aberrant subclavian artery ($n = 3$); and clinical characteristics including hypersensitivity to nickel titanium ($n = 1$), radial artery occlusion ($n = 1$), or previous left common carotid artery interventions ($n = 5$) [33].

Another important anatomic consideration concerning Sentinel insertion eligibility is the presence of vascular tortuosity. Tortuosity hampers access to the filter-landing zone [34–36], increasing device manipulation, contrast use, vessel injury risk, and CEPD insertion failure [35]. Device instructions stipulate that Sentinel should be avoided in patients with "excessive" vessel tortuosity; however, there is no specific definition of what excessive tortuosity means. In our study, the overall prevalence of aortic arch branches tortuosity was 16.4% ($n = 27/165$), with no significant difference in tortuosity distribution between bovine and non-bovine Sentinel groups (17.2% in non-bovine vs. 2% in bovine; $p = 0.412$).

Considering the benefits of cerebral protection during TAVR, even though no randomized trial had found significant stroke or mortality reduction, a propensity-matched cohort study by Seeger et al. identified lower mortality or all-stroke rate 7 days post-TAVR when a CEPD was used (2.1% vs. 6.8%; $p = 0.01$). All-stroke rate was also inferior in protected TAVR (1.4% vs. 4.6%, $p = 0.03$; OR 0.29, 95% CI 0.10-0.93; NNT 31). In multivariable analysis, STS score ($p = 0.02$) and TAVR without cerebral protection device ($p = 0.02$) were independent predictors for the primary endpoint (mortality or stroke) [37]. Two years after this initial study, the same authors evaluated the incidence of procedural stroke within 72 h post-TAVR in a propensity-matched population comprising patients from the SENTINEL US IDE trial [24], the CLEAN-TAVI trial [34], and SENTINEL-Ulm registry (University Hospital of Ulm, Ulm, Germany) ($n = 1306$). The main result showed that the procedural all-stroke rate was significantly lower in the CEPD group compared to the unprotected group (1.88% vs. 5.44%; OR 0.35, 95% CI 0.17-0.72). In addition, the combined outcome of all-cause mortality and all-stroke was significantly lower (2.06% vs. 6.00%; OR 0.34, 95% CI 0.17-0.68) in the protected group [38]. These findings were supported by two recently released propensity scoring match analyses showing benefit in terms of stroke and mortality rate reduction when Sentinel was used [9,10].

Regarding Sentinel's cost-effectiveness, estimations show that the cost of preventing a single stroke or death is around 60,000 USD [39]. As the Sentinel device costs approximately 2800 USD, according to Giustino et al., a total amount of 61,600 USD should be spent to prevent one stroke or death. This value seems to be justifiable given the negative physical, emotional, and economic impact of stroke [40].

6. Limitations

The present analysis reflects a single-center, non-randomized, but prospectively acquired experience. Therefore, all the inherent limitations of such design need to be taken into account. In addition, our results are based on a single specific cerebral embolic protection device and cannot be generalized to other available devices. Despite our small sample size, this report represents the first cohort of patients with bovine aortic arch anatomy successfully treated with TAVR procedure under cerebral protection.

7. Conclusions

This study demonstrated Sentinel insertion feasibility and safety in bovine aortic arch anatomy. No procedural and access complications related to Sentinel deployment were reported. Being aware of the bovine arch prevalence and having the techniques to navigate through it allows operators to successfully use Sentinel in this anatomy.

Supplementary Materials: The following are available online at http://www.mdpi.com/2077-0383/9/12/4118/s1, Table S1: Baseline clinical and aortic valve characteristics in patients who received or not a Sentinel device during a transfemoral TAVR procedure; Movie S1: Sentinel cerebral protection device implanted in a bovine aortic arch anatomy.

Author Contributions: Conceptualization, A.P.T., E.F., P.K.H., M.O.S., L.V., M.G. (Mara Gavazzoni), M.G. (Marco Gennari), L.J., A.A.K., S.B., F.M., and M.T.; Methodology, A.P.T., E.F., P.K.H., and M.T. Formal Analysis, A.P.T., E.F., P.K.H., and M.T. Investigation, A.P.T., E.F., P.K.H., M.O.S., L.V., M.G. (Mara Gavazzoni), M.G. (Marco Gennari), L.J., A.A.K., S.B., F.M., and M.T.; Data Curation, A.P.T.; Writing—Original Draft Preparation, A.P.T., E.F.; Writing—Review & Editing, A.P.T., E.F., P.K.H., M.O.S., L.V., M.G. (Mara Gavazzoni), M.G. (Marco Gennari), L.J., A.A.K., S.B., F.M., and M.T.; Supervision, E.F., P.K.H., and M.T. All authors have read and agreed to the published version of the manuscript.

Funding: This research received no external funding.

Acknowledgments: The authors thank Malik Riva and Leonora Kodzadziku for supporting TAVR procedures.

Conflicts of Interest: Dr. Tagliari received Research Support from Coordenação de Aperfeiçoamento de Pessoal de Nível Superior—Brasil (Capes)—Finance Code 001. Dr. Ferrari is consultant for Edwards Lifesciences and received Grants and Research Support from Edwards Lifescences, Medtronic and Somahlution. Dr. Gavazzoni is consultant for Abbott Vascular and Biotronik. Dr. Gennari is consultant for Medtronic. Dr. Maisano received Grant and/or Research Support from Abbott, Medtronic, Edwards Lifesciences, Biotronik, Boston Scientific Corporation, NVT, Terumo; receives Consulting fees, Honoraria from Abbott, Medtronic, Edwards Lifesciences, Swissvortex, Perifect, Xeltis, Transseptal solutions, Cardiovalve, Magenta; has Royalty Income/IP Rights Edwards Lifesciences and is Shareholder, Cardiogard, Magenta, SwissVortex, Transseptalsolutions, 4 Tech, Perifect. Dr. Taramasso is a consultant for Abbott Vascular, Boston Scientific, and 4tech; and has received fees from Edwards Lifesciences, CoreMedic, Swissvortex, and Mitraltech.

Abbreviations

Bioprosthetic or native aortic scallop intentional laceration to prevent coronary artery obstruction (BASILICA); bovine aortic arch (BAA); cerebral embolic protection device (CEPD); confidence interval (CI); dual-filter-based Sentinel™ Cerebral Protection System (Sentinel); Food and Drug Administration (FDA); interquartile range (IQR); multislice computed tomography (MSCT); odds ratio (OR); relative risk (RR); standard deviation (SD); Society of Thoracic Surgeons/American College of Cardiology (STS/ACC); transcatheter aortic valve replacement (TAVR); The Society of Thoracic Surgeons (STS); Valve Academic Research Consortium (VARC-2).

References

1. Mack, M.J.; Leon, M.B.; Thourani, V.H.; Makkar, R.; Kodali, S.K.; Russo, M.; Kapadia, S.R.; Malaisrie, S.C.; Cohen, D.J.; Pibarot, P.; et al. Transcatheter Aortic-Valve Replacement with a Balloon-Expandable Valve in Low-Risk Patients. *N. Engl. J. Med.* **2019**, *380*, 1695–1705. [CrossRef] [PubMed]
2. Popma, J.J.; Deeb, G.M.; Yakubov, S.J.; Mumtaz, M.; Gada, H.; O'Hair, D.; Bajwa, T.; Heiser, J.C.; Merhi, W.; Kleiman, N.S.; et al. Transcatheter Aortic-Valve Replacement with a Self-Expanding Valve in Low-Risk Patients. *N. Engl. J. Med.* **2019**, *380*, 1706–1715. [CrossRef] [PubMed]
3. Nombela-Franco, L.; Webb, J.G.; De Jaegere, P.P.; Toggweiler, S.; Nuis, R.-J.; Dager, A.E.; Amat-Santos, I.J.; Cheung, A.; Ye, J.; Binder, R.K.; et al. Timing, Predictive Factors, and Prognostic Value of Cerebrovascular Events in a Large Cohort of Patients Undergoing Transcatheter Aortic Valve Implantation. *Circulation* **2012**, *126*, 3041–3053. [CrossRef] [PubMed]
4. Muralidharan, A.; Thiagarajan, K.; Van Ham, R.; Gleason, T.G.; Mulukutla, S.; Schindler, J.T.; Jeevanantham, V.; Thirumala, P.D. Meta-Analysis of Perioperative Stroke and Mortality in Transcatheter Aortic Valve Implantation. *Am. J. Cardiol.* **2016**, *118*, 1031–1045. [CrossRef]
5. Gleason, T.G.; Schindler, J.T.; Adams, D.H.; Reardon, M.J.; Kleiman, N.S.; Caplan, L.R.; Conte, J.V.; Deeb, G.M.; Hughes, G.C.; Chenoweth, S.; et al. The risk and extent of neurologic events are equivalent for high-risk patients treated with transcatheter or surgical aortic valve replacement. *J. Thorac. Cardiovasc. Surg.* **2016**, *152*, 85–96. [CrossRef]
6. Kapadia, S.; Agarwal, S.; Miller, D.C.; Webb, J.G.; Mack, M.; Ellis, S.; Herrmann, H.C.; Pichard, A.D.; Tuzcu, E.M.; Svensson, L.G.; et al. Insights Into Timing, Risk Factors, and Outcomes of Stroke and Transient Ischemic Attack After Transcatheter Aortic Valve Replacement in the PARTNER Trial (Placement of Aortic Transcatheter Valves). *Circ. Cardiovasc. Interv.* **2016**, *9*, 1–10. [CrossRef]
7. Nombela-Franco, L.; Armijo, G.; Tirado-Conte, G. Cerebral embolic protection devices during transcatheter aortic valve implantation: Clinical versus silent embolism. *J. Thorac. Dis.* **2018**, *10*, S3604–S3613. [CrossRef]

8. Naber, C.K.; Ghanem, A.; Abizaid, A.A.; Wolf, A.; Sinning, J.-M.; Werner, N.; Nickenig, G.; Schmitz, T.; Grube, E. First-in-man use of a novel embolic protection device for patients undergoing transcatheter aortic valve implantation. *EuroIntervention* **2012**, *8*, 43–50. [CrossRef]
9. Cohen, D.J. Cerebral Embolic Protection and TAVR Outcomes: Results from the TVT Registry. In Proceedings of the Transcatheter Cardiovascular Therapeutics Conference (TCT), Online, 14–16 October 2020.
10. Megaly, M.; Sorajja, P.; Cavalcante, J.L.; Pershad, A.; Gössl, M.; Abraham, B.; Omer, M.; Elbadawi, A.; Garcia, S. Ischemic Stroke with Cerebral Protection System During Transcatheter Aortic Valve Replacement. *JACC Cardiovasc. Interv.* **2020**, *13*, 2149–2155. [CrossRef]
11. Layton, K.F.; Kallmes, D.F.; Cloft, H.J.; Lindell, E.P.; Cox, V.S. Bovine aortic arch variant in humans: Clarification of a common misnomer. *AJNR Am. J. Neuroradiol.* **2006**, *27*, 1541–1542.
12. Marrocco-Trischitta, M.M.; Alaidroos, M.; Romarowski, R.M.; Secchi, F.; Righini, P.; Glauber, M.; Nano, G. Geometric Pattern of Proximal Landing Zones for Thoracic Endovascular Aortic Repair in the Bovine Arch Variant. *Eur. J. Vasc. Endovasc. Surg.* **2020**, *59*, 808–816. [CrossRef] [PubMed]
13. Macdonald, S.; Lee, R.; Williams, R.; Stansby, G. Towards Safer Carotid Artery Stenting. *Stroke* **2009**, *40*, 1698–1703. [CrossRef] [PubMed]
14. Marrocco-Trischitta, M.M.; Alaidroos, M.; Romarowski, R.; Milani, V.; Ambrogi, F.; Secchi, F.; Glauber, M.; Nano, G. Aortic arch variant with a common origin of the innominate and left carotid artery as a determinant of thoracic aortic disease: A systematic review and meta-analysis. *Eur. J. Cardio-Thoracic Surg.* **2019**, *57*, 422–427. [CrossRef] [PubMed]
15. Wenaweser, P.; Stortecky, S.; Heg, D.; Tueller, D.; Nietlispach, F.; Falk, V.; Pedrazzini, G.; Jeger, R.; Reuthebuch, O.; Carrel, T.; et al. Short-term clinical outcomes among patients undergoing transcatheter aortic valve implantation in Switzerland: The Swiss TAVI registry. *EuroIntervention* **2014**, *10*, 982–989. [CrossRef]
16. Stortecky, S.; Franzone, A.; Heg, D.; Tueller, D.; Noble, S.; Pilgrim, T.; Jeger, R.; Toggweiler, S.; Ferrari, E.; Nietlispach, F.; et al. Temporal trends in adoption and outcomes of transcatheter aortic valve implantation: A SwissTAVI Registry analysis. *Eur. Heart J. Qual. Care Clin. Outcomes* **2018**, *5*, 242–251. [CrossRef]
17. Kappetein, A.-P.; Head, S.J.; Généreux, P.; Piazza, N.; Van Mieghem, N.M.; Blackstone, E.H.; Brott, T.G.; Cohen, D.J.; Cutlip, D.E.; Van Es, G.-A.; et al. Updated standardized endpoint definitions for transcatheter aortic valve implantation: The Valve Academic Research Consortium-2 consensus document (VARC-2). *Eur. J. Cardio-Thoracic Surg.* **2012**, *42*, S45–S60. [CrossRef]
18. Eggebrecht, H.; Schmermund, A.; Voigtländer, T.; Kahlert, P.; Erbel, R.; Mehta, R.H. Risk of stroke after transcatheter aortic valve implantation (TAVI): A meta-analysis of 10,037 published patients. *EuroIntervention* **2012**, *8*, 129–138. [CrossRef]
19. Tchetche, D.; Farah, B.; Misuraca, L.; Pierri, A.; Vahdat, O.; LeReun, C.; Dumonteil, N.; Modine, T.; Laskar, M.; Eltchaninoff, H.; et al. Cerebrovascular Events Post-Transcatheter Aortic Valve Replacement in a Large Cohort of Patients. *JACC Cardiovasc. Interv.* **2014**, *7*, 1138–1145. [CrossRef]
20. Lai, S.-M.; Studenski, S.; Duncan, P.W.; Perera, S. Persisting Consequences of Stroke Measured by the Stroke Impact Scale. *Stroke* **2002**, *33*, 1840–1844. [CrossRef]
21. Daniel, K.; Wolfe, C.D.A.; Busch, M.A.; McKevitt, C. What Are the Social Consequences of Stroke for Working-Aged Adults? *Stroke* **2009**, *40*, e431–e440. [CrossRef]
22. Arnold, S.V.; Lei, Y.; Reynolds, M.R.; Magnuson, E.A.; Suri, R.M.; Tuzcu, E.M.; Petersen, J.L.; Douglas, P.S.; Svensson, L.G.; Gada, H.; et al. Costs of periprocedural complications in patients treated with transcatheter aortic valve replacement: Results from the Placement of Aortic Transcatheter Valve trial. *Circ. Cardiovasc. Interv.* **2014**, *7*, 829–836. [CrossRef] [PubMed]
23. Nuis, R.-J.; Van Mieghem, N.M.; Schultz, C.J.; Moelker, A.; Van Der Boon, R.M.; Van Geuns, R.-J.; Van Der Lugt, A.; Serruys, P.W.; Rodés-Cabau, J.; Van Domburg, R.; et al. Frequency and Causes of Stroke During or After Transcatheter Aortic Valve Implantation. *Am. J. Cardiol.* **2012**, *109*, 1637–1643. [CrossRef] [PubMed]
24. Müller, M.D.; Ahlhelm, F.J.; Von Hessling, A.; Doig, D.; Nederkoorn, P.J.; Macdonald, S.; Lyrer, P.A.; Van Der Lugt, A.; Hendrikse, J.; Stippich, C.; et al. Vascular Anatomy Predicts the Risk of Cerebral Ischemia in Patients Randomized to Carotid Stenting Versus Endarterectomy. *Stroke* **2017**, *48*, 1285–1292. [CrossRef] [PubMed]
25. Kapadia, S.; Kodali, S.; Makkar, R.; Mehran, R.; Lazar, R.M.; Zivadinov, R.; Dwyer, M.G.; Jilaihawi, H.; Virmani, R.; Anwaruddin, S.; et al. Protection Against Cerebral Embolism During Transcatheter Aortic Valve Replacement. *J. Am. Coll. Cardiol.* **2017**, *69*, 367–377. [CrossRef]

26. Van Mieghem, N.M.; El Faquir, N.; Rahhab, Z.; Rodríguez-Olivares, R.; Wilschut, J.; Ouhlous, M.; Galema, T.W.; Geleijnse, M.L.; Kappetein, A.-P.; Schipper, M.E.; et al. Incidence and Predictors of Debris Embolizing to the Brain During Transcatheter Aortic Valve Implantation. *JACC Cardiovasc. Interv.* **2015**, *8*, 718–724. [CrossRef]
27. Van Mieghem, N.M.; Van Gils, L.; Ahmad, H.; Van Kesteren, F.; Van Der Werf, H.W.; Brueren, G.; Storm, M.; Lenzen, M.; Daemen, J.; Heuvel, A.F.V.D.; et al. Filter-based cerebral embolic protection with transcatheter aortic valve implantation: The randomised MISTRAL-C trial. *EuroIntervention* **2016**, *12*, 499–507. [CrossRef]
28. Schmidt, T.; Akdag, O.; Wohlmuth, P.; Thielsen, T.; Schewel, D.; Schewel, J.; Alessandrini, H.; Kreidel, F.; Bader, R.; Romero, M.; et al. Histological Findings and Predictors of Cerebral Debris From Transcatheter Aortic Valve Replacement: The ALSTER Experience. *J. Am. Heart Assoc.* **2016**, *5*. [CrossRef]
29. Gallo, M.; Putzu, A.; Conti, M.; Pedrazzini, G.; Demertzis, S.; Ferrari, E. Embolic protection devices for transcatheter aortic valve replacement. *Eur. J. Cardio-Thoracic Surg.* **2017**, *53*, 1118–1126. [CrossRef]
30. Faggioli, G.; Ferri, M.; Freyrie, A.; Gargiulo, M.; Fratesi, F.; Rossi, C.; Manzoli, L.; Stella, A. Aortic Arch Anomalies are Associated with Increased Risk of Neurological Events in Carotid Stent Procedures. *Eur. J. Vasc. Endovasc. Surg.* **2007**, *33*, 436–441. [CrossRef]
31. Ahn, S.S.; Chen, S.W.; Miller, T.J.; Chen, J.F. What Is the True Incidence of Anomalous Bovine Left Common Carotid Artery Configuration? *Ann. Vasc. Surg.* **2014**, *28*, 381–385. [CrossRef]
32. Rozado, J.; Padron, R.; Alperi, A.; Pascual, I.; Cubero, H.; Ayesta, A.; Avanzas, P.; Moris, C. TAVI Procedures with Sentinel Device in a Bovine Aortic Arch. Neurological Protection during TAVI. In *Eapci Textbook of Percutaneous Interventional Cardiovascular Medicine*; Part II. PCR.; Piazza, N., Cribier, A., De Palma, R., Eds.; Europa Digital & Publishing: Toulouse, France, 2012.
33. Grabert, S.; Schechtl, J.; Nöbauer, C.; Bleiziffer, S.; Lange, R. Patient eligibility for application of a two-filter cerebral embolic protection device during transcatheter aortic valve implantation: Does one size fit all? *Interact. Cardiovasc. Thorac. Surg.* **2020**, *30*, 605–612. [CrossRef]
34. Haussig, S.; Mangner, N.; Dwyer, M.G.; Lehmkuhl, L.; Lücke, C.; Woitek, F.; Holzhey, D.M.; Mohr, F.W.; Gutberlet, M.; Zivadinov, R.; et al. Effect of a Cerebral Protection Device on Brain Lesions Following Transcatheter Aortic Valve Implantation in Patients with Severe Aortic Stenosis. *JAMA* **2016**, *316*, 592–601. [CrossRef] [PubMed]
35. Halkin, A.; Iyer, S.S.; Roubin, G.S.; Vitek, J. Carotid Artery Stenting. In *Textbook of Interventional Cardiovascular Pharmacology*; Kipshidze, N.N., Fareed, J., Moses, J.W., Serruys, P.W., Eds.; Taylor & Francis Ltd.: London, UK, 2007; pp. 555–569.
36. Patel, T.; Shah, S.; Pancholy, S.; Deora, S.; Prajapati, K.; Coppola, J.; Gilchrist, I.C. Working through challenges of subclavian, innominate, and aortic arch regions during transradial approach. *Catheter. Cardiovasc. Interv.* **2014**, *84*, 224–235. [CrossRef] [PubMed]
37. Seeger, J.; Gonska, B.; Otto, M.; Rottbauer, W.; Wöhrle, J. Cerebral Embolic Protection During Transcatheter Aortic Valve Replacement Significantly Reduces Death and Stroke Compared with Unprotected Procedures. *JACC Cardiovasc. Interv.* **2017**, *10*, 2297–2303. [CrossRef] [PubMed]
38. Seeger, J.; Kapadia, S.; Kodali, S.; Linke, A.; Wöhrle, J.; Haussig, S.; Makkar, R.; Mehran, R.; Rottbauer, W.; Leon, M. Rate of peri-procedural stroke observed with cerebral embolic protection during transcatheter aortic valve replacement: A patient-level propensity-matched analysis. *Eur. Heart J.* **2018**, *40*, 1334–1340. [CrossRef] [PubMed]
39. Simsek, C.; Schölzel, B.E.; Heijer, P.D.; Vos, J.; Meuwissen, M.; Branden, B.V.D.; Ijsselmuiden, A. The rationale of using cerebral embolic protection devices during transcatheter aortic valve implantation. *Neth. Heart J.* **2020**, *28*, 249–252. [CrossRef] [PubMed]
40. Giustino, G.; Sorrentino, S.; Mehran, R.; Faggioni, M.; Dangas, G. Cerebral Embolic Protection During TAVR: A Clinical Event Meta-Analysis. *J. Am. Coll. Cardiol.* **2017**, *69*, 465–466. [CrossRef]

Publisher's Note: MDPI stays neutral with regard to jurisdictional claims in published maps and institutional affiliations.

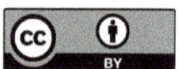

© 2020 by the authors. Licensee MDPI, Basel, Switzerland. This article is an open access article distributed under the terms and conditions of the Creative Commons Attribution (CC BY) license (http://creativecommons.org/licenses/by/4.0/).

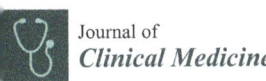

Journal of Clinical Medicine

Review

Preoperative TAVR Planning: How to Do It

Rodrigo Petersen Saadi [1,*], Ana Paula Tagliari [1,2], Eduardo Keller Saadi [1,2,3], Marcelo Haertel Miglioranza [4] and Carisi Anne Polanczyck [1,5]

1. Post Graduate Program in Cardiology and Cardiovascular Science, Hospital de Clínicas de Porto Alegre, Federal University of Rio Grande do Sul, Porto Alegre 90410-000, Brazil; aninhatagliari@yahoo.com.br (A.P.T.); esaadi@terra.com.br (E.K.S.); carisi.anne@gmail.com (C.A.P.)
2. Cardiovascular Surgery Department, Hospital São Lucas da PUC-RS, Porto Alegre 90610-001, Brazil
3. Cardiovascular Surgery Department, Hospital Mãe de Deus, Porto Alegre 90980-481, Brazil
4. EcoHaertel, Echocardiography Department, Hospital Mãe de Deus, Porto Alegre 90980-481, Brazil; marcelohaertel@gmail.com
5. Cardiology Department, Hospital Moinhos de Vento, Porto Alegre 90035-000, Brazil
* Correspondence: rodrigosaadi@terra.com.br; Tel.: +55-51-98182-9424

Abstract: Transcatheter aortic valve replacement (TAVR) is a well-established treatment option for patients with severe symptomatic aortic stenosis (AS) whose procedural efficacy and safety have been continuously improving. Appropriate preprocedural planning, including aortic valve annulus measurements, transcatheter heart valve choice, and possible procedural complication anticipation is mandatory to a successful procedure. The gold standard for preoperative planning is still to perform a multi-detector computed angiotomography (MDCT), which provides all the information required. Nonetheless, 3D echocardiography and magnet resonance imaging (MRI) are great alternatives for some patients. In this article, we provide an updated comprehensive review, focusing on preoperative TAVR planning and the standard steps required to do it properly.

Keywords: TAVR; sizing; planning; MDCT; 3D echocardiography; MRI

1. Introduction

Transcatheter aortic valve replacement (TAVR) has risen as a less invasive alternative for treating severe symptomatic aortic stenosis (AS) in patients at all surgical risk scores [1–7]. Since Alain Cribier pioneered the TAVR procedure in 2002, the advances in this field have been outstanding. Newer generation devices and different types of self and balloon-expandable valves are being released every year, and the results are remarkable improvements in procedural efficacy and safety [8].

One of the key points for a successful TAVR is carefully preprocedural planning, including accurate aortic root and aortic valve diameters measurements. Aortic angulation; aortic annulus minimum, medium and maximum diameters, area, and perimeter; left ventricle outflow tract minimum, medium and maximum diameters, area, and perimeter; sinus of Valsalva diameters; right and left coronary arteries height; sinotubular junction diameters, area, and perimeter; ascending aorta diameters; calcification distribution pattern; and C-arm angulation are all relevant information to perform a procedure properly [9].

The measurements of the aortic root and ascending aorta are used to choose the appropriate transcatheter heart valve type and size and foresee possible procedure-related complications, such as coronary artery obstruction, aortic annulus, and sinotubular junction rupture, paravalvular leak, valve embolization, and pacemaker implantation need. The size of the transcatheter heart valve that will be implanted is chosen based on the aortic annulus perimeter for the self-expandable platforms, and on the aortic annulus area for the balloon-expandable ones [10,11]. Undersizing the aortic annulus may cause paravalvular leak or valve embolization, whereas oversizing may reduce prosthesis durability, cause annulus rupture, and conduction issues leading to pacemaker implantation [12–14].

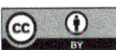

Initially, TAVR sizing was made using 2D echocardiography and/or during the procedure, using graduated pigtail catheters (Figure 1). However, the planning strategy evolved dramatically, especially when 3D technology started to be used since 2D echo frequently undersized the aortic annulus. The current gold standard method to perform valve measurements and preprocedural TAVR planning is the multi-detector computed angiotomography (MDCT), with an appropriate TAVR protocol [15,16]. MDCT measurements can be performed manually, using semi-automated software, or using automated software. Furthermore, the aortic annulus may be measured by magnetic resonance imaging and 3D transesophageal echocardiography. The possibility of a 3D image (MDCT or 3D echo) allowed a more precise measurement.

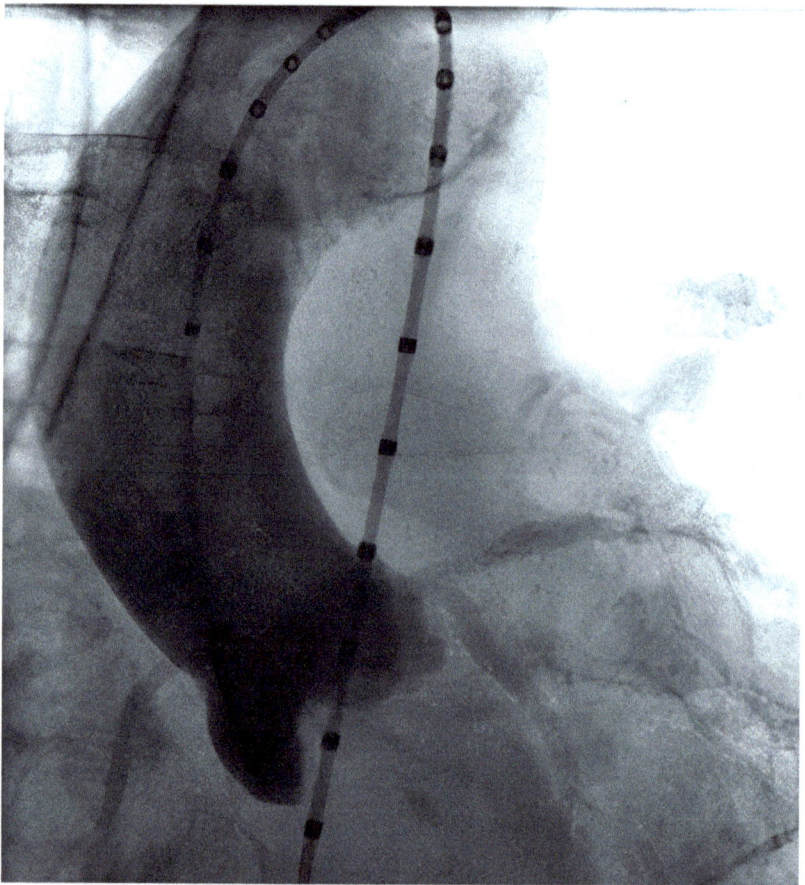

Figure 1. Aortic valve measurement using contrast injection from a pigtail catheter.

Herein, we provided an updated comprehensive review, focusing on preoperative TAVR planning and the standard steps required to do it properly.

2. Aortic Root Assessment

Understanding the aortic root anatomy and the importance of each anatomical feature involved in a TAVR procedure is fundamental to achieving a successful intervention.

2.1. Aortic Annulus

The aortic annulus dimension is fundamental for choosing the appropriate transcatheter heart valve type and size. The aortic annulus is defined as a virtual ring built by joining the points of the basal attachments of the aortic leaflets [17]. It is crucial to understand that the aortic annulus is a 3D structure and that 2D measures may cause mistakes. That is the reason why the gold standard for annulus evaluation is the 3D multiplanar reconstruction (MPR) of MDCT. Three-dimensional echocardiography provides similar measurements compared with MDCT [18]. On the other hand, 2D measures usually undersize the aortic annulus [19].

The aortic annulus perimeter is used to choose the size of self-expandable valves, whereas the aortic annulus area is used for the balloon-expandable ones. It is important to have the correct dimension of the annulus, to avoid oversizing or undersizing the implanted transcatheter heart valve and, therefore, avoid procedural complications (Figure 2).

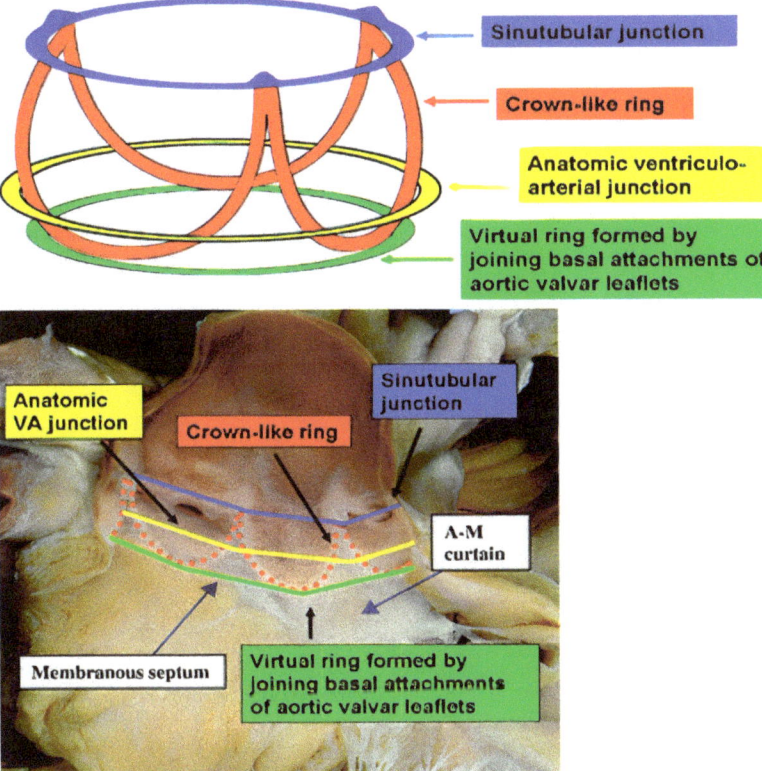

Figure 2. Virtual aortic annulus, sinotubular junction, and coronary arteries anatomy (adapted from Zarayelyan A. et al. [20]).

2.2. Left Ventricle Outflow Tract (LVOT)

The LVOT is a virtual area below the mitral valve. It is a convention to measure LVOT diameters, perimeter, and area 4 mm below the virtual aortic ring. The LVOT is part of the TAVR "landing zone", which includes the aortic annulus, aortic leaflets, and LVOT [14]. It is known that a calcified and non-tubular LVOT is associated with poor outcomes, including paravalvular leak and LVOT rupture risk [21,22]. Thus, proper analysis of the LVOT is mandatory to plan the procedure and prevent possible complications.

2.3. Coronary Arteries Height and Sinus of Valsalva

Coronary obstruction is a life-threatening complication following TAVR, with a mortality rate achieving up to 50%, and an incidence varying from 0.4% to 1.2% [23,24]. Low coronary ostia height and narrow sinus of Valsalva are the two main risk factors for coronary occlusion. The coronaries height is measured by tracing a straight line from the bottom of the coronary ostium until the virtual aortic annulus. The sinus of Valsalva is measured from the middle of the leaflet to the opposite commissure. Coronary arteries with a height less than 10 mm, especially if associated with small sinus of Valsalva (less than 28 mm), are associated with high coronary occlusion risk.

2.4. C-Arm Angulation

A perfect C-arm angulation, avoiding parallax effect, is important to have no optic illusion during the procedure. Parallax is a displacement or difference in the apparent position of an object viewed along two different lines of sight and is measured by the angle or semi-angle of inclination between those two lines. At the beginning of TAVR experience, C-arm angulation was acquired using three pigtails and a considerable degree of contrast injection to align the three aortic leaflets and prevent the aortic annulus parallax effect during TAVR deployment. Nowadays, with preoperative TAVR MDCT planning, it is possible to predict all C-arm angulations required to avoid parallax [25,26]. By unifying all these angulations, a curve is formatted, the so-called aortic valve S curve [27,28]. Before each TAVR, it is important to know the S curve for that patient to optimize the results and prevent unnecessary contrast injections. Two main angulations predictions are mandatory before TAVR: three-sinus coplanar and cusp overlap views. The three-sinus coplanar is the angulation where the three sinuses are aligned and equidistant from each other, being the non-coronary cusp at the left of the image, the right coronary cusp in the middle, and the left coronary cusp at the right. The cusp overlap view is the angulation where the non-coronary cusp is isolated at the left of the image, and the right coronary cusp is overlapping the left coronary cusp at the right part of the image.

2.5. Sinotubular Junction

Sinotubular junction (STJ) diameter and height are especially important for balloon-expandable valves implants since the balloon may injure the STJ in the case of a low STJ. In self-expandable supra-annular devices, valve-in-valve, and TAVR-in-TAVR, a low and narrow STJ can cause sinus sequestration with coronary malperfusion. The STJ height is measured perpendicularly to the annular plane, and the diameter is measured by the standard way [29].

2.6. Ascending Aorta

Assessment of any aortopathy is relevant, especially in patients with bicuspid aortic valve, when the commitment of the aorta is frequent, so measurement of the diameter of ascending aorta is part of the TAVR protocol.

2.7. Peripheral Access Vessels

Peripheral vessel accesses analysis, starting with femoral arteries, is relevant once most TAVR contraindications are related to inadequate accesses. If transfemoral TAVR is unsuitable, the second access of choice is trans left subclavian/axillary artery. If left subclavian/axillary is not indicated, due to inadequate diameter, calcification, or in the presence of a patent left internal mammary artery bypass, the left carotid should be analyzed to use as third transarterial alternative access. Transaortic and transapical are seldom used.

3. Computed Angiotomography (MDCT)

Computed angiotomography (MDCT) is the preferred method to plan a TAVR procedure by most operators [30]. The planning can be performed manually, using semi-automated and automated software. Each one has intra- and inter-observational variabilities, which will be discussed below.

3.1. MDCT Acquisition

The key component for well-acquired MDCT images is an ECG-synchronized MDCT that covers at least the aortic root, followed by non-ECG synchronized images of the aorta, iliac, and femoral vasculature [29]. The ECG-synchronized MDCT of the aortic root is important, because the aortic annulus undergo conformable change throughout the cardiac cycle, being bigger and circular in systole, and oval in diastole. The goal is to measure the greatest possible annular dimension, which can be found during the cardiac systole (20–40% of the cardiac cycle) [31,32].

Regarding radiation, a tube potential of 100 kV is usually indicated for patients weighing <90 kg or with a body mass index (BMI) <30 kg/m^2, whereas a tube potential of 120 kV is indicated for patients weighing >90 kg and with BMI >30 kg/m^2.

Intravenous contrast administration is mandatory. Optimal images require high intra-arterial opacification, and attenuation values should exceed 250 Hounsfield units. MDCT data should be reconstructed as an axial, thin-sliced multiphasic data set, with <1 mm slice thickness. Reconstruction intervals should be spaced at <10% intervals across the acquired portion of the cardiac cycle [29].

A 3D multiplanar reconstruction (MPR) of the aorta, aortic valve, and its structures is mandatory to perform TAVR planning (Figure 3).

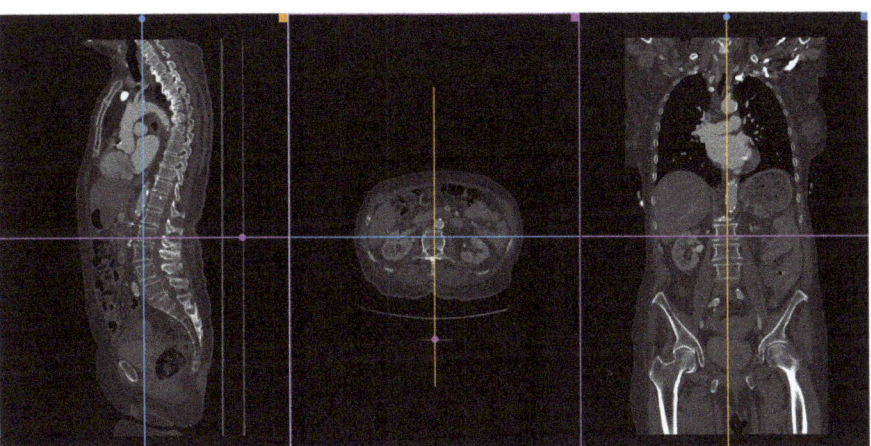

Figure 3. A MPR reconstruction from MDCT images using the Horos® software.

3.2. Available Methods

Many different kinds of software can be used to make appropriate MDCT measurements of the aortic root, coronary ostia, and optimal angiographic deployment projections: manual, semi-automated, and automated. The manual measures are the most used by operators since they can be done by cheap or free software, such as Horos® and Osirix®.

3.2.1. Manual Sizing

The manual TAVR sizing is usually made using the 3D MPR tool of Osirix® or Horos® software. In the MPR mode, we have three correlated images: coronal, sagittal, and transversal. The goal is to perfectly align the virtual aortic annulus, which corresponds to the base of the three aortic cusps. The manual method does not provide information about the steps needed for sizing, and there is no automated report. In 2019, a consensus on MDCT imaging on TAVR describing the main steps was published [29]. This consensus provides further and detailed information about MDCT manual preprocedural planning. The manual measurement takes more time than the semi-automated and automated measures, and its learning curve is bigger. However, when used by experienced professionals, it may provide all the information necessary to perform a safe TAVR procedure.

There are some studies comparing the variability of measurement by different observers. These articles found a strong agreement for aortic annulus and coronary arteries height assessment for experienced observers (at least 2 years of experience) [33,34].

Furthermore, Knobloch et al. and Le Couteulx et al. reported interobserver variability in MDCTs evaluated by observers with different levels of expertise. In the Le Couteulx et al. study, Observer 1 was an expert, whereas Observer 2 was a resident physician with 6 months of practice, and Observer 3 was a trained resident physician with starting experience. Intra- and inter-observer reproducibility were excellent for all aortic annulus dimensions, with an intraclass correlation coefficient ranging, respectively, from 0.84 to 0.98 and from 0.82 to 0.97. Agreement for selection of prosthesis size was almost perfect between the two most experienced observers ($k = 0.82$) and substantial with the inexperienced observer ($k = 0.67$) [35]. In the Knobloch et al. study, Observer 1 was a radiologist with 6 years of experience, Observer 2 was a laboratory technician with 3 years of experience, and Observer 3 was a medical student with no experience. Intra-observer variability did not differ significantly. However, significant differences were found in mean inter-observer variance ($p < 0.001$). They advocate that multi-reader paradigms led to significantly increased precision compared with single readers with different levels of experience [36].

3.2.2. Semi-Automated and Automated Sizing

Semi-automated software are broadly used by TAVR companies and operators around the globe. The most commonly utilized software is the 3MensioValves (3mensio Medical Imaging BV, Maastricht, The Netherlands). However, the drawback of 3MensioVales software is its high cost, preventing its broad use (Figure 4). There is another semi-automated software called ProSizeAV, which is actually a plugin to be used with Horos® or Osirix®. However, this plugin does not have CE or FDA approval, and there are no data proving its efficacy (Figure 5).

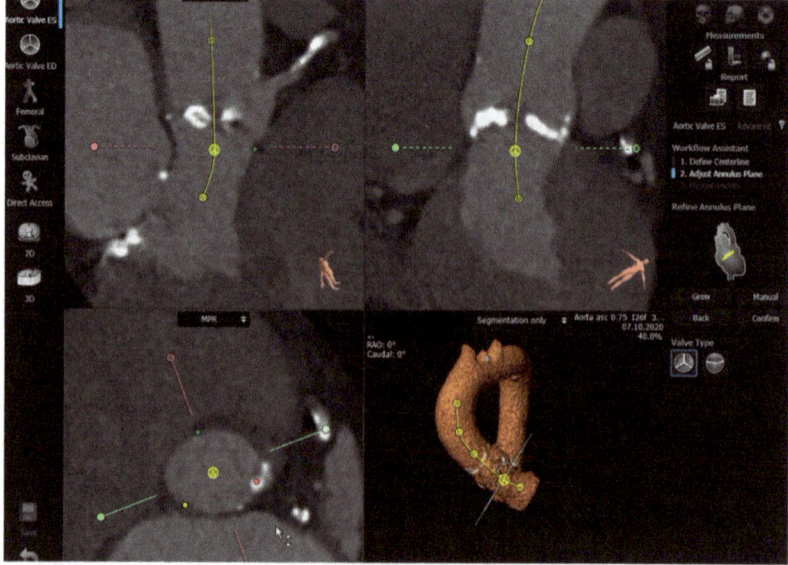

Figure 4. Measurements performed using the 3MensioValves.

ProSize^AV

General:

Name: 14	Examined by: Rodrigo Saadi
Date of Birth: 24 May 1947 (74)	Study Date: Aug 13, 2018
Patient ID: 14	Report Date: Jan 14, 2022

Aortic Annulus Measurements:

Perimeter:	76.7 mm (ø 24.4 mm)
Area:	459.0 mm² (ø 24.2 mm)
Excentricity:	0.15 (22.1 x 26.2 mm)
Aortic Angulation:	50.8°
LCA Distance:	13.8 mm
RCA Distance:	16.7 mm
Cusp Calcification:	Severe (3)
LVOT Calcification:	None (0)
Annulus Calcification:	Mild (1)

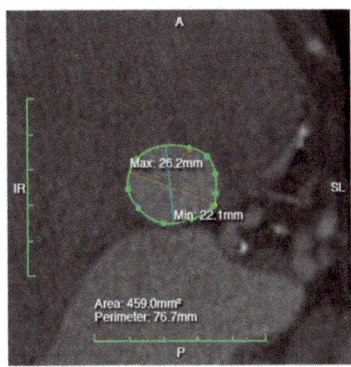

Implantation Plane:

RCC Anterior:	LAO 16° Cranial 19°
LCC Posterior:	RAO 39° Caudal 37°
NCC Posterior:	LAO 71° Cranial 49°
LV View:	RAO 30° Caudal 31°

Access:

Planned Access:	TF Right
Pigtail Access:	TF Left

Comments:
Cusp overlap RAO 9 CAU 10

Figure 5. ProSizeAV report.

There is another available semi-automated (syngo. viaVB20A, Siemens, Munich, Germany) software. In 2018, Horehledova et al. compared the Siemens manual and semi-automated software and demonstrated an excellent inter-software agreement (ICC = 0.93; range 0.90–0.95). The time needed for evaluation using semi-automatic assessment (3 min 24 s) was significantly lower ($p < 0.001$) compared with a fully manual approach (6 min 31 s) [37].

Lou et al. also compared manual, semi-automated, and fully automated measurement of the aortic annulus using Siemens software. Semi-automated analysis required major correction in five patients (4.5%). Mean manual annulus area was significantly smaller than fully automated results ($p < 0.001$), but similar to semi-automated measurements. The frequency of concordant recommendations for valve size increased if a manual analysis was replaced by semi-automated method (60% agreement was improved to 82.4%; 95% confidence interval for the difference [69.1–83.4%]) [38].

4. Echocardiography

Echocardiography is a non-invasive broadly available method used to diagnose cardiac conditions and plan cardiac procedures. The 2D transthoracic echo, at the beginning of TAVR experience, was used to size aortic annulus diameters, perimeter, and area. However, it is known that 2D echo usually underestimates the measures, thus undersizing the aortic annulus, facilitating the occurrence of paravalvular regurgitation and resulting in poor outcomes [19,39,40]. On the other hand, novel 3D transesophageal echo has been evolving and apparently, when correctly used, has a good correlation with MDCT regarding aortic annulus measures and has some advantages, such as not requiring venous contrast [18,41–43]. However, it is important to keep in mind that the aortic annulus measures are fundamental to choosing appropriate transcatheter heart valve size, nonetheless, there are many other important measurements as coronary arteries height, LVOT dimensions, sinus of Valsalva diameter, and ascending aorta which cannot be done properly by any 2D or 3E echo (Figure 6). Furthermore, vascular access cannot be measured by echo as well, and calcium-related artifacts may compromise echocardiography imaging.

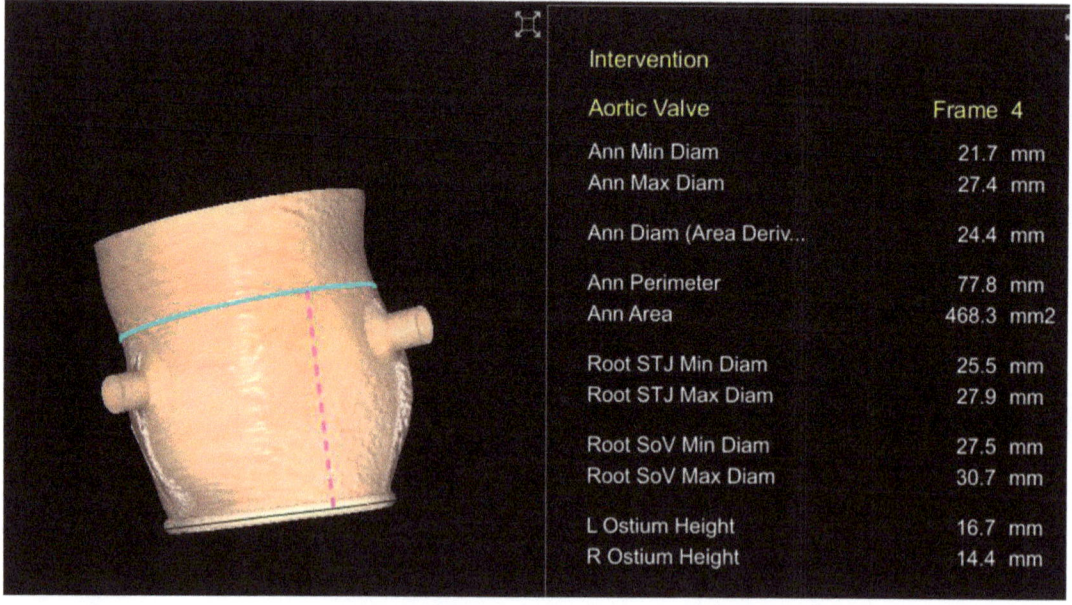

Figure 6. Example of a 3D transesophageal echocardiography aortic root assessment.

3D Transesophageal Echocardiography Annulus Sizing

Elkaryoni et al. published, in 2018, a systematic review and meta-analysis about 3D TEE as an alternative to MDCT for aortic annular sizing. Thirteen studies were included (1228 patients). A strong linear correlation was found between 3D TEE and MDCT measurements of aortic annulus area ($r = 0.84$, $p < 0.001$), mean perimeter ($r = 0.85$, $p < 0.001$), and mean diameter ($r = 0.80$, $p < 0.001$). They concluded the 3D TEE demonstrated a high level of correlation with those evaluated by MDCT, and that 3D TEE is a feasible choice for aortic annulus assessment, with advantages of real-time assessment, lack of contrast, and no radiation exposure [44]. Another systematic review and meta-analysis comparing 3D TEE and MDCT sizing was published by Mork et al., in 2021. In this paper, a total of 889 patients from ten studies were included. Pooled correlation coefficients between 3D TEE and MDCT of annulus area, perimeter, area derived-diameter, perimeter derived-diameter, maximum and minimum diameter measurements were strong 0.89 (95% CI: 0.84–0.92), 0.88 (95% CI: 0.83–0.92), 0.87 (95% CI: 0.77–0.93), 0.87 (95% CI: 0.77–0.93), 0.79 (95% CI: 0.64–0.87), and 0.75 (95% CI: 0.61–0.84) (overall $p < 0.0001$), respectively [45].

In another systematic review and meta-analysis, Rong et al. also reported strong correlation between 3D TEE and MDCT annular area, annular perimeter, annular diameter, and left ventricular outflow tract area measurements (0.86 [95% CI, 0.80–0.90]; 0.89 [CI, 0.82–0.93]; 0.80 [CI, 0.70–0.87]; and 0.78 [CI, 0.61–0.88], respectively) [46].

On the other hand, Vaquerizo et al. reported a single-center cohort study comparing 3D TEE and MDCT, and stated that 3D TEE-derived measurements were significantly smaller compared with MSCT: perimeter (68.6 + 5.9 vs. 75.1 + 5.7 mm, respectively; $p < 0.0001$); area (345.6 + 64.5 vs. 426.9 + 68.9 mm^2, respectively; $p < 0.0001$). The percentage difference between 3D TEE and MSCT measurements was around 9%. Agreement between MSCT- and 3D TEE-based THV sizing (perimeter) occurred in 44% of patients. Using the 3D TEE perimeter annular measurements, up to 50% of patients would have received an inappropriate valve size according to manufacturer-recommended, area-derived sizing algorithms [47].

Similarly, Singh et al. reported 185 patients between 2013 and 2015 and stated that the undersize of echo sizing may reduce even patients' survival. 2D and 3D TEE underestimated the annulus size by −1.49 and −1.32, respectively, and discrepancies >10% between TEE and MDCT were associated with a decrease in post-implant survival [48].

Aortic short axis (upper esophageal, 40–45°), and long axis (mid esophageal 120–140°), are the most used probe positions to evaluate the aortic valve annulus.

5. Magnetic Resonance Imaging

The use of magnetic resonance imaging (MRI) for TAVR planning has been increasing in the last years. Although 3D TEE is an alternative for the aortic annulus sizing for patients who cannot undergo MDCT due to contrast allergy or renal failure, it is not possible to perform all fundamental measures to plan the entire procedure through echo evaluation, and MRI has emerged as a feasible alternative to MDCT [49]. However, MRI is significantly inferior to MDCT defining the presence and extension of valvular and vascular calcium, which is an important feature for TAVR.

In 2016, Ruile et al. compared MDCT with non-contrast MRI for aortic root assessment, and the agreement for hypothetical prosthesis sizing was found in 63 of 67 (94%) of patients. However, accesses were not evaluated in this study [50].

Mayr et al. performed a pilot study in 16 patients comparing MDCT with a dedicated MRI protocol including non-contrast 3D "whole heart" acquisition and contrast-enhanced 3D aortoiliofemoral MRI, and MRI demonstrated a very strong correlation ($r = 0.956$, $p < 0.0001$) and complete consistency between MRI and MDCT regarding the decision for valve size. Vessel luminal diameters and angulation of aortoiliofemoral access also showed very strong correlation ($r = 0.819$ to 0.996, $p < 0.001$) [51]. A total non-contrast MRI protocol for TAVI guidance was developed by the same group. A comparison between MDCT and non-contrast MRI in 26 patients demonstrated a moderate to strong correlation for assessment of minimal vessel diameter for aortoiliofemoral access ($r = 0.572$ for the right external iliac artery to $r = 0.851$ for the thoracic descending aorta, $p = 0.002$ and $p \leq 0.0001$, respectively), with good-to-excellent inter-observer reliability (ICC 0.862 to 0.999, all $p < 0.0001$), whereas mean diameters of the infrarenal aorta and iliofemoral vessels differed significantly (bias 0.37 to 0.98 mm, $p = 0.041$ to <0.0001) (Figure 7) [52].

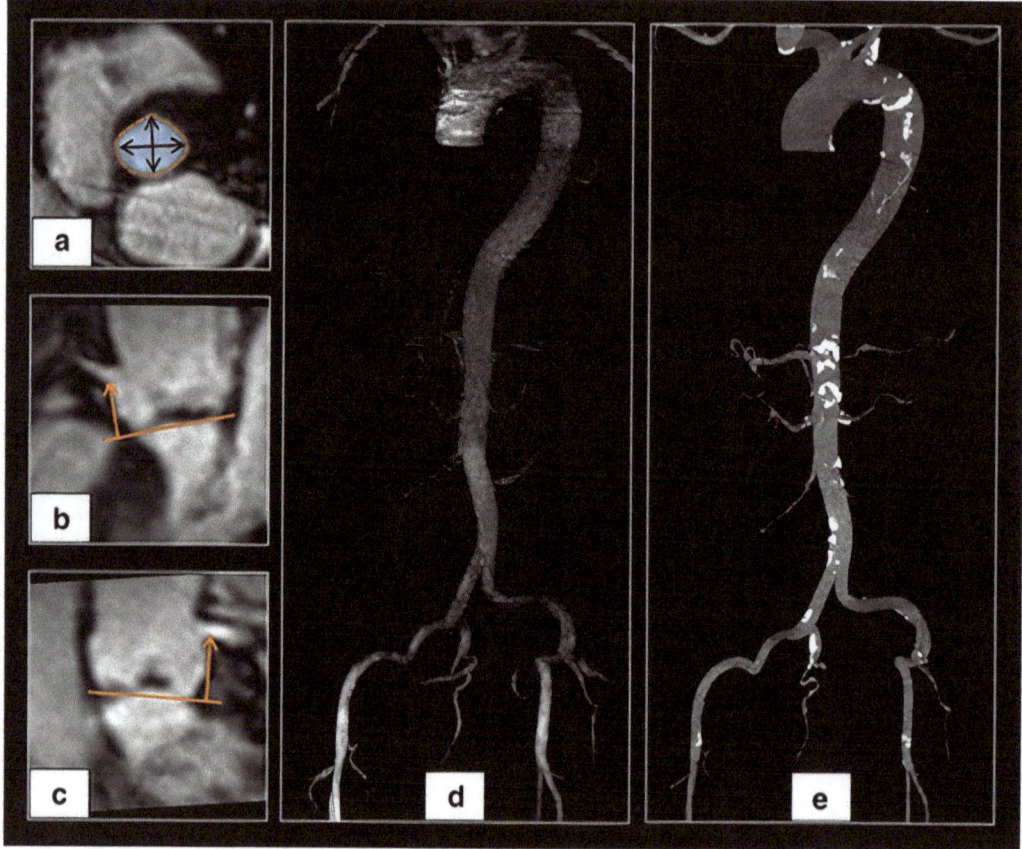

Figure 7. Example of a non-contrast 3D 'whole heart' MRI (**a**) aortic annular, arrows showing the minimum and maximum diameters, (**b**) right coronary and (**c**) left coronary arteries height (orange arrows), (**d**) maximum intensity projection of aortoiliofemoral MRI and (**e**) MDCT image (adapted from Pammiger et al. [52]).

As MRI requires reliable compensation strategies to deal with cardiac and respiratory motion artifacts including ECG triggering and respiratory navigator gating, Pammiger et al. compared a simpler self-navigated with a navigator-gated non-contrast 3D whole-heart MRI and found high to very high correlation for aortic root measurements ($p < 0.0001$), concluding that a self-navigator is feasible and achieve similar results to navigator-gated MRI, with shorter acquisition time [53].

Similarly, Aouad et al. validated a faster single breath-hold MRI acquisition (k-t acceleration to 3D cine b-SSFP MRI) [54].

6. Discussion

Preoperative TAVR imaging planning is fundamental to achieve procedural success. MDCT with 3D MPR remains the gold standard for aortic root and iliofemoral system evaluation. Semi-automated software (3MensioValves and Siemens) play an important role since they have a low inter- and intra-observer variability, whereas the ProSizeAV plugin still demands CE and FDA approval. The drawback of these semi-automated software is still their high cost. Manual measurements provide accurate results when performed by experienced professionals, although they have a longer learning curve compared with semi-automatic software. Totally automated software still need approval to become the gold standard method, since they usually overestimate aortic annulus measures. Furthermore, MDCT provides a full assessment of the aortic root (aortic annulus, LVOT, and sinus of Valsalva dimensions, coronary arteries height, STJ, and ascending aorta evaluation), besides iliofemoral or alternative accesses (axillary/subclavian, carotid, direct aortic, transapical and transcaval) evaluation.

Although 2D images, such as 2D echocardiography, underestimate aortic annulus dimensions, 3D TEE has proved to be an excellent alternative to MDCT to perform aortic annulus sizing and appropriate transcatheter heart valve selection. The major advantage of 3D echo is that it is a minimally invasive exam, which does not need contrast injection or radiation. However, although it is feasible to measure aortic annulus and LVOT dimensions with 3D echo, usually it is not possible to properly size coronary arteries height, and it is not precise for MDCT to measure sinus of Valsalva and ascending aorta diameters. Furthermore, the access vessels cannot be evaluated as well.

Magnetic resonance imaging has arisen as an alternative for patients who cannot receive iodine intravenous contrast. The correlation between MDCT and MRI for aortic root dimensions is excellent. However, for peripheral accesses evaluation, historically, gadolinium contrast used to be administered. Today, it is possible to evaluate the access with MRI without gadolinium administration, nonetheless, the vessels' diameters do not match perfectly. The disadvantages of MRI are its high cost, more time to acquire the image, and less experience of the operators to perform the measurements. This imaging method will certainly increase in the next years.

7. Conclusions

Careful preprocedural planning is mandatory to achieve a successful TAVR procedure and avoid serious complications. There are many ways to acquire and evaluate the anatomical details required to perform a safe TAVR planning (aortic annulus, LVOT, sinus of Valsalva, coronary arteries, STJ, ascending aorta, and access sites evaluation) including 3D echo, MDCT, and MRI. Although MDCT is still the gold standard, it is important to be familiarized with alternative methods and know the pros and cons of each one, in order to choose the most appropriate method or a combination of them for each specific patient.

Funding: This study was funded by Hospital de Clínicas de Porto Alegre (Fundo de Incentivo à Pesquisa e Eventos; FIPE/HCPA, number 2020-0343,) and Postgraduate Program in Health Sciences: Cardiology and Cardiovascular Sciences/PPG, UFRGS.

Conflicts of Interest: Tagliari A.P. had received a research grant from the Coordenação de Aperfeiçoamento de Pessoal de Nível Superior—Brasil (CAPES)—Finance Code 001. Saadi E.K. is a proctor in TAVI for Medtronic, Edwards and Abbott.

References

1. Kapadia, S.R.; Leon, M.B.; Makkar, R.R.; Tuzcu, E.M.; Svensson, L.G.; Kodali, S.; Webb, J.G.; Mack, M.J.; Douglas, P.S.; Thourani, V.H.; et al. 5-year outcomes of transcatheter aortic valve replacement compared with standard treatment for patients with inoperable aortic stenosis (PARTNER 1): A randomised controlled trial. *Lancet* **2015**, *385*, 2485–2491. [CrossRef]
2. Reardon, M.J.; Van Mieghem, N.M.; Popma, J.J.; Kleiman, N.S.; Sondergaard, L.; Mumtaz, M.; Adams, D.H.; Deeb, G.M.; Maini, B.; Gada, H.; et al. Surgical or transcatheter aortic-valve replacement in intermediate-risk patients. *N. Engl. J. Med.* **2017**, *376*, 1321–1331. [CrossRef] [PubMed]
3. Mack, M.J.; Leon, M.B.; Thourani, V.H.; Makkar, R.; Kodali, S.K.; Russo, M.; Kapadia, S.R.; Malaisrie, S.C.; Cohen, D.J.; Pibarot, P.; et al. Transcatheter aortic-valve replacement with a balloon-expandable valve in low-risk patients. *N. Engl. J. Med.* **2019**, *380*, 1695–1705. [CrossRef] [PubMed]
4. Popma, J.J.; Deeb, G.M.; Yakubov, S.J.; Mumtaz, M.; Gada, H.; O'Hair, D.; Bajwa, T.; Heiser, J.C.; Merhi, W.; Kleiman, N.S.; et al. Transcatheter aortic-valve replacement with a self-expanding valve in low-risk patients. *N. Engl. J. Med.* **2019**, *380*, 1706–1715. [CrossRef] [PubMed]
5. Leon, M.B.; Smith, C.R.; Mack, M.; Miller, D.C.; Moses, J.W.; Svensson, L.G.; Tuzcu, E.M.; Webb, J.G.; Fontana, G.P.; Makkar, R.R.; et al. Transcatheter Aortic-Valve Implantation for Aortic Stenosis in Patients Who Cannot Undergo Surgery. *N. Engl. J. Med.* **2016**, *363*, 1511–1520. [CrossRef] [PubMed]
6. Barker, C.M.; Reardon, M.J. The CoreValve US Pivotal Trial. *Semin. Thorac. Cardiovasc. Surg.* **2014**, *26*, 179–186. [CrossRef]

7. Leon, M.B.; Smith, C.R.; Mack, M.J.; Herrmann, H.C.; Doshi, D.; Cohen, D.J.; Pichard, A.D.; Kapadia, S.; Dewey, T.; Babaliaros, V.; et al. Transcatheter or Surgical Aortic-Valve Replacement in Intermediate-Risk Patients. *N. Engl. J. Med.* **2016**, *374*, 1609–1620. [CrossRef]
8. Généreux, P.; Head, S.J.; Wood, D.A.; Kodali, S.K.; Williams, M.R.; Paradis, J.M.; Spaziano, M.; Kappetein, A.P.; Webb, J.G.; Cribier, A.; et al. Transcatheter aortic valve implantation 10-year anniversary: Review of current evidence and clinical implications. *Eur. Heart J.* **2012**, *33*, 2388–2400. [CrossRef]
9. Blanke, P.; Euringer, W.; Baumann, T.; Reinöhl, J.; Schlensak, C.; Langer, M.; Pache, G. Combined assessment of aortic root anatomy and aortoiliac vasculature with dual-source CT as a screening tool in patients evaluated for transcatheter aortic valve implantation. *Am. J. Roentgenol.* **2010**, *195*, 872–881. [CrossRef]
10. Schwarz, F.; Lange, P.; Zinsser, D.; Greif, M.; Boekstegers, P.; Schmitz, C.; Reiser, M.F.; Kupatt, C.; Becker, H.C. CT-Angiography–Based Evaluation of the Aortic Annulus for Prosthesis Sizing in Transcatheter Aortic Valve Implantation (TAVI)–Predictive Value and Optimal Thresholds for Major Anatomic Parameters. *PLoS ONE* **2014**, *9*, e103481. [CrossRef]
11. Kasel, A.M.; Cassese, S.; Bleiziffer, S.; Amaki, M.; Hahn, R.T.; Kastrati, A.; Sengupta, P.P. Standardized imaging for aortic annular sizing: Implications for transcatheter valve selection. *JACC Cardiovasc. Imaging* **2013**, *6*, 249–262. [CrossRef]
12. Horehledova, B.; Mihl, C.; Hendriks, B.M.F.; Eijsvoogel, N.G.; Vainer, J.; Veenstra, L.F.; Wildberger, J.E.; Das, M. Do CTA measurements of annular diameter, perimeter and area result in different TAVI prosthesis sizes? *Int. J. Cardiovasc. Imaging* **2018**, *34*, 1819–1829. [CrossRef] [PubMed]
13. Bleakley, C.; Monaghan, M.J. The Pivotal Role of Imaging in TAVR Procedures. *Curr. Cardiol. Rep.* **2018**, *20*, 9. [CrossRef] [PubMed]
14. Latsios, G.; Gerckens, U.; Buellesfeld, L.; Mueller, R.; John, D.; Yuecel, S.; Syring, J.; Sauren, B.; Grube, E. "Device landing zone" calcification, assessed by MSCT, as a predictive factor for pacemaker implantation after TAVI. *Catheter. Cardiovasc. Interv.* **2010**, *76*, 431–439. [CrossRef] [PubMed]
15. Hayashida, K.; Bouvier, E.; Lefèvre, T.; Hovasse, T.; Morice, M.C.; Chevalier, B.; Romano, M.; Garot, P.; Mylotte, D.; Farge, A.; et al. Impact of CT-guided valve sizing on post-procedural aortic regurgitation in transcatheter aortic valve implantation. *EuroIntervention* **2012**, *8*, 546–555. [CrossRef] [PubMed]
16. Lehmkuhl, L.; Foldyna, B.; Von Aspern, K.; Lücke, C.; Grothoff, M.; Nitzsche, S.; Kempfert, J.; Haensig, M.; Rastan, A.; Walther, T.; et al. Inter-individual variance and cardiac cycle dependency of aortic root dimensions and shape as assessed by ECG-gated multi-slice computed tomography in patients with severe aortic stenosis prior to transcatheter aortic valve implantation: Is it crucial for. *Int. J. Cardiovasc. Imaging* **2013**, *29*, 693–703. [CrossRef] [PubMed]
17. Gilard, M.; Boschat, J. *Transcatheter Aortic Valve Implantation*; Mayo Clinic: Rochester, MN, USA, 2016; ISBN 9783319396118.
18. Dima, C.N.; Gaspar, M.; Mornos, C.; Mornos, A.; Deutsch, P.; Cioloca, H.; Cerbu, S.; Dinu, M.; Hoinoiu, B.; Luca, C.T.; et al. Three-dimensional transesophageal echocardiography as an alternative to multidetector computed tomography in aortic annular diameter measurements for transcatheter aortic valve implantation. *Biology* **2021**, *10*, 132. [CrossRef]
19. Altiok, E.; Koos, R.; Schröder, J.; Brehmer, K.; Hamada, S.; Becker, M.; Mahnken, A.H.; Almalla, M.; Dohmen, G.; Autschbach, R.; et al. Comparison of two-dimensional and three-dimensional imaging techniques for measurement of aortic annulus diameters before transcatheter aortic valve implantation. *Heart* **2011**, *97*, 1578–1584. [CrossRef]
20. Zarayelyan, A. Dynamic Anatomy of Aortic Root and Its Potential Role in TAVR Prostheses Further Development and Modification. *Br. J. Med. Med. Res.* **2015**, *5*, 1534–1546. [CrossRef]
21. Condado, J.F.; Corrigan, F.E.; Lerakis, S.; Parastatidis, I.; Stillman, A.E.; Binongo, J.N.; Stewart, J.; Mavromatis, K.; Devireddy, C.; Leshnower, B.; et al. Anatomical risk models for paravalvular leak and landing zone complications for balloon-expandable transcatheter aortic valve replacement. *Catheter. Cardiovasc. Interv.* **2017**, *90*, 690–700. [CrossRef]
22. Mauri, V.; Frohn, T.; Deuschl, F.; Mohemed, K.; Kuhr, K.; Reimann, A.; Körber, M.I.; Schofer, N.; Adam, M.; Friedrichs, K.; et al. Impact of device landing zone calcification patterns on paravalvular regurgitation after transcatheter aortic valve replacement with different next-generation devices. *Open Heart* **2020**, *7*, e001164. [CrossRef] [PubMed]
23. Akinseye, O.A.; Jha, S.K.; Ibebuogu, U.N. Clinical outcomes of coronary occlusion following transcatheter aortic valve replacement: A systematic review. *Cardiovasc. Revascularization Med.* **2018**, *19*, 229–236. [CrossRef] [PubMed]
24. Ribeiro, H.B.; Sarmento-Leite, R.; Siqueira, D.A.A.; Carvalho, L.A.; Mangione, J.A.; Rodés-Cabau, J.; Perin, M.A.; de Brito, F.S. Obstrução coronária após implante por cateter de prótese valvar aórtica. *Arq. Bras. Cardiol.* **2014**, *102*, 93–96. [CrossRef] [PubMed]
25. Mehier, B.; Dubourg, B.; Eltchaninoff, H.; Durand, E.; Tron, C.; Cribier, A.; Michelin, P.; Dacher, J.N. MDCT planning of trans catheter aortic valve implantation (TAVI): Determination of optimal c-arm angulation. *Int. J. Cardiovasc. Imaging* **2020**, *36*, 1551–1557. [CrossRef]
26. Gurvitch, R.; Wood, D.A.; Leipsic, J.; Tay, E.; Johnson, M.; Ye, J.; Nietlispach, F.; Wijesinghe, N.; Cheung, A.; Webb, J.G. Multislice computed tomography for prediction of optimal angiographic deployment projections during transcatheter aortic valve implantation. *JACC Cardiovasc. Interv.* **2010**, *3*, 1157–1165. [CrossRef] [PubMed]
27. Ben-Shoshan, J.; Alosaimi, H.; Lauzier, P.T.; Pighi, M.; Talmor-Barkan, Y.; Overtchouk, P.; Martucci, G.; Spaziano, M.; Finkelstein, A.; Gada, H.; et al. Double S-Curve Versus Cusp-Overlap Technique: Defining the Optimal Fluoroscopic Projection for TAVR With a Self-Expanding Device. *JACC Cardiovasc. Interv.* **2021**, *14*, 185–194. [CrossRef]
28. Tchétché, D.; Siddiqui, S. Optimizing Fluoroscopic Projections for TAVR: Any Difference Between the Double S-Curve and the Cusp-Overlap Technique? *JACC Cardiovasc. Interv.* **2021**, *14*, 195–197. [CrossRef]

29. Blanke, P.; Weir-McCall, J.R.; Achenbach, S.; Delgado, V.; Hausleiter, J.; Jilaihawi, H.; Marwan, M.; Norgaard, B.L.; Piazza, N.; Schoenhagen, P.; et al. Computed tomography imaging in the context of transcatheter aortic valve implantation (TAVI)/transcatheter aortic valve replacement (TAVR): An expert consensus document of the Society of Cardiovascular Computed Tomography. *J. Cardiovasc. Comput. Tomogr.* **2019**, *13*, 1–20. [CrossRef]

30. Chiocchi, M.; Ricci, F.; Pasqualetto, M.; D'Errico, F.; Benelli, L.; Pugliese, L.; Cavallo, A.U.; Forcina, M.; Presicce, M.; De Stasio, V.; et al. Role of computed tomography in transcatheter aortic valve implantation and valve-in-valve implantation: Complete review of preprocedural and postprocedural imaging. *J. Cardiovasc. Med.* **2020**, *21*, 182–191. [CrossRef]

31. Suchá, D.; Tuncay, V.; Prakken, N.H.J.; Leiner, T.; Van Ooijen, P.M.A.; Oudkerk, M.; Budde, R.P.J. Does the aortic annulus undergo conformational change throughout the cardiac cycle? A systematic review. *Eur. Heart J. Cardiovasc. Imaging* **2015**, *16*, 1307–1317. [CrossRef]

32. Jurencak, T.; Turek, J.; Kietselaer, B.L.J.H.; Mihl, C.; Kok, M.; van Ommen, V.G.V.A.; van Garsse, L.A.F.M.; Nijssen, E.C.; Wildberger, J.E.; Das, M. MDCT evaluation of aortic root and aortic valve prior to TAVI. What is the optimal imaging time point in the cardiac cycle? *Eur. Radiol.* **2015**, *25*, 1975–1983. [CrossRef]

33. Schmidkonz, C.; Marwan, M.; Klinghammer, L.; Mitschke, M.; Schuhbaeck, A. Interobserver variability of CT angiography for evaluation of aortic annulus dimensions prior to transcatheter aortic valve implantation. *Eur. J. Radiol.* **2014**, *83*, 1672–1678. [CrossRef]

34. Schuhbaeck, A.; Achenbach, S.; Pflederer, T.; Marwan, M.; Schmid, J.; Nef, H.; Rixe, J.; Hecker, F.; Schneider, C.; Lell, M.; et al. Reproducibility of aortic annulus measurements by computed tomography. *Eur. Radiol.* **2014**, *24*, 1878–1888. [CrossRef] [PubMed]

35. Le Couteulx, S.; Caudron, J.; Dubourg, B.; Cauchois, G.; Dupré, M.; Michelin, P.; Durand, E.; Eltchaninoff, H.; Dacher, J.N. Multidetector computed tomography sizing of aortic annulus prior to transcatheter aortic valve replacement (TAVR): Variability and impact of observer experience. *Diagn. Interv. Imaging* **2018**, *99*, 279–289. [CrossRef] [PubMed]

36. Knobloch, G.; Sweetman, S.; Bartels, C.; Raval, A.; Gimelli, G.; Jacobson, K.; Lozonschi, L.; Kohmoto, T.; Osaki, S.; François, C.; et al. Inter- and intra-observer repeatability of aortic annulus measurements on screening CT for transcatheter aortic valve replacement (TAVR): Implications for appropriate device sizing. *Eur. J. Radiol.* **2018**, *105*, 209–215. [CrossRef] [PubMed]

37. Horehledova, B.; Mihl, C.; Schwemmer, C.; Hendriks, B.M.F.; Eijsvoogel, N.G.; Kietselaer, B.L.J.H.; Wildberger, J.E.; Das, M. Aortic root evaluation prior to transcatheter aortic valve implantation—Correlation of manual and semi-automatic measurements. *PLoS ONE* **2018**, *13*, e0199732. [CrossRef]

38. Lou, J.; Obuchowski, N.A.; Krishnaswamy, A.; Popovic, Z.; Flamm, S.D.; Kapadia, S.R.; Svensson, L.G.; Bolen, M.A.; Desai, M.Y.; Halliburton, S.S.; et al. Manual, semiautomated, and fully automated measurement of the aortic annulus for planning of transcatheter aortic valve replacement (TAVR/TAVI): Analysis of interchangeability. *J. Cardiovasc. Comput. Tomogr.* **2015**, *9*, 42–49. [CrossRef]

39. Hansson, N.C.; Thuesen, L.; Hjortdal, V.E.; Leipsic, J.; Andersen, H.R.; Poulsen, S.H.; Webb, J.G.; Christiansen, E.H.; Rasmussen, L.E.; Krusell, L.R.; et al. Three-dimensional multidetector computed tomography versus conventional 2-dimensional transesophageal echocardiography for annular sizing in transcatheter aortic valve replacement: Influence on postprocedural paravalvular aortic regurgitation. *Catheter. Cardiovasc. Interv.* **2013**, *82*, 977–986. [CrossRef]

40. Athappan, G.; Patvardhan, E.; Tuzcu, E.M.; Svensson, L.G.; Lemos, P.A.; Fraccaro, C.; Tarantini, G.; Sinning, J.M.; Nickenig, G.; Capodanno, D.; et al. Incidence, predictors, and outcomes of aortic regurgitation after transcatheter aortic valve replacement: Meta-analysis and systematic review of literature. *J. Am. Coll. Cardiol.* **2013**, *61*, 1585–1595. [CrossRef]

41. Husser, O.; Holzamer, A.; Resch, M.; Endemann, D.H.; Nunez, J.; Bodi, V.; Schmid, C.; Riegger, G.A.J.; Gössmann, H.; Hamer, O.; et al. Prosthesis sizing for transcatheter aortic valve implantation—Comparison of three dimensional transesophageal echocardiography with multislice computed tomography. *Int. J. Cardiol.* **2013**, *168*, 3431–3438. [CrossRef]

42. Ebuchi, K.; Yoshitani, K.; Kanemaru, E.; Fujii, T.; Tsukinaga, A.; Shimahara, Y.; Ohnishi, Y. Measurement of the Aortic Annulus Area and Diameter by Three-Dimensional Transesophageal Echocardiography in Transcatheter Aortic Valve Replacement. *J. Cardiothorac. Vasc. Anesth.* **2019**, *33*, 2387–2393. [CrossRef] [PubMed]

43. Maia, J.; Ladeiras-Lopes, R.; Guerreiro, C.; Carvalho, M.; Fontes-Carvalho, R.; Braga, P.; Sampaio, F. Accuracy of three-dimensional echocardiography in candidates for transcatheter aortic valve replacement. *Int. J. Cardiovasc. Imaging* **2020**, *36*, 291–298. [CrossRef] [PubMed]

44. Elkaryoni, A.; Nanda, N.C.; Baweja, P.; Arisha, M.J.; Zamir, H.; Elgebaly, A.; Altibi, A.M.A.; Sharma, R. Three-dimensional transesophageal echocardiography is an attractive alternative to cardiac multi-detector computed tomography for aortic annular sizing: Systematic review and meta-analysis. *Echocardiography* **2018**, *35*, 1626–1634. [CrossRef]

45. Mork, C.; Wei, M.; Jiang, W.; Ren, J.; Ran, H. Aortic annular sizing using novel software in three-dimensional transesophageal echocardiography for transcatheter aortic valve replacement: A systematic review and meta-analysis. *Diagnostics* **2021**, *11*, 751. [CrossRef]

46. Rong, L.Q.; Hameed, I.; Salemi, A.; Rahouma, M.; Khan, F.M.; Wijeysundera, H.C.; Angiolillo, D.J.; Shore-Lesserson, L.; Biondi-Zoccai, G.; Girardi, L.N.; et al. Three-Dimensional Echocardiography for Transcatheter Aortic Valve Replacement Sizing: A Systematic Review and Meta-Analysis. *J. Am. Heart Assoc.* **2019**, *8*, e013463. [CrossRef]

47. Vaquerizo, B.; Spaziano, M.; Alali, J.; Mylote, D.; Theriault-Lauzier, P.; Alfagih, R.; Martucci, G.; Buithieu, J.; Piazza, N. Three-dimensional echocardiography vs. computed tomography for transcatheter aortic valve replacement sizing. *Eur. Heart J. Cardiovasc. Imaging* **2016**, *17*, 15–23. [CrossRef] [PubMed]

48. Singh, S.; Rutkowski, P.S.; Dyachkov, A.; Iyer, V.S.; Pourafkari, L.; Nader, N.D. A discrepancy between CT angiography and transesophageal echocardiographic measurements of the annular size affect long-term survival following trans-catheter aortic valve replacement. *J. Cardiovasc. Thorac. Res.* **2021**, *13*, 208–215. [CrossRef]
49. Lopez-Mattei, J.C.; Shah, D.J. When to consider cardiovascular magnetic resonance in patients undergoing transcatheter aortic valve replacement? *Curr. Opin. Cardiol.* **2013**, *28*, 505–511. [CrossRef]
50. Ruile, P.; Blanke, P.; Krauss, T.; Dorfs, S.; Jung, B.; Jander, N.; Leipsic, J.; Langer, M.; Neumann, F.J.; Pache, G. Pre-procedural assessment of aortic annulus dimensions for transcatheter aortic valve replacement: Comparison of a non-contrast 3D MRA protocol with contrast-enhanced cardiac dual-source CT angiography. *Eur. Heart J. Cardiovasc. Imaging* **2016**, *17*, 458–466. [CrossRef]
51. Mayr, A.; Klug, G.; Reinstadler, S.J.; Feistritzer, H.J.; Reindl, M.; Kremser, C.; Kranewitter, C.; Bonaros, N.; Friedrich, G.; Feuchtner, G.; et al. Is MRI equivalent to CT in the guidance of TAVR? A pilot study. *Eur. Radiol.* **2018**, *28*, 4625–4634. [CrossRef]
52. Pamminger, M.; Klug, G.; Kranewitter, C.; Reindl, M.; Reinstadler, S.J.; Henninger, B.; Tiller, C.; Holzknecht, M.; Kremser, C.; Bauer, A.; et al. Non-contrast MRI protocol for TAVI guidance: Quiescent-interval single-shot angiography in comparison with contrast-enhanced CT. *Eur. Radiol.* **2020**, *30*, 4847–4856. [CrossRef] [PubMed]
53. Pamminger, M.; Kranewitter, C.; Kremser, C.; Reindl, M.; Reinstadler, S.J.; Henninger, B.; Reiter, G.; Piccini, D.; Tiller, C.; Holzknecht, M.; et al. Self-navigated versus navigator-gated 3D MRI sequence for non-enhanced aortic root measurement in transcatheter aortic valve implantation. *Eur. J. Radiol.* **2021**, *137*, 109573. [CrossRef] [PubMed]
54. Aouad, P.; Jarvis, K.B.; Botelho, M.F.; Serhal, A.; Blaisdell, J.; Collins, L.; Giri, S.; Kim, D.; Markl, M.; Ricciardi, M.J.; et al. Aortic annular dimensions by non-contrast MRI using k–t accelerated 3D cine b-SSFP in pre-procedural assessment for transcatheter aortic valve implantation: A technical feasibility study. *Int. J. Cardiovasc. Imaging* **2021**, *37*, 651–661. [CrossRef] [PubMed]

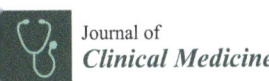

Review

Atrial Functional Tricuspid Regurgitation as a Distinct Pathophysiological and Clinical Entity: No Idiopathic Tricuspid Regurgitation Anymore

Diana R. Florescu [1,2], Denisa Muraru [2,3], Valentina Volpato [2,3], Mara Gavazzoni [2], Sergio Caravita [2,4], Michele Tomaselli [2,3], Pellegrino Ciampi [2,5], Cristina Florescu [1], Tudor A. Bălșeanu [1], Gianfranco Parati [2,3] and Luigi P. Badano [2,3,*]

1. Faculty of Medicine, University of Medicine and Pharmacy of Craiova, 200349 Craiova, Romania; dianarflorescu@yahoo.com (D.R.F.); cristina.t.florescu@umfcv.ro (C.F.); adrian.balseanu@umfcv.ro (T.A.B.)
2. Department of Cardiology, Istituto Auxologico Italiano, IRCCS, 20145 Milan, Italy; d.muraru@auxologico.it (D.M.); valevolpato@hotmail.it (V.V.); gavazzonimara@gmail.com (M.G.); s.caravita@auxologico.it (S.C.); m.tomaselli5@campus.unimib.it (M.T.); pellegrino.ciampi.rc@gmail.com (P.C.); gianfranco.parati@unimib.it (G.P.)
3. Department of Medicine and Surgery, University of Milano-Bicocca, 20126 Milan, Italy
4. Department of Management, Information and Production Engineering, University of Bergamo, 24044 Dalmine, Italy
5. Department of Cardiovascular and Pneumological Sciences, Catholic University of the Sacred Heart, 20123 Rome, Italy
* Correspondence: luigi.badano@unimib.it; Tel.: +39-375-6119209

Abstract: Functional tricuspid regurgitation (FTR) is a strong and independent predictor of patient morbidity and mortality if left untreated. The development of transcatheter procedures to either repair or replace the tricuspid valve (TV) has fueled the interest in the pathophysiology, severity assessment, and clinical consequences of FTR. FTR has been considered to be secondary to tricuspid annulus (TA) dilation and leaflet tethering, associated to right ventricular (RV) dilation and/or dysfunction (the "classical", ventricular form of FTR, V-FTR) for a long time. Atrial FTR (A-FTR) has recently emerged as a distinct pathophysiological entity. A-FTR typically occurs in patients with persistent/permanent atrial fibrillation, in whom an imbalance between the TA and leaflet areas results in leaflets malcoaptation, associated with the dilation and loss of the sphincter-like function of the TA, due to right atrium enlargement and dysfunction. According to its distinct pathophysiology, A-FTR poses different needs of clinical management, and the various interventional treatment options will likely have different outcomes than in V-FTR patients. This review aims to provide an insight into the anatomy of the TV, and the distinct pathophysiology of A-FTR, which are key concepts to understanding the objectives of therapy, the choice of transcatheter TV interventions, and to properly use pre-, intra-, and post-procedural imaging.

Keywords: tricuspid regurgitation; atrial functional tricuspid regurgitation; transcatheter tricuspid valve interventions; echocardiography; three-dimensional echocardiography; multimodality imaging

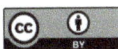

1. Introduction

Functional tricuspid regurgitation (FTR), secondary to tricuspid annulus (TA) dilation, tricuspid valve (TV) leaflet tethering, or a combination of both, resulting in leaflet malcoaptation [1], accounts for ~90% of all cases of TR [2,3]. FTR represents a progressive valvular condition that plays a strong and independent role in patient morbidity and mortality [4–8]. Several studies have demonstrated that, if left untreated, FTR can independently worsen patient outcomes and quality of life [4,9,10]. Furthermore, the development of transcatheter procedures to either repair or replace the TV [11], as valuable treatment alternatives in patients considered at high surgical risk, has further contributed to the increased interest in the pathophysiology, severity assessment, and clinical consequences of FTR [12–17].

FTR has been traditionally considered secondary to the dilation and/or dysfunction of the right ventricle (RV), mainly associated to pulmonary hypertension. Only recently, atrial FTR (A-FTR) has been recognized as a distinct pathophysiological entity, and its peculiar mechanisms have begun to being elucidated [18–23]. A-FTR is typically characterized by the dilation, and either the decrease or loss of the sphincter function of the TA, associated with the dilation and the dysfunction of the right atrium (RA), in patients with persistent/permanent atrial fibrillation (AF) [21,24,25]. These geometrical and functional changes determine an imbalance between the TA and leaflet areas, resulting in malcoaptation of the TV leaflets, even in the presence of normal RV size and function (type I of the Carpentier classification [26,27]). Given the distinct pathophysiological cascade leading to significant FTR development, A-FTR might pose different needs of clinical management [28], and the various interventional treatment options will likely have different outcomes than in the classical ventricular form of FTR (V-FTR, type IIIb of the Carpentier classification) [29,30]. Moreover, the transcatheter tricuspid valve interventions (TTVI) in A-FTR mainly have the goal to decrease the size of the TA, and require specific criteria of anatomic feasibility to plan the procedure [31–33].

Accordingly, the aim of this review is to provide an insight into the anatomy of the TV, and the pathophysiology of A-FTR, which are key concepts to understanding the objectives of therapy, the choice of TTVI, and to properly use pre-, intra-, and post-procedural imaging [32].

2. Anatomy and Pathophysiology of A-FTR

The TV is a complex structure that includes the TA, the TV leaflets, and a sub-valvular apparatus (chordae and papillary muscles). Both the anatomic integrity of the TV apparatus and the normal shape and function of the right heart chambers are needed for the correct functioning of the valve [31,34,35].

The healthy TA has a dynamic, three-dimensional (3D) saddle-shaped elliptical geometry (Figure 1) [34–37], characterized by higher antero-septal and postero-lateral parts and lower antero-lateral and postero-septal parts [37].

The size of the TA is larger during diastole and smaller during systole. In pathological conditions of TA dilation, it tends to become more planar and circular [34]. The anterior and posterior parts of the TA are muscular, whereas the septal part is more fibrous. Consequently, the portion of the TA that is the least involved in the remodeling process is the septal one, the dilation mostly occurring in the antero-posterior direction, and leading to the progressive distancing of the aortic valve and the antero-posterior commissure [34].

However, the prevalence of significant FTR is extremely variable with the same degree of RA and TA dilation, and TA dilation secondary to RA remodeling in patients with persistent/permanent AF is not always associated with the development of significant FTR [38]. The imbalance between the degree of TA enlargement and the severity of A-FTR in some patients might partly be explained by the molecular adaptive mechanisms of the leaflet tissue that impact the amount of leaflet growth in response to the remodeling of the RA and the dilation of the TA, similar to those described in V-FTR [39,40]. Afilalo et al. [39] showed that in V-FTR, the remodeling and pressure overload of the RV are associated with a significant increase of the TV leaflet areas. The difference between the extent of TV leaflet areas adaptation in response to TA and RA dilation could be a key factor in the pathophysiological cascade that leads to the development and progression of A-FTR. Moreover, Utsunomiya et al. [19] showed that the posterior dilation of the RA that causes posterior TV plane displacement is not efficiently compensated by the TV leaflet adaptation. These mechanisms might explain why despite similar extent of RA dilation, some of the patients present with only trivial/mild A-FTR [21].

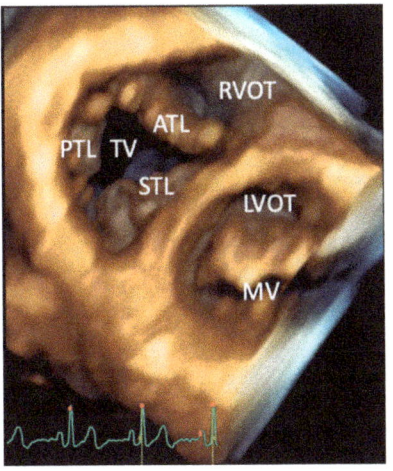 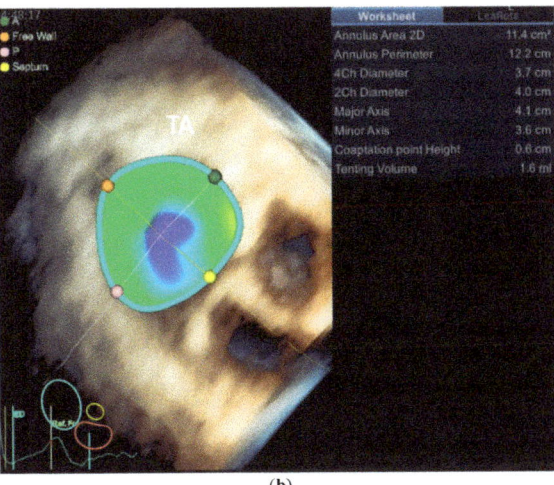

Figure 1. Transthoracic 3DE volume rendering of the tricuspid valve. (**a**) Anatomy of the tricuspid valve seen from the ventricular perspective and its relationships with adjacent structures; (**b**) Quantitative assessment of the tricuspid annulus. The colored dots on the annulus are used for anatomic orientation. Abbreviations: 2Ch, 2-chamber view; 2D, two-dimensional echocardiography; 3DE, three-dimensional echocardiography; 4Ch, 4-chamber view; A, anterior; ATL, anterior tricuspid leaflet; LVOT, left ventricular outflow tract; MV, mitral valve; P, posterior; PTL, posterior tricuspid leaflet; RVOT, right ventricular outflow tract; STL, septal tricuspid leaflet; TA, tricuspid annulus; TV, tricuspid valve.

Although several studies have elegantly described the pathophysiological mechanisms of A-FTR (previously-referred to as "idiopathic" or "isolated" TR), it represents nevertheless an overlooked consequence of persistent/permanent AF. A-FTR is characterized by TA remodeling associated with RA enlargement, and normal/mildly abnormal RV size and function, especially in the initial stages of the disease [18]. Yamasaki et al. [41] hypothesized that severe A-FTR is caused by the loss of TV leaflets' systolic coaptation in the context of TA and RA dilation. Muraru et al. [24,42] demonstrated that the RA plays a substantial role in determining TA size in FTR patients, including A-FTR. Guta et al. [21] have further contributed to understanding the pathophysiology of A-FTR by showing that RA minimum volume is the main determinant of TA area at end-diastole in AF patients, and that it determines A-FTR severity, while leaflet tethering plays a far less important role in the process. Furthermore, Utsunomiya et al. [43] showed that TA area was more closely correlated with RA maximum volume than with RV end-systolic volume in AF patients, and that the only predictor of A-FTR severity was TA area at mid-systole. In contrast, both RA and RV volumes were found to be independent predictors of severe A-FTR according to Najib et al. [44]. RV enlargement is usually detected in more advanced stages of A-FTR, with longer disease progression, as the dilation of the RV is usually a late event in A-FTR, as reported by Nemoto et al. [45]. Finally, the shape of the RV is markedly different in patients with A-FTR and V-FTR [23]. In A-FTR the RV remodeling pattern resembles a conical shape, with isolated enlargement of the inflow portion of the RV, and without significant chamber dilation or dysfunction compared to controls. Conversely, in V-FTR the RV becomes spherical or elliptic, with significantly increased basal and mid-cavity RV diameters and volumes, and significantly decreased RV function compared to controls [23]. Therefore, RV size assessment by two-dimensional echocardiography (2DE) linear methods, such as RV basal diameter, has important limitations in patients with A-FTR, and should be replaced by three-dimensional echocardiography (3DE) volumetric measurement.

3. TTVIs in A-FTR

Although still under development and underused in clinical practice, TV interventions should be considered in patients with severe symptomatic FTR, in the absence of severe left ventricular or RV dysfunction, or severe pulmonary hypertension (class IIa) [17,29], and according to current guidelines [16,46], RV dilation is a criterion for severe FTR. However, it has recently been reported that patients with severe A-FTR might present with normal RV size, and a dilated RV might be found in patients with less than severe A-FTR [23]. Therefore, A-FTR severity grading should be carefully performed, and absence of RV enlargement should not be considered an exclusion criterion of severe A-FTR. Moreover, FTR severity is not linearly associated with prognosis [47], demonstrating that the recommended indications for TV interventions should take into consideration the etiology of FTR [16]. In a recent study, patients with severe FTR treated with TTVIs had better 1 year prognosis compared to patients undergoing only medical treatment [48]. In patients with indications for TV interventions, diuretic therapy is useful in the presence of right-sided heart failure, and rhythm control strategies might decrease A-FTR severity in patients with AF [24,43,49–51]. Wang et al. [50] demonstrated that catheter ablation (CA) for AF and sinus rhythm (SR) maintenance lead to TR improvement in FTR patients without significant TV tethering (tethering height < 6 mm). These findings are supported by the study by Markman et al. [51] that show a significant reduction (of at least one grade) of TR severity in 64% of patients after CA for AF. Lastly, Itakura et al. [52] showed how the reduction in RA size following the restoration of SR by CA correlated with the decrease in FTR severity in patients with persistent AF. However, although cardioversion and/or ablation of AF might be beneficial in patients with A-FTR, these therapies should not delay the referral for intervention in patients with indications [16].

In patients referred for TTVIs, the parameters used for TR grading often have far greater values than the lower thresholds currently recommended to identify severe TR [53,54], and among all patients with functional atrioventricular valve regurgitation of various causes, patients with A-FTR can particularly have extremely severe annular dilation, making catheter-guided interventions challenging and controversial in end-stage forms [55]. These findings have highlighted the need for a novel grading system that could illustrate the continuum of TR severity [56]. A group of experts proposed the introduction of two new TR categories, massive and torrential TR, by extending the current cut-off values for severe TR [13,57], and their significance has been demonstrated in several studies [13,15,54,58]. The systematic combined use of vena contracta (VC) width and effective regurgitant orifice area (EROA) to identify severe (VC width $\geq$ 7 mm and EROA < 80 mm^2) and torrential TR (VC width $\geq$ 7 mm and EROA $\geq$ 80 mm^2) has been useful in predicting patient outcomes in significant FTR [59]. Since massive to torrential A-FTR is characterized by prominent annular dilation associated with significant tethering of the leaflets, Utsunomiya et al. [19] suggested that the most suitable patients for TR annuloplasty are those with severe FTR. Therefore, the updated proposed FTR severity grading could impact the timing of TV interventions, especially since they are mostly performed too late, in end-stage forms. Subsequently, TTVIs may improve the prognosis of patients with severe A-FTR, especially as an early treatment, before the development of massive to torrential FTR.

The feasibility, safety, and efficacy of TTVIs have been demonstrated in recent studies [53,60,61]. The best technique and choice of intervention are based on an accurate pre-procedural assessment consisting of multimodality imaging evaluation [31,62,63], yet relying mainly on echocardiography, and the identification of the exact mechanism of TR. To confirm the indication of TTVI and to select the type and size of the device used, accurate measurement of the TA done using 3D imaging (echocardiography, multidetector cardiac computed tomography- CCT, or cardiac magnetic resonance- CMR) is key [64]. Furthermore, a deep understanding of the anatomic relationships between the TV and various essential surrounding structures such as the right coronary artery, the conduction tissue, the aortic valve, and the coronary sinus (CS) are of paramount importance in planning, guiding, and monitoring of TTVIs [31,65,66].

3.1. Echocardiography

The state-of-the-art echocardiographic evaluation of the TV and quantification of the severity of FTR should imply: (1) confirming the presence of pathological FTR; (2) assessing the morphology of the TV; (3) identifying the mechanisms of FTR (annular dilation, leaflet tethering, cardiac implanted electronic device interference, etc.); (4) distinguishing between A-FTR and V-FTR; (5) assessing the severity of FTR and quantifying its hemodynamic impact [67].

In clinical routine practice, 2DE and Doppler echocardiography are recommended by guidelines for TR evaluation [26,68,69]. When quantifying TR severity, different parameters (structural, qualitative, semi-quantitative, or quantitative) should be evaluated (Figure 2), and grading of FTR severity based on a sole parameter is not recommended [26,65,68,69].

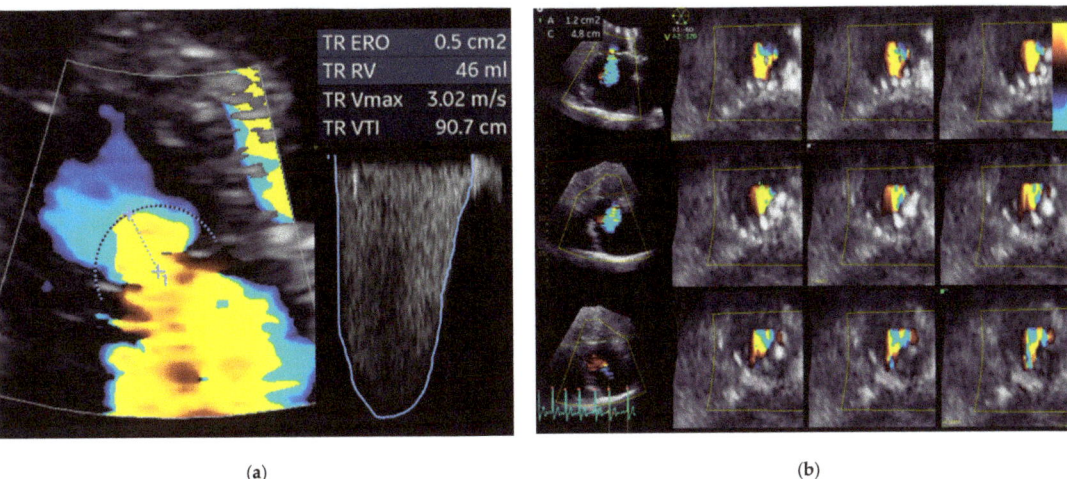

Figure 2. Quantitative assessment of functional tricuspid regurgitation severity by Color-Doppler echocardiography. (**a**) 2D PISA method. (**b**) 3D vena contracta area. Abbreviations: 2D, two-dimensional echocardiography; 3D, three-dimensional echocardiography; A, area; C, circumference; ERO, effective regurgitant orifice area; RV, right ventricle; TR, tricuspid regurgitation; Vmax, maximal regurgitant velocity; VTI, velocity-time integral.

The majority of Doppler methods used for the assessment of left-sided valvular heart disease are applicable when evaluating FTR. However, the TR jet has lower pressure and velocity (the main determinants of the jet momentum) compared to mitral regurgitation [13]. Jet flow and thus color Doppler jet area are governed mainly by the conservation of momentum which is flow (Q) × velocity (V). If Q = effective regurgitant orifice area (EROA) × V, and jet momentum (M) = Q × V, then M = EROA × V^2. Thus, for the same EROA, the regurgitant volume (RegVol) of a TR jet with a velocity of 2.5 m/s (as frequently recorded in patients without pulmonary hypertension) could be a quarter of the color jet area of a mitral regurgitant jet with a velocity of 5.0 m/s.

Moreover, in patients with A-FTR qualitative signs of TR severity may be misleading: the assumption that the absence of RV dilation usually indicates milder degrees of FTR does not stand true, and the systolic hepatic vein flow reversal could represent the RA dysfunction, and not necessarily FTR severity. Finally, due to the geometrical assumptions regarding single plane VC measurement, and EROA calculation using the PISA method, and since for the same EROA, the RegVol can be quite different with different pressure gradients [40,70], severity quantification in A-FTR is challenging. However, averaged VC width, and VC area by 3DE might overcome the limitations of other semi-quantitative or quantitative parameters that assume the regurgitant orifice is flat and circular, and could be used for A-FTR severity grading when indices provide discordant results [16,70,71].

Structural parameters (TV morphology, TA size, RV, and RA size) need to be evaluated and 3DE is the most accurate echocardiography technique for this task (Figure 3) [70,72]. 3DE allows to precisely identify the number, morphology, and motion of the different TV leaflets [40,69,73–75], which is key to select the optimal devices for transcatheter repair procedures [76].

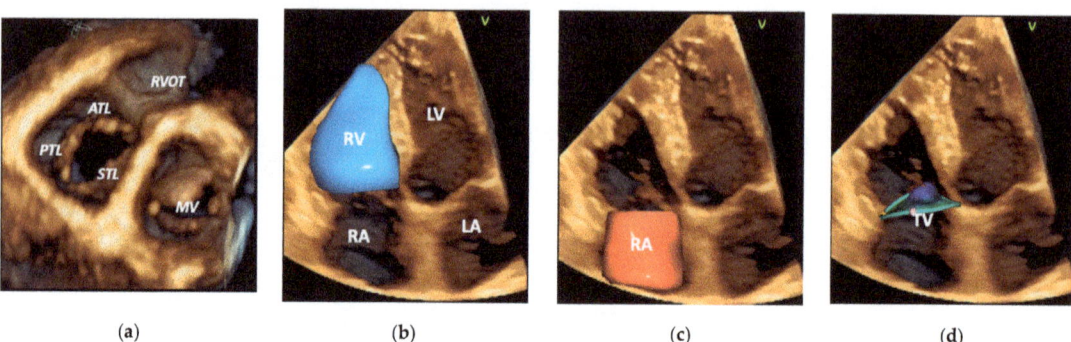

Figure 3. Utility of transthoracic 3DE to assess patients with tricuspid regurgitation. (**a**) Tricuspid valve functional anatomy. (**b**) Right ventricular volume and ejection fraction. (**c**) Right atrial size and function. (**d**) Tricuspid annulus geometry and valve tenting volume and height. Abbreviations: 3DE, three-dimensional echocardiography; ATL, anterior tricuspid leaflet; LA, left atrium; LV, left ventricle; MV, mitral valve; PTL, posterior tricuspid leaflet; RA, right atrium; RV, right ventricle; RVOT, right ventricular outflow tract; STL, septal tricuspid leaflet; TV, tricuspid valve.

Additionally, 3DE can easily visualize the structures surrounding the TV, which may serve as landmarks for TV interventions or may have implications for TR, such as the inferior and superior vena cava, the CS inflow, the RV outflow tract, the ascending aorta [32,70].

Due to the complex, 3D configuration and variable spatial orientation of the TA, and since both the 2DE view and the timing of the measurement during the cardiac cycle significantly influence TA size [77,78], 3DE should be the first-line modality for TA sizing in patients with FTR. Since the TA dilates more antero-posteriorly in FTR [79], the greatest TA is unlikely to be identified in the 2D apical 4-chamber view as recommended by the current guidelines [36,40,73]. Furthermore, slight variations in transducer position from apical 4-chamber to RV-focused view results in relatively large differences in TA diameter measurements, and both the absence of anatomical landmarks, as well as the non-circular shape, make 2DE TA linear dimension less reproducible across different studies made in the same patient [36,73]. 3DE provides a precise assessment of the actual TA dimensions (linear, non-planar area, and perimeter), eliminating the geometrical assumptions and absence of anatomical landmarks that characterize 2DE [36,80,81].

A semi-automated 3DE dedicated software for the quantification of TV size and morphology has recently been developed (Figure 4) [36]. The feasibility of TA measurements using this software is high, even in presence of irregular heart rhythms such as AF, and preliminary validation of this software has already been reported [82]. This software package provides various important parameters for TV characterization which are key elements in recognizing the prevalent mechanism of FTR and properly selecting the device used to treat TR [81] (i.e.,: 2D and 3D TA area, TA perimeter, 4- and 2-chamber systolic and diastolic diameters, major and minor axis, sphericity index, longitudinal displacement of the TA during the cardiac cycle, leaflets coaptation point height, tenting volume, maximal tenting height [42]).

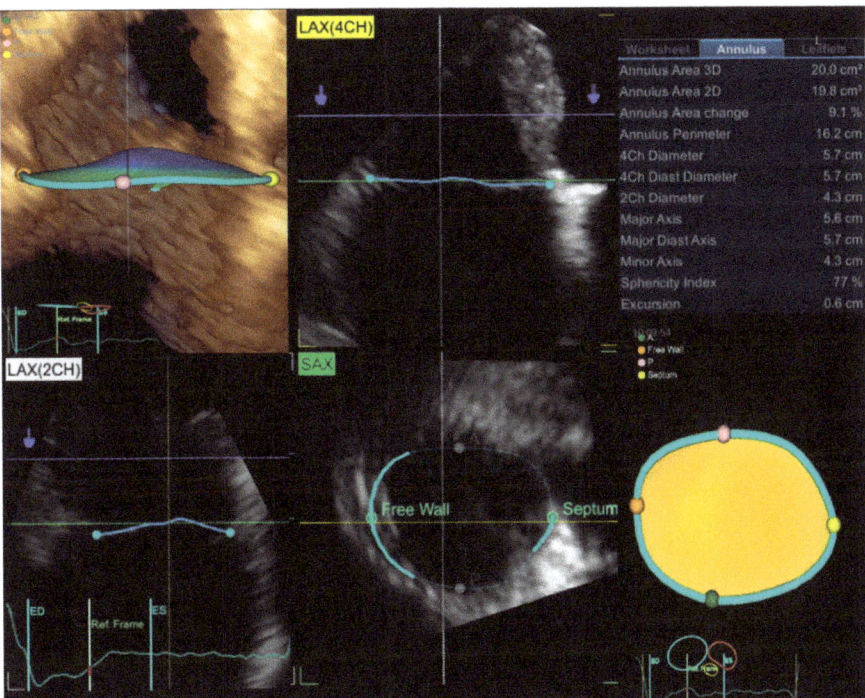

Figure 4. Evaluation of tricuspid annular size and shape by 4D Auto TVQ software ((EchoPac v204, GE, Horten, Norway). Abbreviations: 2Ch, apical 2-chamber view; 2D, two-dimensional echocardiography; 3D, three-dimensional echocardiography; 4Ch, apical 4-chamber view; A, anterior; ED, end-diastole; ES, end-systole; LAX, long axis; P, posterior; SAX, short axis.

While 2DE may also significantly underestimate right heart chambers' sizes due to foreshortening or geometrical assumptions, 3DE-derived methods allow a more precise and reliable measure of both the RV and the RA [72,83,84].

Lastly, several echocardiographic features have been correlated with procedural failure, suboptimal results, or worse outcomes after transcatheter edge-to-edge TV repair, and they should be assessed when considering patient eligibility. These factors are the presence of more severe leaflets tethering, higher tenting volume, greater coaptation depth (>1 cm), large TR coaptation gap size (>7.2 mm), and non-central/non anteroseptal TR jet [60,61,85,86]. The number of TV leaflets will also affect TTVIs' outcomes [87]. Conversely, conventional echocardiographic parameters used to assess RV function and systolic pulmonary artery pressure may not predict clinical outcomes after transcatheter valve repair [88].

3.2. Cardiac Magnetic Resonance, Cardiac Computed Tomography, and Fusion Imaging

The reference imaging technique for evaluating RV size and systolic function, which are important elements in distinguishing between A-FTR and V-FTR, is CMR. Moreover, CMR can provide accurate TR severity grading based on the measurement of the RegVol and the regurgitant fraction, indirectly calculated by subtracting the pulmonic forward volume from the RV stroke volume [68], or directly measured by the use of either standard phase-contrast sequences [89,90], or by innovative 4D-flow velocity-encoded approaches, using whole-heart free-breathing sequences [91,92]. However, CMR is not well suited for assessing the TV leaflets due to their thinness. Conversely, CCT, that is characterized by high spatial resolution, is not only the ideal method to assess TA dimensions and the anatomic considerations that are fundamental when planning transcatheter procedures targeting the TA [2,3], but also allows visualization of TV leaflets, precise assessment of RV dimensions and sub-valvular structures—trabeculations, papillary muscles, moderator band, and direct measurement of EROA by multiplanar reformations analysis [32,93,94].

CMR and CCT acquisitions and postprocessing can be hampered by motion artifacts in AF patients. However, the use of new pulse sequences and imaging reconstruction algorithms allow real-time free-breathing cine sequences with good spatial and temporal resolution, and can provide precise results in the CMR evaluation of the right heart chambers [95–97]. Similarly, CCT data acquisition impacts the quality of the images, and it is of paramount significance. An optimal contrast enhancement of the right heart using a dedicated CCT contrast protocol [98] allows the acquisition of images of good quality even in the challenging scenarios of AF. Moreover, the dedicated CCT protocols used to study the TV [99] limit the use of contrast media, avoid artifacts, and provide a homogeneous opacification of the right heart. Accordingly, CCT has emerged as a standard imaging modality that provides incremental value in establishing patient eligibility and proper device sizing in the setting of TTVI [64], and it represents an ideal alternative to CMR for the measurement of right heart dimensions in patients with noncompatible intracardiac devices or contraindications to CMR [83,100].

Finally, although CCT is the method of choice for assessing TA dimensions [32,37,101], reevaluating TA dimensions and TR severity by TEE at the start of the procedure is of paramount importance since TR severity and TA size are dynamic and load-dependent. TEE is also used to identify anatomic markers that are not visible at fluoroscopy, such as the CS or the venae cavae [22,32]. Furthermore, fluoroscopy is required to position wires and guiding catheters during TTVIs. However, fluoroscopy does not allow the visualization of the TV or landmark structures. Therefore, fusion imaging (superimposing echocardiographic or CCT images on fluoroscopic projections) represents a novel alternative for imaging patients undergoing TTVIs [102–105].

4. Conclusions

A-FTR is a distinct pathophysiological and clinical entity, with different needs of clinical management as well as choice of TV intervention, and most likely with different outcomes than V-FTR. Defining the etiology of FTR, and distinguishing between A-FTR and V-FTR plays a crucial role in the management and selection of the patients for TTVIs. Multimodality imaging is key for confirming the indication for the interventions, the guiding and monitoring of TTVIs, and in the assessment and follow-up of the results of the procedure.

Author Contributions: Conceptualization, D.R.F. and L.P.B.; methodology, D.R.F. and L.P.B.; formal analysis, D.M. and M.G.; investigation, D.R.F., M.T., and C.F.; resources, P.C. and S.C.; data curation, D.R.F., V.V., P.C., S.C., C.F., and T.A.B.; writing—original draft preparation, D.R.F.; writing—review and editing, all authors; visualization, L.P.B.; supervision, L.P.B.; project administration, L.P.B., D.M. All authors have read and agreed to the published version of the manuscript.

Funding: This research received no external funding.

Institutional Review Board Statement: Not applicable.

Informed Consent Statement: Not applicable.

Data Availability Statement: No new data were created or analyzed in this study. Data sharing is not applicable to this article.

Conflicts of Interest: The authors declare no conflict of interest.

References

1. Badano, L.P.; Muraru, D.; Enriquez-Sarano, M. Assessment of functional tricuspid regurgitation. *Eur. Heart J.* **2013**, *34*, 1875–1884. [CrossRef] [PubMed]
2. Asmarats, L.; Taramasso, M.; Rodés-Cabau, J. Tricuspid valve disease: Diagnosis, prognosis and management of a rapidly evolving field. *Nat. Rev. Cardiol.* **2019**, *16*, 538–554. [CrossRef] [PubMed]
3. Prihadi, E.A.; Delgado, V.; Leon, M.B.; Enriquez-Sarano, M.; Topilsky, Y.; Bax, J.J. Morphologic Types of Tricuspid Regurgitation: Characteristics and Prognostic Implications. *JACC Cardiovasc. Imaging* **2019**, *12*, 491–499. [CrossRef]
4. Benfari, G.; Antoine, C.; Miller, W.L.; Thapa, P.; Topilsky, Y.; Rossi, A.; Michelena, H.I.; Pislaru, S.; Enriquez-Sarano, M. Excess Mortality Associated with Functional Tricuspid Regurgitation Complicating Heart Failure With Reduced Ejection Fraction. *Circulation* **2019**, *140*, 196–206. [CrossRef]
5. Prihadi, E.A.; van der Bijl, P.; Gursoy, E.; Abou, R.; Mara Vollema, E.; Hahn, R.T.; Stone, G.W.; Leon, M.B.; Ajmone Marsan, N.; Delgado, V.; et al. Development of significant tricuspid regurgitation over time and prognostic implications: New insights into natural history. *Eur. Heart J.* **2018**, *39*, 3574–3581. [CrossRef] [PubMed]
6. Wang, N.; Fulcher, J.; Abeysuriya, N.; McGrady, M.; Wilcox, I.; Celermajer, D.; Lal, S. Tricuspid regurgitation is associated with increased mortality independent of pulmonary pressures and right heart failure: A systematic review and meta-analysis. *Eur. Heart J.* **2019**, *40*, 476–484. [CrossRef]
7. Chorin, E.; Rozenbaum, Z.; Topilsky, Y.; Konigstein, M.; Ziv-Baran, T.; Richert, E.; Keren, G.; Banai, S. Tricuspid regurgitation and long-term clinical outcomes. *Eur. Heart J. Cardiovasc. Imaging* **2020**, *21*, 157–165. [CrossRef]
8. Spinka, G.; Bartko, P.E.; Heitzinger, G.; Prausmüller, S.; Pavo, N.; Frey, M.K.; Arfsten, H.; Genger, M.; Hengstenberg, C.; Hülsmann, M.; et al. Natural Course of Nonsevere Secondary Tricuspid Regurgitation. *J. Am. Soc. Echocardiogr.* **2021**, *34*, 13–19. [CrossRef]
9. Messika-Zeitoun, D.; Verta, P.; Gregson, J.; Pocock, S.J.; Boero, I.; Feldman, T.E.; Abraham, W.T.; Lindenfeld, J.; Bax, J.; Leon, M.; et al. Impact of tricuspid regurgitation on survival in patients with heart failure: A large electronic health record patient-level database analysis. *Eur. J. Heart Fail.* **2020**, *22*, 1803–1813. [CrossRef]
10. Nath, J.; Foster, E.; Heidenreich, P.A. Impact of Tricuspid Regurgitation on Long-Term Survival. *J. Am. Coll. Cardiol.* **2004**, *43*, 405–409. [CrossRef]
11. Voci, D.; Pozzoli, A.; Miura, M.; Gavazzoni, M.; Gülmez, G.; Scianna, S.; Zuber, M.; Maisano, F.; Taramasso, M. Developments in transcatheter tricuspid valve therapies. *Expert Rev. Cardiovasc. Ther.* **2019**, *17*, 841–856. [CrossRef]
12. Kebed, K.Y.; Addetia, K.; Henry, M.; Yamat, M.; Weinert, L.; Besser, S.A.; Mor-Avi, V.; Lang, R.M. Refining Severe Tricuspid Regurgitation Definition by Echocardiography with a New Outcomes-Based "Massive" Grade. *J. Am. Soc. Echocardiogr.* **2020**, *33*, 1087–1094. [CrossRef] [PubMed]
13. Santoro, C.; Marco Del Castillo, A.; González-Gómez, A.; Monteagudo, J.M.; Hinojar, R.; Lorente, A.; Abellás, M.; Vieitez, J.M.; Garcia Martin, A.; Casas Rojo, E.; et al. Mid-term outcome of severe tricuspid regurgitation: Are there any differences according to mechanism and severity? *Eur. Heart J. Cardiovasc. Imaging* **2019**, *20*, 1035–1042. [CrossRef]
14. Vieitez, J.M.; Monteagudo, J.M.; Mahia, P.; Perez, L.; Lopez, T.; Marco, I.; Perone, F.; González, T.; Sitges, M.; Bouzas, A.; et al. New insights of tricuspid regurgitation: A large-scale prospective cohort study. *Eur. Heart J. Cardiovasc. Imaging* **2021**, *22*, 196–202. [CrossRef] [PubMed]
15. Muraru, D.; Previtero, M.; Ochoa-Jimenez, R.C.; Guta, A.C.; Figliozzi, S.; Gregori, D.; Bottigliengo, D.; Parati, G.; Badano, L.P. Prognostic validation of partition values for quantitative parameters to grade functional tricuspid regurgitation severity by conventional echocardiography. *Eur. Heart J. Cardiovasc. Imaging* **2021**, *22*, 155–165. [CrossRef] [PubMed]
16. Vahanian, A.; Beyersdorf, F.; Praz, F.; Milojevic, M.; Baldus, S.; Bauersachs, J.; Capodanno, D.; Conradi, L.; De Bonis, M.; De Paulis, R.; et al. 2021 ESC/EACTS Guidelines for the management of valvular heart disease. *Eur. Heart J.* **2021**, *60*, 727–800. [CrossRef]
17. Otto, C.M.; Nishimura, R.A.; Bonow, R.O.; Carabello, B.A.; Erwin, J.P., 3rd; Gentile, F.; Jneid, H.; Krieger, E.V.; Mack, M.; McLeod, C.; et al. 2020 ACC/AHA Guideline for the Management of Patients with Valvular Heart Disease. *J. Am. Coll. Cardiol.* **2021**, *212*, e131–e135. [CrossRef]
18. Muraru, D.; Guta, A.C.; Ochoa-Jimenez, R.C.; Bartos, D.; Aruta, P.; Mihaila, S.; Popescu, B.A.; Iliceto, S.; Basso, C.; Badano, L. Functional Regurgitation of Atrioventricular Valves and Atrial Fibrillation: An Elusive Pathophysiological Link Deserving Further Attention. *J. Am. Soc. Echocardiogr.* **2020**, *33*, 42–53. [CrossRef]
19. Utsunomiya, H.; Harada, Y.; Susawa, H.; Ueda, Y.; Izumi, K.; Itakura, K.; Hidaka, T.; Shiota, T.; Nakano, Y.; Kihara, Y. Tricuspid valve geometry and right heart remodelling: Insights into the mechanism of atrial functional tricuspid regurgitation. *Eur. Heart J. Cardiovasc. Imaging* **2020**, *21*, 1068–1078. [CrossRef]
20. Silbiger, J.J. Atrial functional tricuspid regurgitation: An underappreciated cause of secondary tricuspid regurgitation. *Echocardiography* **2019**, *36*, 954–957. [CrossRef]
21. Guta, A.C.; Badano, L.P.; Tomaselli, M.; Mihalcea, D.; Bartos, D.; Parati, G.; Muraru, D. The pathophysiological link between right atrial remodeling and functional tricuspid regurgitation in patients with atrial fibrillation. A three-dimensional echocardiography study. *J. Am. Soc. Echocardiogr.* **2021**, *34*, 585–594.e1. [CrossRef]
22. Praz, F.; Muraru, D.; Kreidel, F.; Lurz, P.; Hahn, R.T.; Delgado, V.; Senni, M.; von Bardeleben, R.S.; Nickenig, G.; Hausleiter, J.; et al. Transcatheter treatment for tricuspid valve disease. *EuroIntervention* **2021**, *17*, 791–808. [CrossRef]

23. Florescu, D.R.; Muraru, D.; Florescu, C.; Volpato, V.; Caravita, S.; Perger, E.; Bălșeanu, T.A.; Parati, G.; Badano, L.P. Right heart chambers geometry and function in patients with the atrial and the ventricular phenotypes of functional tricuspid regurgitation. *Eur. Heart J. Cardiovasc. Imaging* **2021**. Epub ahead of print. [CrossRef] [PubMed]
24. Muraru, D.; Caravita, S.; Guta, A.C.; Muraru, D.; Caravita, S.; Guta, A.C.; Mihalcea, D.; Branzi, G.; Parati, G.; Badano, L.P. Functional Tricuspid Regurgitation and Atrial Fibrillation: Which Comes First, the Chicken or the Egg? *Case* **2020**, *4*, 458. [CrossRef]
25. Ortiz-Leon, X.A.; Posada-Martinez, E.L.; Trejo-Paredes, M.C.; Ivey-Miranda, J.B.; Pereira, J.; Crandall, I.; DaSilva, P.; Bouman, E.; Brooks, A.; Gerardi, C.; et al. Understanding tricuspid valve remodelling in atrial fibrillation using three-dimensional echocardiography. *Eur. Heart J. Cardiovasc. Imaging* **2020**, *21*, 747–755. [CrossRef]
26. Lancellotti, P.; Tribouilloy, C.; Hagendorff, A.; Popescu, B.A.; Edvardsen, T.; Pierard, L.A.; Badano, L.; Zamorano, J.L. Recommendations for the echocardiographic assessment of native valvular regurgitation: An executive summary from the European Association of Cardiovascular Imaging. *Eur. Heart J. Cardiovasc. Imaging* **2013**, *14*, 611–644. [CrossRef]
27. Lancellotti, P.; Moura, L.; Pierard, L.A.; Agricola, E.; Popescu, B.A.; Tribouilloy, C.; Hagendorff, A.; Monin, J.L.; Badano, L.; Zamorano, J.L. European association of echocardiography recommendations for the assessment of valvular regurgitation. Part 2: Mitral and tricuspid regurgitation (native valve disease). *Eur. J. Echocardiogr.* **2010**, *11*, 307–332. [CrossRef] [PubMed]
28. Shibata, T.; Takahashi, Y.; Fujii, H.; Morisaki, A.; Abe, Y. Surgical considerations for atrial functional regurgitation of the mitral and tricuspid valves based on the etiological mechanism. *Gen. Thorac. Cardiovasc. Surg.* **2021**, *69*, 1041–1049. [CrossRef] [PubMed]
29. Baumgartner, H.; Falk, V.; Bax, J.J.; De Bonis, M.; Hamm, C.; Holm, P.J.; Iung, B.; Lancellotti, P.; Lansac, E.; Rodriguez Muñoz, D.; et al. 2017 ESC/EACTS Guidelines for the Management of Valvular Heart Disease. *Eur. J. Cardio-Thorac. Surg.* **2017**, *52*, 616–664. [CrossRef]
30. Badano, L.; Pardo, A.; Muraru, D.; Zamorano, J. Acquired tricuspid valve diseases. In *Hurst's the Heart*, 15th ed.; Fuster, V., Harrington, R., Narula, J., Eapen, Z., Eds.; McGraw-Hill Education: New York, NY, USA, 2021.
31. Prihadi, E.A.; Delgado, V.; Hahn, R.T.; Leipsic, J.; Min, J.K.; Bax, J.J. Imaging Needs in Novel Transcatheter Tricuspid Valve Interventions. *JACC Cardiovasc. Imaging* **2018**, *11*, 736–754. [CrossRef]
32. Agricola, E.; Asmarats, L.; Maisano, F.; Cavalcante, J.L.; Liu, S.; Milla, F.; Meduri, C.; Rodés-Cabau, J.; Vannan, M.; Pibarot, P. Imaging for Tricuspid Valve Repair and Replacement. *JACC Cardiovasc. Imaging* **2021**, *14*, 61–111. [CrossRef] [PubMed]
33. Hahn, R.T.; Nabauer, M.; Zuber, M.; Nazif, T.M.; Hausleiter, J.; Taramasso, M.; Pozzoli, A.; George, I.; Kodali, S.; Bapat, V.; et al. Intraprocedural Imaging of Transcatheter Tricuspid Valve Interventions. *JACC Cardiovasc. Imaging* **2019**, *12*, 532–553. [CrossRef] [PubMed]
34. Fukuda, S.; Saracino, G.; Matsumura, Y.; Daimon, M.; Tran, H.; Greenberg, N.L.; Hozumi, T.; Yoshikawa, J.; Thomas, J.D.; Shiota, T. Three-dimensional geometry of the tricuspid annulus in healthy subjects and in patients with functional tricuspid regurgitation: A real-time, 3-dimensional echocardiographic study. *Circulation* **2006**, *114*, I492–I498. [CrossRef]
35. Anwar, A.M.; Geleijnse, M.L.; Soliman, O.I.I.; McGhie, J.S.; Frowijn, R.; Nemes, A.; van den Bosch, A.E.; Galema, T.W.; Ten Cate, F.J. Assessment of normal tricuspid valve anatomy in adults by real-time three-dimensional echocardiography. *Int. J. Cardiovasc. Imaging* **2007**, *23*, 717–724. [CrossRef] [PubMed]
36. Addetia, K.; Muraru, D.; Veronesi, F.; Jenei, C.; Cavalli, G.; Besser, S.A.; Mor-Avi, V.; Lang, R.M.; Badano, L.P. 3-Dimensional Echocardiographic Analysis of the Tricuspid Annulus Provides New Insights Into Tricuspid Valve Geometry and Dynamics. *JACC Cardiovasc. Imaging* **2019**, *12*, 401–412. [CrossRef]
37. Khalique, O.K.; Cavalcante, J.L.; Shah, D.; Guta, A.C.; Zhan, Y.; Piazza, N.; Muraru, D. Multimodality Imaging of the Tricuspid Valve and Right Heart Anatomy. *JACC Cardiovasc. Imaging* **2019**, *12*, 516–531. [CrossRef] [PubMed]
38. Topilsky, Y.; Maltais, S.; Medina Inojosa, J.; Oguz, D.; Michelena, H.; Maalouf, J.; Mahoney, D.W.; Enriquez-Sarano, M. Burden of Tricuspid Regurgitation in Patients Diagnosed in the Community Setting. *JACC Cardiovasc. Imaging* **2019**, *12*, 433–442. [CrossRef]
39. Afilalo, J.; Grapsa, J.; Nihoyannopoulos, P.; Beaudoin, J.; Gibbs, J.S.; Channick, R.N.; Langleben, D.; Rudski, L.G.; Hua, L.; Handschumacher, M.D.; et al. Leaflet Area as a Determinant of Tricuspid Regurgitation Severity in Patients with Pulmonary Hypertension. *Circ. Cardiovasc. Imaging* **2015**, *8*, e002714. [CrossRef] [PubMed]
40. Badano, L.P.; Hahn, R.; Zanella, H.; Araiza Garaygordobil, D.; Ochoa-Jimenez, R.C.; Muraru, D. Morphological Assessment of the Tricuspid Apparatus and Grading Regurgitation Severity in Patients With Functional Tricuspid Regurgitation: Thinking Outside the Box. *JACC Cardiovasc. Imaging* **2019**, *12*, 652–664. [CrossRef]
41. Yamasaki, N.; Kondo, F.; Kubo, T.; Okawa, M.; Matsumura, Y.; Kitaoka, H.; Yabe, T.; Furuno, T.; Doi, Y. Severe tricuspid regurgitation in the aged: Atrial remodeling associated with long-standing atrial fibrillation. *J. Cardiol.* **2006**, *48*, 315–323.
42. Muraru, D.; Addetia, K.; Guta, A.C.; Ochoa-Jimenez, R.C.; Genovese, D.; Veronesi, F.; Basso, C.; Iliceto, S.; Badano, L.P.; Lang, R.M. Right atrial volume is a major determinant of tricuspid annulus area in functional tricuspid regurgitation: A three-dimensional echocardiographic study. *Eur. Heart J. Cardiovasc. Imaging* **2020**, *22*, 660–669. [CrossRef] [PubMed]
43. Utsunomiya, H.; Itabashi, Y.; Mihara, H.; Berdejo, J.; Kobayashi, S.; Siegel, R.J.; Shiota, T. Functional Tricuspid Regurgitation Caused by Chronic Atrial Fibrillation: A Real-Time 3-Dimensional Transesophageal Echocardiography Study. *Circ. Cardiovasc. Imaging* **2017**, *10*, 1–11. [CrossRef]
44. Najib, M.Q.; Vinales, K.L.; Vittala, S.S.; Challa, S.; Lee, H.R.; Chaliki, H.P. Predictors for the Development of Severe Tricuspid Regurgitation with Anatomically Normal Valve in Patients with Atrial Fibrillation. *Echocardiography* **2012**, *29*, 140–146. [CrossRef]

45. Nemoto, N.; Lesser, J.R.; Pedersen, W.R.; Sorajja, P.; Spinner, E.; Garberich, R.F.; Vock, D.M.; Schwartz, R.S. Pathogenic structural heart changes in early tricuspid regurgitation. *J. Thorac. Cardiovasc. Surg.* **2015**, *150*, 323–330. [CrossRef] [PubMed]
46. Otto, C.M.; Nishimura, R.A.; Bonow, R.O.; Carabello, B.A.; Erwin, J.P., 3rd; Gentile, F.; Jneid, H.; Krieger, E.V.; Mack, M.; McLeod, C.; et al. 2020 ACC/AHA Guideline for the Management of Patients With Valvular Heart Disease: Executive Summary: A Report of the American College of Cardiology/American Heart Association Joint Committee on Clinical Practice Guidelines. *J. Am. Coll. Cardiol.* **2021**, *77*, 450–500. [CrossRef]
47. Federico Fortuni, M.D.; Marlieke FDietz, M.D.; Edgard APrihadi, M.D.; Pieter van der Bijl, M.D.; Gaetano MDe Ferrari, M.D.; Jeroen JBax, M.D.; Victoria Delgado, M.D.; Nina Ajmone Marsan, M.P. Ratio between vena contracta width and tricuspid annular diameter: Prognostic value in secondary tricuspid regurgitation. *J. Am. Soc. Echocardiogr.* **2021**, *34*, 944–954. [CrossRef]
48. Taramasso, M.; Benfari, G.; van der Bijl, P.; Alessandrini, H.; Attinger-Toller, A.; Biasco, L.; Lurz, P.; Braun, D.; Brochet, E.; Connelly, K.A.; et al. Transcatheter Versus Medical Treatment of Patients With Symptomatic Severe Tricuspid Regurgitation. *J. Am. Coll. Cardiol.* **2019**, *74*, 2998–3008. [CrossRef]
49. Fender, E.A.; Zack, C.J.; Nishimura, R.A. Isolated tricuspid regurgitation: Outcomes and therapeutic interventions. *Heart* **2018**, *104*, 798–806. [CrossRef]
50. Wang, J.; Li, S.; Ye, Q.; Ma, X.; Zhao, Y.; Han, J.; Li, Y.; Zheng, S.; Liu, K.; He, M.; et al. Catheter ablation or surgical therapy in moderate-severe tricuspid regurgitation caused by long-standing persistent atrial fibrillation. Propensity score analysis. *J. Cardiothorac. Surg.* **2020**, *15*, 277. [CrossRef]
51. Markman, T.M.; Plappert, T.; de Feria Alsina, A.; Levin, M.; Amankwah, N.; Sheth, S.; Gertz, Z.M.; Schaller, R.D.; Marchlinski, F.E.; Rame, J.E.; et al. Improvement in tricuspid regurgitation following catheter ablation of atrial fibrillation. *J. Cardiovasc. Electrophysiol.* **2020**, *31*, 2883–2888. [CrossRef] [PubMed]
52. Itakura, K.; Hidaka, T.; Nakano, Y.; Utsunomiya, H.; Kinoshita, M.; Susawa, H.; Harada, Y.; Izumi, K.; Kihara, Y. Successful catheter ablation of persistent atrial fibrillation is associated with improvement in functional tricuspid regurgitation and right heart reverse remodeling. *Heart Vessel.* **2020**, *35*, 842–851. [CrossRef] [PubMed]
53. Hahn, R.T.; Meduri, C.U.; Davidson, C.J.; Lim, S.; Nazif, T.M.; Ricciardi, M.J.; Rajagopal, V.; Ailawadi, G.; Vannan, M.A.; Thomas, J.D.; et al. Early Feasibility Study of a Transcatheter Tricuspid Valve Annuloplasty: SCOUT Trial 30-Day Results. *J. Am. Coll. Cardiol.* **2017**, *69*, 1795–1806. [CrossRef]
54. Miura, M.; Alessandrini, H.; Alkhodair, A.; Attinger-Toller, A.; Biasco, L.; Lurz, P.; Braun, D.; Brochet, E.; Connelly, K.A.; de Bruijn, S.; et al. Impact of Massive or Torrential Tricuspid Regurgitation in Patients Undergoing Transcatheter Tricuspid Valve Intervention. *JACC Cardiovasc. Interv.* **2020**, *13*, 1999–2009. [CrossRef] [PubMed]
55. Rodés-Cabau, J.; Hahn, R.T.; Latib, A.; Laule, M.; Lauten, A.; Maisano, F.; Schofer, J.; Campelo-Parada, F.; Puri, R.; Vahanian, A. Transcatheter Therapies for Treating Tricuspid Regurgitation. *J. Am. Coll. Cardiol.* **2016**, *67*, 1829–1845. [CrossRef] [PubMed]
56. Hahn, R.T.; Zamorano, J.L. The need for a new tricuspid regurgitation grading scheme. *Eur. Heart J. Cardiovasc. Imaging* **2017**, *18*, 1342–1343. [CrossRef] [PubMed]
57. Go, Y.Y.; Dulgheru, R.; Lancellotti, P. The Conundrum of Tricuspid Regurgitation Grading. *Front. Cardiovasc. Med.* **2018**, *5*, 3–6. [CrossRef]
58. Peri, Y.; Sadeh, B.; Sherez, C.; Hochstadt, A.; Biner, S.; Aviram, G.; Ingbir, M.; Nachmany, I.; Topaz, G.; Flint, N.; et al. Quantitative assessment of effective regurgitant orifice: Impact on risk stratification, and cut-off for severe and torrential tricuspid regurgitation grade. *Eur. Heart J. Cardiovasc. Imaging* **2020**, *21*, 768–776. [CrossRef] [PubMed]
59. Fortuni, F.; Dietz, M.F.; Prihadi, E.A.; van der Bijl, P.; De Ferrari, G.M.; Knuuti, J.; Bax, J.J.; Delgado, V.; Marsan, N.A. Prognostic Implications of a Novel Algorithm to Grade Secondary Tricuspid Regurgitation. *JACC Cardiovasc. Imaging* **2021**, *14*, 1085–1095. [CrossRef] [PubMed]
60. Taramasso, M.; Gavazzoni, M.; Pozzoli, A.; Dreyfus, G.D.; Bolling, S.F.; George, I.; Kapos, I.; Tanner, F.C.; Zuber, M.; Maisano, F. Tricuspid Regurgitation: Predicting the Need for Intervention, Procedural Success, and Recurrence of Disease. *JACC Cardiovasc. Imaging* **2019**, *12*, 605–621. [CrossRef] [PubMed]
61. Taramasso, M.; Alessandrini, H.; Latib, A.; Asami, M.; Attinger-Toller, A.; Biasco, L.; Braun, D.; Brochet, E.; Connelly, K.A.; Denti, P.; et al. Outcomes After Current Transcatheter Tricuspid Valve Intervention: Mid-Term Results From the International TriValve Registry. *JACC Cardiovasc. Interv.* **2019**, *12*, 155–165. [CrossRef]
62. Volpato, V.; Badano, L.P.; Figliozzi, S.; Florescu, D.R.; Parati, G.; Muraru, D. Multimodality cardiac imaging and new display options to broaden our understanding of the tricuspid valve. *Curr. Opin. Cardiol.* **2021**, *36*, 1085–1095. [CrossRef] [PubMed]
63. Caravita, S.; Figliozzi, S.; Florescu, D.R.; Volpato, V.; Oliverio, G.; Tomaselli, M.; Torlasco, C.; Muscogiuri, G.; Cernigliaro, F.; Parati, G.; et al. Recent advances in multimodality imaging of the tricuspid valve. *Expert Rev. Med. Devices* **2021**, *18*, 1069–1081. [CrossRef]
64. Praz, F.; Khalique, O.K.; dos Reis Macedo, L.G.; Pulerwitz, T.C.; Jantz, J.; Wu, I.Y.; Kantor, A.; Patel, A.; Vahl, T.; Bapat, V.; et al. Comparison between Three-Dimensional Echocardiography and Computed Tomography for Comprehensive Tricuspid Annulus and Valve Assessment in Severe Tricuspid Regurgitation: Implications for Tricuspid Regurgitation Grading and Transcatheter Therapies. *J. Am. Soc. Echocardiogr. Off. Publ. Am. Soc. Echocardiogr.* **2018**, *31*, 1190–1202.e3. [CrossRef]
65. Hahn, R.T. State-of-the-art review of echocardiographic imaging in the evaluation and treatment of functional tricuspid regurgitation. *Circ. Cardiovasc. Imaging* **2016**, *9*, 1–15. [CrossRef]

66. Asmarats, L.; Puri, R.; Latib, A.; Navia, J.L.; Rodés-Cabau, J. Transcatheter Tricuspid Valve Interventions. *J. Am. Coll. Cardiol.* **2018**, *71*, 2935–2956. [CrossRef]
67. Patrizio, L.; Luis, Z.J.; Habib Gilbert, B.L. *The EACVI Textbook of Echocardiography*; Oxford University Press: Oxford, UK, 2017; Available online: https://www.oupjapan.co.jp/en/node/16697 (accessed on 8 October 2021).
68. Zoghbi, W.A.; Adams, D.; Bonow, R.O.; Enriquez-Sarano, M.; Foster, E.; Grayburn, P.A.; Hahn, R.T.; Han, Y.; Hung, J.; Lang, R.M.; et al. Recommendations for Noninvasive Evaluation of Native Valvular Regurgitation: A Report from the American Society of Echocardiography Developed in Collaboration with the Society for Cardiovascular Magnetic Resonance. *J. Am. Soc. Echocardiogr.* **2017**, *30*, 303–371. [CrossRef]
69. Zaidi, A.; Oxborough, D.; Augustine, D.X.; Bedair, R.; Harkness, A.; Rana, B.; Robinson, S.; Badano, L.P. Echocardiographic assessment of the tricuspid and pulmonary valves: A practical guideline from the British Society of Echocardiography. *Echo Res. Pract.* **2020**, *7*, G95–G122. [CrossRef]
70. Hahn, R.T.; Thomas, J.D.; Khalique, O.K.; Cavalcante, J.L.; Praz, F.; Zoghbi, W.A. Imaging Assessment of Tricuspid Regurgitation Severity. *JACC Cardiovasc. Imaging* **2019**, *12*, 469–490. [CrossRef] [PubMed]
71. Abdellaziz, D.; Geraldine, O.; Nadira, H.; Eleonora, A.; Jing, Y.; Hahn, R.T. Quantifying Tricuspid Regurgitation Severity. *JACC Cardiovasc. Imaging* **2019**, *12*, 560–562. [CrossRef]
72. Addetia, K.; Muraru, D.; Badano, L.P.; Lang, R.M. New Directions in Right Ventricular Assessment Using 3-Dimensional Echocardiography. *JAMA Cardiol.* **2019**, *4*, 936–944. [CrossRef] [PubMed]
73. Muraru, D.; Hahn, R.T.; Soliman, O.I.; Faletra, F.F.; Basso, C.; Badano, L.P. 3-Dimensional Echocardiography in Imaging the Tricuspid Valve. *JACC Cardiovasc. Imaging* **2019**, *12*, 500–515. [CrossRef]
74. Hahn, R.T.; Weckbach, L.T.; Noack, T.; Hamid, N.; Kitamura, M.; Bae, R.; Lurz, P.; Kodali, S.K.; Sorajja, P.; Hausleiter, J.; et al. Proposal for a Standard Echocardiographic Tricuspid Valve Nomenclature. *JACC Cardiovasc. Imaging* **2021**, *14*, 1299–1305. [CrossRef]
75. Muraru, D.; Badano, L.P.; Sarais, C.; Soldà, E.; Iliceto, S. Evaluation of tricuspid valve morphology and function by transthoracic three-dimensional echocardiography. *Curr. Cardiol. Rep.* **2011**, *13*, 242–249. [CrossRef]
76. Karagodin, I.; Yamat, M.; Addetia, K.; Lang, R.M. Visualization of Number of Tricuspid Valve Leaflets Using Three-Dimensional Transthoracic Echocardiography. *J. Am. Soc. Echocardiogr. Off. Publ. Am. Soc. Echocardiogr.* **2021**, *34*, 449–450. [CrossRef]
77. Miglioranza, M.H.; Mihăilă, S.; Muraru, D.; Cucchini, U.; Iliceto, S.; Badano, L.P. Dynamic changes in tricuspid annular diameter measurement in relation to the echocardiographic view and timing during the cardiac cycle. *J. Am. Soc. Echocardiogr. Off. Publ. Am. Soc. Echocardiogr.* **2015**, *28*, 226–235. [CrossRef]
78. Miglioranza, M.H.; Mihăilă, S.; Muraru, D.; Cucchini, U.; Iliceto, S.; Badano, L.P. Variability of Tricuspid Annulus Diameter Measurement in Healthy Volunteers. *JACC Cardiovasc. Imaging* **2015**, *8*, 864–866. [CrossRef] [PubMed]
79. Ton-Nu, T.T.; Levine, R.A.; Handschumacher, M.D.; Dorer, D.J.; Yosefy, C.; Fan, D.; Hua, L.; Jiang, L.; Hung, J. Geometric determinants of functional tricuspid regurgitation: Insights from 3-dimensional echocardiography. *Circulation* **2006**, *114*, 143–149. [CrossRef] [PubMed]
80. Volpato, V.; Lang, R.M.; Yamat, M.; Veronesi, F.; Weinert, L.; Tamborini, G.; Muratori, M.; Fusini, L.; Pepi, M.; Genovese, D.; et al. Echocardiographic Assessment of the Tricuspid Annulus: The Effects of the Third Dimension and Measurement Methodology. *J. Am. Soc. Echocardiogr. Off. Publ. Am. Soc. Echocardiogr.* **2019**, *32*, 238–247. [CrossRef]
81. Badano, L.; Caravita, S.; Rella, V.; Guida, V.; Parati, G.; Muraru, D. The Added Value of 3-Dimensional Echocardiography to Understand the Pathophysiology of Functional Tricuspid Regurgitation. *JACC Cardiovasc. Imaging* **2021**, *14*, 683–689. [CrossRef]
82. Mihalcea, D.; Guta, A.C.; Caravita, S.; Parati, G.; Vinereanu, D.; Badano, L.P.; Muraru, D. Sex, body size and right atrial volume are the main determinants of tricuspid annulus geometry in healthy volunteers. A 3D echo study using a novel, commercially-available dedicated software package. *Eur. Heart J.* **2020**, *41* (Suppl. 2). [CrossRef]
83. Muraru, D.; Spadotto, V.; Cecchetto, A.; Romeo, G.; Aruta, P.; Ermacora, D.; Jenei, C.; Cucchini, U.; Iliceto, S.; Badano, L.P. New speckle-tracking algorithm for right ventricular volume analysis from three-dimensional echocardiographic data sets: Validation with cardiac magnetic resonance and comparison with the previous analysis tool. *Eur. Heart J. Cardiovasc. Imaging* **2016**, *17*, 1279–1289. [CrossRef]
84. Moreno, J.; de Isla, L.P.; Campos, N.; Guinea, J.; Domínguez-Perez, L.; Saltijeral, A.; Lennie, V.; Quezada, M.; de Agustín, A.; Marcos-Alberca, P.; et al. Right atrial indexed volume in healthy adult population: Reference values for two-dimensional and three-dimensional echocardiographic measurements. *Echocardiography* **2013**, *30*, 667–671. [CrossRef] [PubMed]
85. Besler, C.; Orban, M.; Rommel, K.P.; Braun, D.; Patel, M.; Hagl, C.; Borger, M.; Nabauer, M.; Massberg, S.; Thiele, H.; et al. Predictors of Procedural and Clinical Outcomes in Patients With Symptomatic Tricuspid Regurgitation Undergoing Transcatheter Edge-to-Edge Repair. *JACC Cardiovasc. Interv.* **2018**, *11*, 1119–1128. [CrossRef] [PubMed]
86. Lurz, P.; Besler, C.; Noack, T.; Forner, A.F.; Bevilacqua, C.; Seeburger, J.; Rommel, K.P.; Blazek, S.; Hartung, P.; Zimmer, M.; et al. Transcatheter treatment of tricuspid regurgitation using edge-to-edge repair: Procedural results, clinical implications and predictors of success. *EuroIntervention* **2018**, *14*, e290–e297. [CrossRef] [PubMed]
87. Kitamura, M.; Kresoja, K.P.; Besler, C.; Leontyev, S.; Kiefer, P.; Rommel, K.P.; Otto, W.; Forner, A.F.; Ender, J.; Holzhey, D.M.; et al. Impact of Tricuspid Valve Morphology on Clinical Outcomes After Transcatheter Edge-to-Edge Repair. *JACC Cardiovasc. Interv.* **2021**, *14*, 1616–1618. [CrossRef]

88. Karam, N.; Mehr, M.; Taramasso, M.; Besler, C.; Ruf, T.; Connelly, K.A.; Weber, M.; Yzeiraj, E.; Schiavi, D.; Mangieri, A.; et al. Value of Echocardiographic Right Ventricular and Pulmonary Pressure Assessment in Predicting Transcatheter Tricuspid Repair Outcome. *JACC Cardiovasc. Interv.* **2020**, *13*, 1251–1261. [CrossRef]
89. Kramer, C.M.; Barkhausen, J.; Bucciarelli-Ducci, C.; Flamm, S.D.; Kim, R.J.; Nagel, E. Standardized cardiovascular magnetic resonance imaging (CMR) protocols: 2020 update. *J. Cardiovasc. Magn. Reson.* **2020**, *22*, 17. [CrossRef]
90. Gatehouse, P.; Rolf, M.; Graves, M.; Hofman, M.B.; Totman, J.; Werner, B.; Quest, R.A.; Liu, Y.; von Spiczak, J.; Dieringer, M. Flow measurement by cardiovascular magnetic resonance: A multi-centre multi-vendor study of background phase offset errors that can compromise the accuracy of derived regurgitant or shunt flow measurements. *J. Cardiovasc. Magn. Reson.* **2010**, *12*, 5. [CrossRef]
91. Feneis, J.F.; Kyubwa, E.; Atianzar, K.; Cheng, J.Y.; Alley, M.T.; Vasanawala, S.S.; Demaria, A.N.; Hsiao, A. 4D flow MRI quantification of mitral and tricuspid regurgitation: Reproducibility and consistency relative to conventional MRI. *J. Magn. Reson. Imaging JMRI* **2018**, *48*, 1147–1158. [CrossRef]
92. Kamphuis, V.P.; Westenberg, J.J.M.; van den Boogaard, P.J.; Clur, S.A.B.; Roest, A.A.W. Direct assessment of tricuspid regurgitation by 4D flow cardiovascular magnetic resonance in a patient with Ebstein's anomaly. *Eur. Heart J. Cardiovasc. Imaging* **2018**, *19*, 587. [CrossRef]
93. Kabasawa, M.; Kohno, H.; Ishizaka, T.; Ishida, K.; Funabashi, N.; Kataoka, A.; Matsumiya, G. Assessment of functional tricuspid regurgitation using 320-detector-row multislice computed tomography: Risk factor analysis for recurrent regurgitation after tricuspid annuloplasty. *J. Thorac. Cardiovasc. Surg.* **2014**, *147*, 312–320. [CrossRef] [PubMed]
94. Lopes, B.B.C.; Hashimoto, G.; Bapat, V.N.; Sorajja, P.; Scherer, M.D.; Cavalcante, J.L. Cardiac Computed Tomography and Magnetic Resonance Imaging of the Tricuspid Valve: Preprocedural Planning and Postprocedural Follow-up. *Interv. Cardiol. Clin.* **2022**, *11*, 27–40. [CrossRef] [PubMed]
95. Therkelsen, S.K.; Groenning, B.A.; Svendsen, J.H.; Jensen, G.B. Atrial and ventricular volume and function in persistent and permanent atrial fibrillation, a magnetic resonance imaging study. *J. Cardiovasc. Magn. Reson. Off. J. Soc. Cardiovasc. Magn. Reson.* **2005**, *7*, 465–473. [CrossRef] [PubMed]
96. Kocaoglu, M.; Pednekar, A.S.; Wang, H.; Alsaied, T.; Taylor, M.D.; Rattan, M.S. Breath-hold and free-breathing quantitative assessment of biventricular volume and function using compressed SENSE: A clinical validation in children and young adults. *J. Cardiovasc. Magn. Reson.* **2020**, *22*, 54. [CrossRef] [PubMed]
97. Xue, H.; Kellman, P.; Larocca, G.; Arai, A.E.; Hansen, M.S. High spatial and temporal resolution retrospective cine cardiovascular magnetic resonance from shortened free breathing real-time acquisitions. *J. Cardiovasc. Magn. Reson.* **2013**, *15*, 102. [CrossRef] [PubMed]
98. Pulerwitz, T.C.; Khalique, O.K.; Leb, J.; Hahn, R.T.; Nazif, T.M.; Leon, M.B.; George, I.; Vahl, T.P.; D'Souza, B.; Bapat, V.N.; et al. Optimizing Cardiac CT Protocols for Comprehensive Acquisition Prior to Percutaneous MV and TV Repair/Replacement. *JACC Cardiovasc. Imaging* **2020**, *13*, 836–850. [CrossRef] [PubMed]
99. Pappalardo, O.A.; Votta, E.; Selmi, M.; Luciani, G.B.; Redaelli, A.; Delgado, V.; Bax, J.J.; Ajmone Marsan, N. 4D MDCT in the assessment of the tricuspid valve and its spatial relationship with the right coronary artery: A customized tool based on computed tomography for the planning of percutaneous procedures. *J. Cardiovasc. Comput. Tomogr.* **2020**, *14*, 520–523. [CrossRef]
100. Surkova, E.; Muraru, D.; Iliceto, S.; Badano, L.P. The use of multimodality cardiovascular imaging to assess right ventricular size and function. *Int. J. Cardiol.* **2016**, *214*, 54–69. [CrossRef]
101. Hell, M.M.; Emrich, T.; Kreidel, F.; Kreitner, K.F.; Schoepf, U.J.; Münzel, T.; von Bardeleben, R.S. Computed tomography imaging needs for novel transcatheter tricuspid valve repair and replacement therapies. *Eur. Heart J. Cardiovasc. Imaging* **2021**, *22*, 601–610. [CrossRef]
102. Faletra, F.F.; Pedrazzini, G.; Pasotti, E.; Murzilli, R.; Leo, L.A.; Moccetti, T. Echocardiography–X-Ray Image Fusion. *JACC Cardiovasc. Imaging* **2016**, *9*, 1114–1117. [CrossRef]
103. Pascual, I.; Pozzoli, A.; Taramasso, M.; Maisano, F.; Ho, E.C. Fusion imaging for transcatheter mitral and tricuspid interventions. *Ann. Transl. Med.* **2020**, *8*, 965. [CrossRef] [PubMed]
104. Fortuni, F.; Marques, A.I.; Bax, J.J.; Ajmone Marsan, N.; Delgado, V. Echocardiography-computed tomography fusion imaging for guidance of transcatheter tricuspid valve annuloplasty. *Eur. Heart J. Cardiovasc. Imaging* **2020**, *21*, 937–938. [CrossRef] [PubMed]
105. Anastasius, M.; Tang, G.H.L.; Love, B.; Krishnamoorthy, P.; Sharma, S.; Kini, A.; Lerakis, S. A Novel Hybrid Imaging Approach for Guidance of Percutaneous Transcatheter Tricuspid Valve Edge-to-Edge Repair. *J. Am. Soc. Echocardiogr. Off. Publ. Am. Soc. Echocardiogr.* **2021**, *34*, 567–568. [CrossRef] [PubMed]

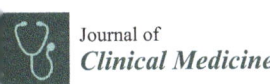

Review

Imaging in Transcatheter Mitral Valve Replacement: State-of-Art Review

Manuel Barreiro-Perez *, Berenice Caneiro-Queija, Luis Puga, Rocío Gonzalez-Ferreiro, Robert Alarcon, Jose Antonio Parada, Andrés Iñiguez-Romo and Rodrigo Estevez-Loureiro

Cardiology Department, University Hospital Alvaro Cunqueiro, Galicia Sur Health Research Institute (IISGS), 36213 Vigo, Pontevedra, Spain; bcanque@gmail.com (B.C.-Q.); luis.romeu.puga@gmail.com (L.P.); ferreiro_44@hotmail.com (R.G.-F.); dr.alarcon1587@hotmail.com (R.A.); chechocat94@gmail.com (J.A.P.); andres.iniguez.romo@sergas.es (A.I.-R.); roiestevez@hotmail.com (R.E.-L.)
* Correspondence: manuelbarreiroperez@gmail.com; Tel.: +34-98-681-1111 (ext. 514332)

Abstract: Mitral regurgitation is the second-most frequent valvular heart disease in Europe and it is associated with high morbidity and mortality. Recognition of MR should encourage the assessment of its etiology, severity, and mechanism in order to determine the best therapeutic approach. Mitral valve surgery constitutes the first-line therapy; however, transcatheter procedures have emerged as an alternative option to treat inoperable and high-risk surgical patients. In patients with suitable anatomy, the transcatheter edge-to-edge mitral leaflet repair is the most frequently applied procedure. In non-reparable patients, transcatheter mitral valve replacement (TMVR) has appeared as a promising intervention. Thus, currently TMVR represents a new treatment option for inoperable or high-risk patients with degenerated or failed bioprosthetic valves (valve-in-valve); failed repairs, (valve-in-ring); inoperable or high-risk patients with native mitral valve anatomy, or those with severe annular calcifications, or valve-in-mitral annular calcification. The patient selection requires multimodality imaging pre-procedural planning to select the best approach and device, study the anatomical landing zone and assess the risk of left ventricular outflow tract obstruction. In the present review, we aimed to highlight the main considerations for TMVR planning from an imaging perspective; before, during, and after TMVR.

Keywords: structural heart intervention; transcatheter mitral valve replacement; mitral regurgitation; transoesophageal echocardiography; cardiac computed tomography

1. Introduction

Mitral regurgitation (MR) is the second-most frequent valvular heart disease encountered in clinical practice in Europe [1], and it is associated with high morbidity and mortality [2]. Recognition of MR should encourage the assessment of its etiology, severity, and mechanism in order to determine the best therapeutic approach [3].

Mitral valve surgery constitutes the first-line therapy for patients with symptomatic severe MR [3]; however, up to 50% of those affected are not referred for surgery due to high risks [4].

In recent years, transcatheter procedures have emerged as an alternative option to treat inoperable and high-risk surgical patients [5]. The edge-to-edge leaflet repair system (TEER) represents the most frequently applied percutaneous transcatheter mitral valve procedure. In patients with suitable anatomy, it can be successful and safe [6]. The current European Valvular Heart Disease Management guidelines [3] give Class IIb recommendations for transcatheter mitral valve repair in symptomatic patients with severe primary MR despite optimal medical therapy, reasonable life expectancy but prohibitive surgical risk; and Class IIa recommendations for symptomatic patients with severe secondary MR fulfilling the anatomical inclusion criteria who are not eligible for surgery. However, due to the complexity and heterogeneity of mitral valve anatomy and pathology, some patients do

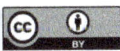

not meet the eligibility criteria for TEER and repair may be ineffective (rheumatic etiology, endocarditis-related valve disease, prior MV surgery, cleft or perforated mitral leaflets, lack of secondary chordal support, posterior leaflet length < 7 mm, leaflet gap > 2 mm, presence of severe calcifications in the grasping area, transmitral pressure gradient > 4 mmHg or MV area < 3.5 cm^2) [7].

Transcatheter mitral valve replacement (TMVR) has appeared as a promising intervention that may overcome some of the current limitations associated with TEER [8]. However, some limitations, such as apical access and the associated thoracotomy marked early experiences with TMVR. The development of transseptal TMVR, by means of improved technology in delivery systems, has allowed TMVR to grow. Transseptal access has shown that it is effective, safe, and also offers less morbidity and recovery time compared to the trans-apical approach [9]. Thus, currently TMVR represents a new treatment option for inoperable or high-risk patients with degenerated or failed bioprosthetic valves, valve-in-valve (ViV); failed repairs, valve-in-ring (ViR); inoperable or high-risk patients with native MV anatomy, or those with severe annular calcifications, or valve-in-mitral annular calcification (ViMAC) [10].

Despite the advancements, TMVR implies a not negligible risk of periprocedural and post-procedural complications [11], and still faces significant disadvantages [12]. The procedure is still not suitable for all, and the most common causes of TMVR exclusion are frailty, severe tricuspid regurgitation, prior aortic valve therapy, mitral anatomical exclusion, severe MAC, and the risk of left ventricular outflow tract (LVOT) obstruction [12].

In the present review, we aimed to highlight the main considerations for TMVR planning from an imaging perspective. This study reviews the role that multimodality cardiac imaging plays before, during, and after TMVR.

2. Imaging Overview

Advances in imaging have enabled the TMVR technique to evolve. Cardiovascular imaging has become a key player in diagnosis, pre-procedural planning, procedural guidance, and follow-up in TMVR therapies. Moreover, a patient-centered structural intervention team with the interventional and the imaging parties well familiarized with each other's tools, skills, language, and procedures are essential for a successful intervention [10].

A pre-procedure cardiac imaging examination, through multimodality imaging, is crucial to identify the severity, etiology, and mechanisms of MR; the coexistence with any degree of mitral stenosis or any other valvular abnormality, and to determine patient eligibility according to the anatomic measurements and anatomic variables used for every specific device. Also, the pre-TVMR cardiac imaging examination should help to predict the risk of potential procedural complications and their likelihood and to localize the most suitable points for access and puncture [12].

Pre-procedural transthoracic echocardiography (TTE) is mandatory and should be the first cardiac imaging examination for patients with a suspicion of mitral valve disease, as it is noninvasive and provides a first characterization of the magnitude and etiology of the mitral valve disease.

Beyond TTE, both transesophageal echocardiography (TEE) and cardiac computed tomography (CCT) modalities are the cornerstones for successful TMVR procedures [13,14]. TEE has the superiority of temporal resolution, hence, is the method of choice for mitral valve function and leaflet characterization. On the other hand, CCT is a non-invasive imaging technique with high isotropic spatial resolution and excellent calcification definition, offering ideal capabilities for a higher accuracy for 3D sizing and procedural simulation [10]. This multimodality imaging approach is, at the time, the gold standard for TMVR [15]. Table 1 shows the advantages and the preferred method for screening, peri-intervention assessment, and post-procedural follow-up.

Echocardiography screening is the first step to assess the indications for a valvular intervention. It includes characterization of the valvular disease mechanism, grading, as well as its impact on heart size and function. Moreover, evaluation of right heart cavities and pulmonary hypertension are important prognostic factors that should be noted [10]. Potential contraindications should also be sought, such as active endocarditis, intracardiac thrombus, or severe patient-prosthesis mismatch [16]. Determining the acoustic window quality and optimizing patient position are also important steps since procedural guidance relies on TEE imaging. 3D-TEE with multiplane reconstruction is a vitally important tool for the correct assessment of valvular or prosthetic valve anatomy, although acoustic shadowing due to extensive calcification, prosthetic heart valves, or annuloplasty rings may hinder a complete analysis of sub-valvular apparatus or LVOT. During the procedure, the echocardiographer will provide continuous image guidance with TEE in close collaboration with the interventional team. Bicaval, aortic short-axis and four-chamber views may help to select the appropriate septal puncture site (the ideal position usually slightly superior and posterior from the midpoint of the interatrial septum). TEE is also used to guide the advancement and positioning of the TMVR prosthesis within the native MV annulus. Simultaneous bicommissural-LVOT and 3D views are highly valuable for final adjustments, which are performed based on TEE image. Immediately after TMVR deployment TEE may help to assess perivalvular leak (PVL), residual MR, mitral gradients, rule out LVOT obstruction and gradients measurements.

Table 1. Suggested assessment steps for TMVR with preferred modalities.

Assessment Steps	TEE	CT
Screening		
Valve disease mechanism	+++	+
Chambers size	+++	++
LV/RV function and pulmonary hypertension	+++	+
Valve disease grading	+++	-
Calcification extension	+	+++
Contra-indications assessment		
Endocarditis	+++	+
Thrombus	+++	+++
Severe patient-prosthesis mismatch	+++	-
Peri-intervention		
Vascular access	-	+++
Annulus sizing	++	+++
Fusion imaging	++	+++
Interatrial septum assessment/transeptal punction planning	+++	+++
Fluoroscopic projection estimation	-	+++
Neo-LVOT size estimation	+	+++
3D simulation/printing	+	+++
Procedural guidance/Device deployment	+++	-
Post-procedural		
Prosthetic valve function	+++	+
Paravalvular leak	+++	++
Vascular complications	-	+++

+++ Preferred method; ++ alternative method; + incomplete assessment; - not possible.

Cardiac computed tomography (CCT) is considered to be essential for TMVR planning. Contrast-enhanced thin-sliced electrocardiography-gated CCT is mandatory. The use of retrospective gating covering the whole cardiac cycle with a 5–10% R-R interval reconstruction is highly recommended, and mandatory to cover the whole systolic phase [17]. CCT offers an isotropic sub-millimeter spatial resolution, facilitating accurate mitral geometry assessment and annular sizing [12]. CCT is employed to evaluate patient suitability according to all TMVR systems' official recommendations. There are some common anatomic points routinely evaluated for all TMVR valve systems, although other CCT-based measures are device-specific, leading to different CCT workup and evaluation algorithms for each valve system. The most relevant aspects of CCT evaluation before TVMR are mitral annulus measurements (intercommissural and anterior-posterior diameters, inter-trigone distance, perimeter, area and calcification assessment), mitral leaflets (length, thickness and calcification), interatrial septum anatomy, left atrial and left ventricle anatomy and LVOT characteristics (aorto-mitral angle, baseline area at systole and diastole and neo-LVOT assessment after virtual valve implantation) [10,12].

CCT also provides a detailed and clear definition of the extent and severity of annular calcium. Some measures such as maximal height and thickness of the observed calcification, the circumferential extension and trigone and leaflets involvement are used for the planning and stratification of TMVR embolization risk.

LVOT obstruction following TMVR is one of the most feared, and potentially fatal, complications. Therefore, recommendations have been issued regarding neo-LVOT estimation to screen and prevent this complication [18]. The neo-LVOT is the result of the dislodgment of the anterior leaflet of the mitral valve toward the ventricular septum [19]. The CCT virtual valve implantation and the evaluation of the neo-LVOT area on a 3D dedicated software best predicts the risk of LVOT obstruction (Figure 1). The predicted neo-LVOT is measured at mid-late-systole as the narrowest 2-dimensional area between the virtual valve and the ventricular septum [20]. Predicted neo-LVOT area < 200 mm^2 identifies patients at risk of significant LVOT obstruction; and a neo-LVOT area < 170 mm^2 has been shown to predict LVOT obstruction with 96.2% sensitivity and 92.3% specificity. Other observed features related to LVOT obstruction are the presence of a bulky septum (>15 mm thickness or <17.8 mm annulus-to-septal distance), an acute aorto-mitral angle (<110°), an elongated anterior mitral leaflet (>25 mm) and the presence of left ventricle small cavity size (end-diastolic diameter <48 mm), hypertrophy (LV mass index >105 g/m^2) or preserved ejection fraction [14,18]. Preemptive LVOT obstruction avoidance strategies have been reported in selected high-risk cases such as alcoholic septal ablation or LAMPOON techniques (base-to-tip [21]; tip-to-base or reverse LAMPOON [22], or anterograde LAMPOON [23]), although data regarding outcomes in large series are missing. A pre-procedural LVOT management algorithm has been recently published [19].

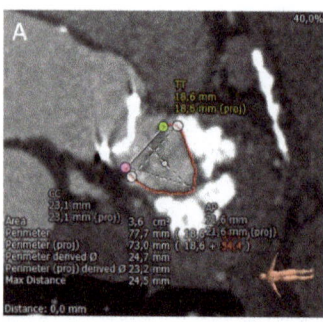 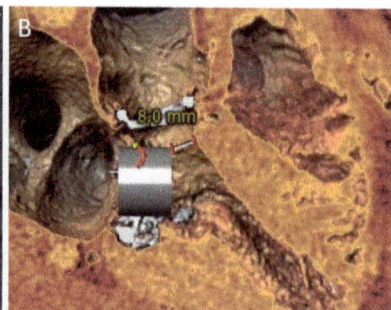 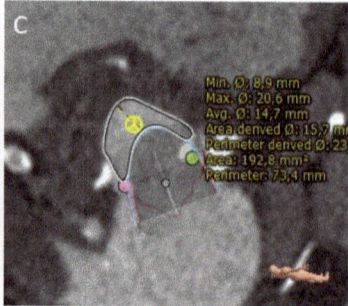

Figure 1. TMVR valve-in-MAC pre-procedural planning. (**A**) Mitral annular calcification with a 180° extension in the posterior and lateral aspect of mitral annulus. Internal dimensions can be noted on the image (TT: inter-trigone diameter; AP: anterior-posterior diameter; area and perimeter). (**B**) Three-dimensional virtual valve implantation (SAPIEN 3 23 mm) with a distance neo-valve to interventricular septum of 8 mm. (**C**) Neo-LVOT area according to the virtual valve implantation (Area 193 mm^2).

Furthermore, it facilitates procedure planning allowing for fluoroscopic projection estimation (en-face, two-chamber and three-chamber views) and access planning (Figure 2). CCT may help to select the most suitable location for transeptal (distance to mitral annular plane, thickness and morphology) or transapical puncture site (most appropriate intercostal space, distance from apex to mitral annular plane and trajectory avoiding any disturbance with papillary muscles). An abdominal-pelvic venous phase CT scan may be useful to evaluate vein diameters and tortuosity for a transeptal approach case.

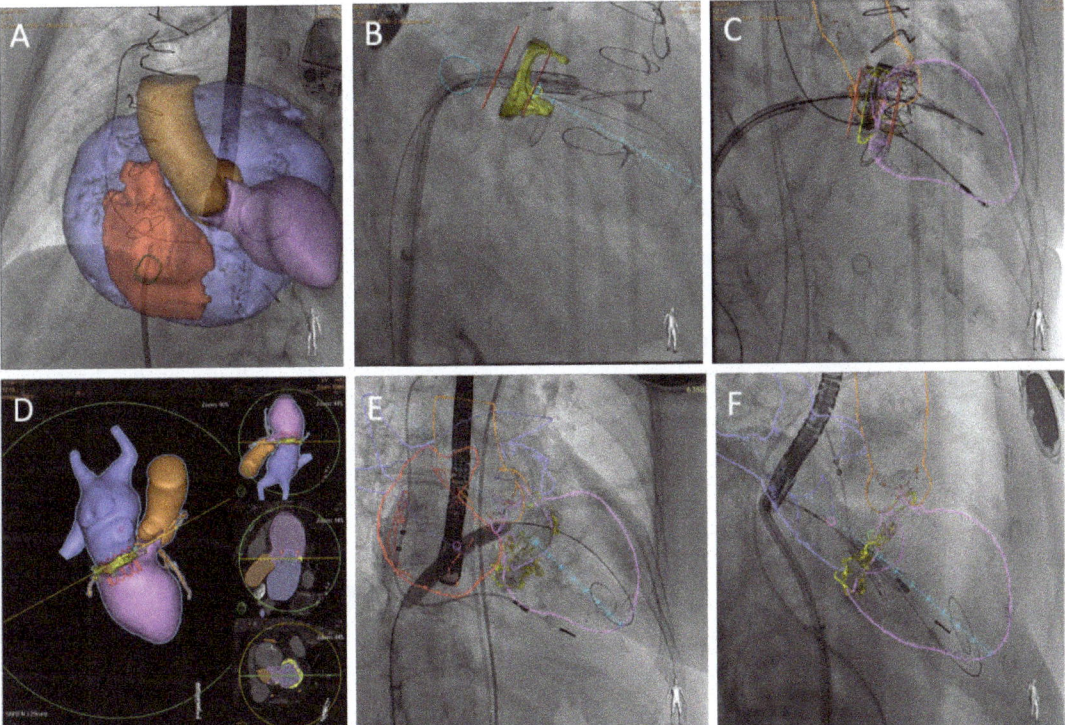

Figure 2. CT-fluoroscopy fusion imaging. The superior row shows a TMVR valve-in-valve procedure in a patient with extreme left atrium enlargement and modified projection required for transeptal puncture (**A**). Markers (red lines) may be over-imposed to fluoroscopy imaging to guide depth deployment (**B**,**C**). Inferior row, TMVR valve-in-MAC CT preprocedural planning (**D**), interatrial septal balloon dilatation (**E**) and initial phase of THV deployment with coaxial projection to mitral annulus (**F**).

3. TMVR: ViV, ViR, ViMAC

Reoperation in degenerated mitral surgical heart valves (SHV) or in failed surgical repair has a high mortality and morbidity risk. TMVR has demonstrated good outcomes for degenerated bioprosthetic valves (ViV) and acceptable results in failed mitral repair (ViR); making adequate patient selection, pre-procedural planning, and operator experience necessary. Transcatheter valve-in-valve implantation in the mitral and tricuspid position may be considered in selected patients at high risk for surgical reintervention according to the actual European guidelines [3].

Mitral annular calcification (MAC) is a degenerative age-dependent process leading to MR or mitral stenosis in severe cases. It has been linked to cardiovascular risk factors and other pathologies [24]. MAC patients tend to be poor candidates for mitral surgery due to technical challenges and the risk of complications.

Currently, experiences have been described with MAC disease using aortic THV and dedicated mitral THV devices [25].

3.1. Procedural Description

Procedural steps are described in detail in the literature [26]. Briefly, the TMVR procedure is usually performed under general anesthesia with TEE and fluoroscopic guidance. Regarding approaches, the transseptal and transapical represented the preferred ones. For vascular access, there is a general consensus that ultrasound guidance is considered the standard of care [27].

There is a growing interest in the transseptal approach, as it is the less invasive option. The anatomic target for the transseptal puncture varies by procedure [28]. In general, the preferred transseptal site puncture for TMVR procedures is mid-to-superior and posterior to the center of the fossa ovalis (approximately 3.5–4.0 cm over the mitral plane). Once the sheath enters the left atrium a 0.032-inch exchange wire is placed in the upper left pulmonary vein, if possible. Next, crossing the mitral valve is facilitated by the flexible Agilis catheter (St Jude Medical, St Paul, Minnesota) using a 5-Fr diagnostic catheter mounted on a standard 0.035-inch exchange wire. Then, a pigtail catheter is delivered into the left ventricle and a J-preshaped stiff wire (such the Safari wire, Boston Scientific) is advanced through. Afterward, the Agilis catheter is withdrawn and the atrial septum is dilated using 12–16 mm peripheral balloons. For the transseptal approach, the SAPIEN (Edwards Lifesciences, Irvine, CA, USA) valves are the most used transcatheter heart valves (THV). The SAPIEN 3, with a lower profile and smaller sheath, provides several advantages. In this case, the THV prosthesis must be mounted for antegrade implantation. Septal crossing is usually done under fluoroscopic and TEE guidance with no push. Positioning THV is executed in the projection perpendicular to the plane of the mitral annulus, carefully advancing the valve near the mitral orifice with the objective of 20–30% of the THV toward the left atrium and 70–80% toward the left ventricle. The implantation depth is adjusted so the external skirt of SAPIEN 3 connects throughout the landing zone. A more ventricular final position may provide better hemodynamic performance with less valvular gradient, but a higher risk of LVOT obstruction. On the other hand, a more atrial final position may provide lower neo-LVOT gradients, but a higher residual paravalvular and prosthetic embolization likelihood. TEE guidance plays an important role to define the appropriate landing zone. A THV valve is deployed by slowly balloon inflation under rapid ventricular pacing (140 beats/min is usually adequate). Post-deployment assessment with TEE is required to confirm optimal function (presence, severity and mechanisms of PVL, transmitral gradients and leaflets motion).

On the other hand, transapical approach provides easy and direct access to the mitral valve. The procedure requires general anesthesia and a transapical approach through the left mini-thoracotomy. The procedure is mainly executed under TEE guidance. Pre-dilatation of the mitral valve apparatus with balloon valvuloplasty catheter is done at the discretion of the local team. A 34Fr sheath is advanced over a soft 0.035 wire into the left atrium. The implant device is advanced into the sheath and then positioned at the level of mitral annulus. Pacing is not needed for deployment in some dedicated mitral THV devices but is still necessary for aortic THV employed for TMVR.

3.2. Clinical Results and Published Evidence

Observational data for ViV TMVR has demonstrated good outcomes for degenerated bioprosthetic valves with adequate patient selection, pre-procedural planning, and operator experience. Transcatheter valve-in-valve implantation in the mitral and tricuspid position may be considered in selected patients at high risk for surgical reintervention according to the actual European guidelines [3]. However, TMVR for ViR and ViMAC is associated with a higher risk of procedural complications and increased mortality following TMVR compared to ViV.

Recently, data from the TMVR multicenter registry was published by Yoon et al. [29] evaluating procedural success and outcomes in this patient population. 521 high-risk patients (STS 9%) were evaluated, with 322 ViV patients, 141 ViR patients, and 58 ViMAC patients. The majority of access was transapical; however, 39.5% were transseptal. Ninety percent used the balloon-expandable Sapien valve. Technical success was 89.1%, and a second valve implant was most frequently needed in ViR followed by ViMAC and ViV (12.1%, 5.2%, 2.5%, respectively). At 30 days, there was a higher residual significant MR in ViR (18.5%) and ViMAC (13.8%) compared to ViV (5.6%) procedures, probably due to a higher rate of PVL after TVMR. Patients with residual MR are known to have higher mortality. All-cause mortality was lower in ViR (9.9%; 30,6%) and ViV (6.2%; 14,0%) at both 30 days and 1 year respectively; compared with worse results with ViMAC (34.5%; 62.8%) [30].

TMVR ViMAC early experience with off-label use of aortic balloon-expandable THV is exposed in two retrospective registries [30,31] showing high 30 day and one year mortality (25–35% and 54–63%, respectively). The first prospective, multicenter clinical trial for ViMAC using balloon-expandable aortic THV has been recently published [32] showing lower mortality rates at 30 day and one year than previously reported (6.7% and 26%, in order). Considering the Tendyne valve in MAC patients, initial experience has indicated high procedure success and without procedure mortality. Nonetheless, the authors recognized a highly selected patient population [33]. Unlike ViV and ViR, which are more consolidated procedures and included in clinical care and guidelines recommendations; ViMAC is in an early phase of development and it should be reserved for selected patients in highly experienced centers.

No significant difference in mortality, stroke, valve embolization or need for conversion to surgery was observed in transseptal compared to transapical access. However, TMVR via transseptal access was associated with a lower rate of life-threatening or fatal bleeding.

3.3. Imaging Key Aspects

During deployment of a THV within a surgical ring, bioprosthetic valve, or MAC, the principal imaging concerns are device size selection, implantation depth, device coaxially respect to mitral annulus, and complete expansion within the constraining tissue (native or prosthetic).

(I) Valve-in-Valve: The essential parameters by CCT are SHV dimensions assessment (internal diameter, height, projection into left ventricle), SHV tissue-type (lower risk of LVOT obstruction with porcine SHVs) and prediction of neo-LVOT area. The internal diameter of the surgical heart valve determined by CT scan helps to choose the optimal THV size because the goal is to achieve a conical shape of the THV after implantation [34,35]. CT measurements are highly dependent on image quality, acquisition and reconstruction technique, prosthetic material opacity, and associated blooming, as well as measurement technique; but a precise sizing of the landing zone decreases valve embolization or migration. CT imaging is helpful to confirm surgical heart valve (SHV) size or to establish SHV size in patients with an unclear surgical history. Imaging-derived measurements maybe not be equivalent to the stent's true internal diameter, thus it can change for thickening and calcification of degenerated leaflets [36]. A smartphone app has been developed, and is available for different platforms, to assist SHV size selection before TMVR ViV [37,38].

The TMVR ViV procedure is guided by 3D-TEE (Figure 3) (transeptal puncture, coaxially alignment) and fluoroscopy (depth deployment). Immediately after THV deployment TEE is crucial to rule out LVOT obstruction, residual paravalvular regurgitation and THV hemodynamic performance (transvalvular gradient, intra-prosthetic residual regurgitation).

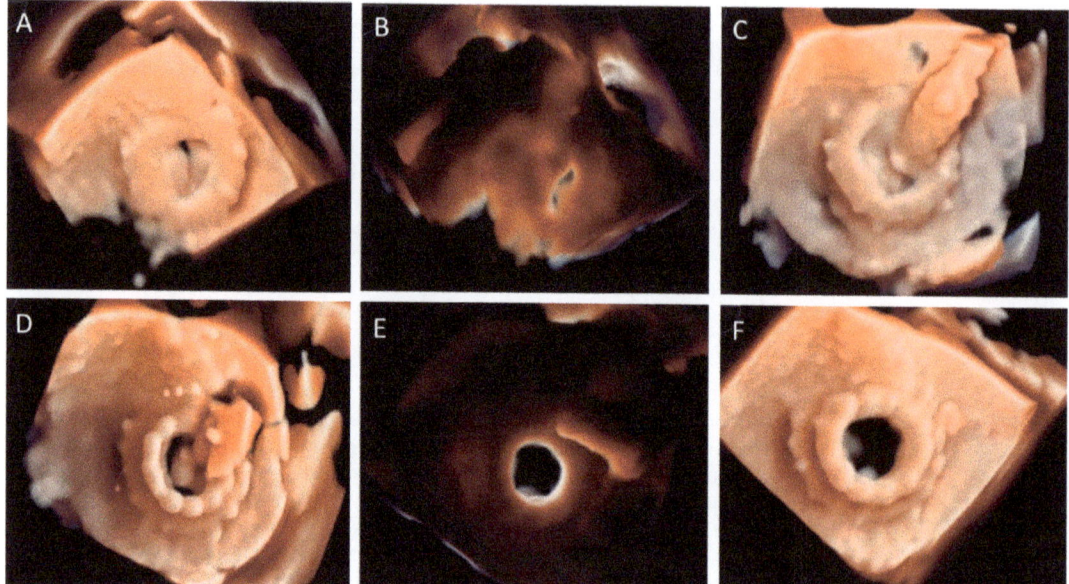

Figure 3. Three-dimensional transoesophageal echocardiography with photo-realistic rendering during TMVR valve-in-valve procedure. (**A**) En-face view of a degenerated mitral surgical prosthetic valve, with severe prosthetic stenosis. (**B**) Same image with light source place behind mitral prosthetic valve during diastole. Prosthetic leaflets thickening and mobility reduction can be easily noted. (**C**) THV positioning inside SHV. (**D**) Balloon-expandable THV deployment. (**E**) Immediate result after deployment. Same image configuration than (**B**), significant improvement in diastolic opening can be noted. (**F**) TMVR ViV final result en-face view.

(II) Valve-in-Ring: There are multiple types of surgical MV annuloplasty rings and not all are suitable for a TMVR ViR procedure. To conform an acceptable landing zone, the surgical ring must become complete and circular or nearly circular. CT imaging is helpful to assess ring shape and type, internal dimensions (diameters, area and perimeter), leaflets calcification, length of anterior leaflet and predicted neo-LVOT area. It is important to note that, according to THV size selection, the ring shape may change from oval to circular after TMVR, increasing its area. The intraprocedural TEE monitoring is employed to guide the THV approach (transeptal puncture and alignment) and to exclude complications as ring dehiscence or anterior leaflet displacement into LVOT after THV deployment.

(III) Valve-in-MAC: CCT is complementary to echocardiography and has been the imaging modality of choice to evaluate patients for TMVR ViMAC [6]. *The appropriate pre-procedural patient selection for Valve-in-MAC requires expertise, is time-consuming and it has to be on consideration several anatomical aspects. In the previous published series, only 33% of evaluated cases for ViMAC were finally acceptable for the TVMR procedure* [20]. First, CCT evaluation of mitral calcification comprises (i) description of quality: brittle, caseous or vastly dense calcium; (ii) distribution: circumferential or noncircumferential; and (iii) severity (based on semiquantitative approach): fleck-like (mild), coalescing (moderate) and bulky/protruding (severe). Furthermore, to grade the severity of MAC and predict valve embolization, a CT-based score has been proposed [33]. A score ≥ 7 points defines severe MAC. The presence of bilateral commissural calcification, as well as some anterior calcification, provides a better anchoring for ViMAC; a recommendation of 270° of contact is considered sufficient to achieve complete sealing. Multi-intensity thick-slab projections facilitate anatomy understanding to trace the area and perimeter measures. Determination of the landing zone (contact between the THV and the annular calcification) is often done at mid-to-late systole by tracing a 3D ellipsoid at the leaflet-annular insertion [19]. It also requires 3D image simulation of the device implantation. The extension and severity of calcification on the mitral annulus are used to determine the degree of THV oversizing. Some authors recommend a 10–25% degree of oversizing to prevent PVL and late migration of the valve [14]. CCT is also fundamental to estimate the risk of LVOT obstruction. Predicted neo-LVOT area < 200 mm^2 identifies patients at risk of significant LVOT obstruction demanding an adjunctive procedure, such as LAMPOON or septal reduction with transcoronary alcohol to ensure a safe procedure. Neo-LVOT area <100 mm^2 identifies very high-risk patients where ViMAC should be avoided. Besides the neo-LVOT area, other anatomical features have been recently related to neo-LVOT obstruction after TVMR ViMAC; systolic LVOT area, indexed neo-LVOT, expected LVOT area reduction, and virtual THV to septum distance [39]. The procedure is guided by TEE and is highly valuable for ruling out complications after THV deployment as anterior leaflet displacement into LVOT, assessing the risk of embolization, or detecting residual paravalvular regurgitation.

4. Valve in Native Mitral Valve Replacement

TMVR on native anatomy has several challenges because the mitral valve apparatus is a very complex dynamic system involving several structures, interacting with the left ventricle, the left atrium and the aortic valve [40,41]. The first is related to the size of the mitral annulus, usually dilated in chronic MR. Complete sealing and stable anchorage of the prosthesis to prevent embolization or displacement represent major concerns of TMVR and pose a challenge due to the large anatomical variability between organic and functional MR. Furthermore, due to the proximity to the aortic valve and the LVOT, TMVR poses an important risk for LVOT obstruction, and is associated with poor clinical outcomes. There is a wide range of TMVR devices at various stages of development. Table 2 shows some TMVR for native anatomy devices with reported clinical data.

Table 2. Transcatheter mitral valve replacement devices.

Device	Intrepid	Tendyne	Tiara	EVOQUE	HighLife	SAPIEN M3
Patients, n	50	109	79	14	15	45
Etiology of MR						
Organic	16	11	8.9	28.6	27	55.6
Functional	72	89	62	21.4	73	35.6
Mixed	12		29.1	50		8.9
LVEF, %	43 ± 12	47.2	37 ± 9	54	38	44
Approach	TA	TA	TA	TF	TA	TF
Device implant success	98	97.2	92.4	92.9	72.7	88.9
30-day mortality	14 (n = 7)	5.5 (n = 6)	11.3 (n = 8)	7.1 (n = 1)	20 (n = 3)	2.2 (n = 1)
Residual MR						
None/mild	100	99	92.5	93	100	92.7
Moderate/severe	0	1	7.5	7	0	7.3
LVOT obstruction	0	0	0	7.1 (n = 1)	6.6 (n = 1)	0

Values are mean (range), mean ± SD, median [interquartile range], n (%), or n. MR: mitral regurgitation; LVEF: left ventricle ejection fraction; LVOT: left ventricle outflow tract; TA: transapical; TF: transfemoral.

The most employed TMVR for native anatomy is the Tendyne device (Abbott, Menlo Park, California). This device is fully repositionable, retrievable and designed to be implanted using a transapical approach. The Tendyne system consists of two self-expandable nitinol frames (inner and outer stent) and a valve formed by three porcine pericardial tissue leaflets sewn onto the circular inner stent. The inner valve is sutured to the outer stent that is coated in porcine pericardium with a polyethylene terephthalate (PET) fabric cuff that provides the sealing surface within the native annulus. The outer stent is designed with a D-shape to fit the mitral annulus and facilitate the orientation of the straight edge against the aortic-mitral continuity. This prosthesis is sutured to an ultra-high molecular weight polyethylene tether designed to stabilize the valve after deployment, which is fixed to an epicardial pad of polyether ether ketone button covered in PET fabric through the left ventricular apex.

4.1. Procedural Description and Imaging Key Aspects

A standardized TEE and CCT evaluation of the mitral valve apparatus is required to determine anatomic suitability and appropriate valve sizing for Tendyne implantation with special attention to mitral annular dimensions (septal-lateral, inter-commissural dimensions and entire perimeter), left ventricular dimensions (measured in the 3-chamber view or the short axis view along the septal-lateral direction) and neo-LVOT evaluation (Figure 4).

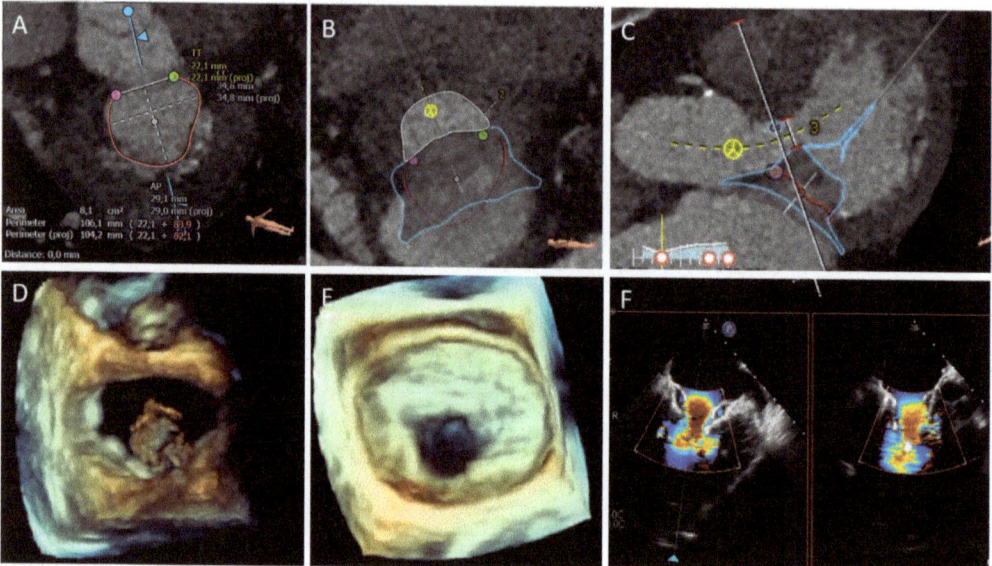

Figure 4. TMVR in native mitral anatomy with Tendyne (Abbott Medical) system. (**A**) Mitral annular dimension assessed with cardiac CT. (**B,C**) Neo-LVOT area after virtual valve implantation with specific Tendyne system design. (**D**) Three-dimensional TEE en-face view of initial THV device deployment and orientation. (**E**) Final result after complete deployment on 3D-TEE and in 2D-TEE color doppler on simultaneous bicommissural and LVOT views (**F**).

The device is implanted under general anesthesia through a left mini-thoracotomy using a transapical approach, using 2D and 3D TEE imaging guidance. The access site and orthogonal annular trajectory are determined from pre-procedural CCT and intraoperative echo imaging. A standard 0.035-inch wire is inserted into the left atrium and a balloon tip catheter is advanced to the left atrium to ensure that the guidewire is not entrapped in the mitral subvalvular apparatus. A 34-Fr sheath is then placed over the wire into the left atrium. The valve prosthesis is delivered through the sheath and partially deployed in the left atrium, until the outer valve expands up to approximately 85% of its final size. The D-shaped outer stent is aligned with the straight edge oriented anteriorly against the aortic-mitral continuity by rotating the device, using TEE guidance. The delivery sheath is then retracted to deploy the remainder of the prosthesis in an intra-annular position. The length and tension of the tether are adjusted to optimize the seating of prosthesis for MR reduction and to minimize the risk of device displacement.

4.2. Clinical Results

The first two temporary valve implants were reported by Lutter et al. [42] in 2013 (before proceeding with conventional mitral valve surgery), and the first-in-human definitive implant was performed in 2014 [43]. Since then, the Tendyne system has accumulated the most extensive clinical data to date. The experience in the first 100 patients revealed promising results, with an implant success of 96%, with no need for emergency surgery or mortality during the procedure [44]. The 30-day mortality rate was 5.5% and the most frequent complication was hemorrhagic, at 20% of cases. At one year, mortality was 26% (cardiac death accounted for the majority of the deaths [22/26; 85%]), disabling stroke was 3%, and the need for reoperation to adjust the strap tension was 3%. There were no cases of embolization or device migration, although there was an incidence of 6% of device thrombosis (within the first 35 cases, when anticoagulation was not specified by the study protocol). MR was absent in 98.4% of patients at one year follow-up. No patients had LVOT obstruction or significant mitral stenosis. At one year improvement in symptoms and quality of life were evident: 88.5% of survivors were in NYHA functional class I or II (34.0% at baseline; $p < 0.0001$) and the KCCQ increased by ≥ 5 points in 81.3% and by ≥ 10 points in 73.4%. The device has also shown promise for the treatment of MR in the setting of severe MAC [36]. Nine patients were successfully treated, with relief of MR in all patients and without procedural deaths. At one year, the survival rate was 78% and the MR remained absent in all treated patients.

The SUMMIT trial (Clinical Trial to Evaluate the Safety and Effectiveness of Using the Tendyne Mitral Valve System for the Treatment of Symptomatic MR; NCT03433274) is investigating the safety and clinical benefits of the Tendyne system compared to the Mitraclip system in patients with symptomatic moderate-severe MR suitable for transcatheter edge-to-edge repair (randomized cohort). In addition, there are two other single-arm cohorts, which will evaluate the Tendyne system for the treatment of severe MR with or without MAC. Tendyne received CE mark approval in January 2020 (the first transcatheter mitral valve replacement device approved for clinical use in Europe).

Employing the Tendyne system, a new option has been reported for a failed TEER in a patient non-candidate for a new TEER procedure or MV surgery. The ELASTA-Clip is a feasible and safe transcatheter electrosurgical detachment of failed TEER clips from the anterior leaflet followed by Tendyne implantation [45].

Very recently, 30-day outcomes of an early feasibility trial with a novel TMVR system have been presented [46]. The Intrepid TMVR is a novel device designed in order to treat patients with severe MR through femoral access with 35Fr sheath. Initial results, despite including a very selected population, are promising. In a cohort of advanced-age patients with mainly primary MR and mildly impaired LVEF, there are no deaths, strokes or reinterventions at 30 days. Significant improvement in NYHA functional class has been also reported. Nonetheless, around 50% of patients had significant major bleeding events due to access site major vascular complications. There is a promising landscape for this device but at this moment only preliminary data are available.

5. Conclusions

TMVR represents a new treatment option for inoperable or high-risk patients with symptomatic severe MR in different anatomical scenarios (ViV, ViR, ViMAC, and native TMVR). Cardiac multimodality imaging (3D-TEE and CT) is crucial for detailed pre-procedural planning, intraprocedural monitoring and successful outcomes.

Author Contributions: Conceptualization, M.B.-P.; methodology, M.B.-P.; Writing-original draft preparation, M.B.-P., L.P., B.C.-Q., R.G.-F., R.A. and J.A.P.; writing-review and editing, M.B.-P., L.P., B.C.-Q., R.G.-F., R.A. and J.A.P.; visualization, all authors; supervision, M.B.-P., A.I.-R. and R.E.-L. All authors have read and agreed to the published version of the manuscript.

Funding: This research received no external funding.

Institutional Review Board Statement: Not applicable.

Informed Consent Statement: Not applicable.

Data Availability Statement: Not applicable.

Conflicts of Interest: Barreiro-Perez and Estévez-Loureiro are proctors for Abbott Medical.

Abbreviations

MR	mitral regurgitation
TEER	Transcatheter edge-to-edge mitral valve repair
TMVR	Transcatheter mitral valve replacement
ViV	Valve-in-valve
ViR	Valve-in-ring
ViMAC	Valve-in-mitral annulus calcification
LVOT	Left ventricular outflow tract
TTE	transthoracic echocardiography
TEE	transesophageal echocardiography
CCT	cardiac computed tomography
PVL	Paravalvular leak closure
LAMPOON	Intentional laceration of the anterior mitral leaflet to prevent LVOT obstruction
THV	transcatheter heart valve
PET	polyethylene terephthalate
SHV	surgical heart valve

References

1. Cahill, T.J.; Prothero, A.; Wilson, J.; Kennedy, A.; Brubert, J.; Masters, M.; Newton, J.D.; Dawkins, S.; Enriquez-Sarano, M.; Prendergast, B.D.; et al. Community prevalence, mechanisms and outcome of mitral or tricuspid regurgitation. *Heart* **2021**, *107*, 1003–1009. [CrossRef] [PubMed]
2. Agricola, E.; Ielasi, A.; Oppizzi, M.; Faggiano, P.; Ferri, L.; Calabrese, A.; Vizzardi, E.; Alfieri, O.; Margonato, A. Long-term prognosis of medically treated patients with functional mitral regurgitation and left ventricular dysfunction. *Eur. J. Heart Fail.* **2009**, *11*, 581–587. [CrossRef] [PubMed]
3. Vahanian, A.; Beyersdorf, F.; Praz, F.; Milojevic, M.; Baldus, S.; Bauersachs, J.; Capodanno, D.; Conradi, L.; De Bonis, M.; De Paulis, R.; et al. 2021 ESC/EACTS Guidelines for the management of valvular heart disease. *Eur. Heart J.* **2021**, *60*, 727–800.
4. Mirabel, M.; Iung, B.; Baron, G.; Messika-Zeitoun, D.; Détaint, D.; Vanoverschelde, J.-L.; Butchart, E.G.; Ravaud, P.; Vahanian, A. What are the characteristics of patients with severe, symptomatic, mitral regurgitation who are denied surgery? *Eur. Heart J.* **2007**, *28*, 1358–1365. [CrossRef]
5. Sorajja, P.; Cavalcante, J.L.; Gössl, M. The need for transcatheter mitralvalve replacement. *J. Am. Coll. Cardiol.* **2019**, *73*, 1247–1249. [CrossRef] [PubMed]
6. Feldman, T.; Foster, E.; Glower, D.D.; Glower, D.G.; Kar, S.; Rinaldi, M.J.; Fail, P.S.; Smalling, R.W.; Siegel, R.; Rose, G.A.; et al. EVEREST II Investigators. Percutaneous repair or surgery for mitral regurgitation. *N. Engl. J. Med.* **2011**, *364*, 1395–1406. [CrossRef] [PubMed]
7. Beigel, R.; Wunderlich, N.C.; Kar, S.; Siegel, R.J. The evolution of percutaneous mitral valve repair therapy: Lessons learned and implications for patient selection. *J. Am. Coll. Cardiol.* **2014**, *64*, 2688–2700. [CrossRef] [PubMed]
8. Rawish, E.; Schmidt, T.; Eitel, I.; Frerker, C. Current status of catheter-based mitral valve replacement. *Curr. Cardiol. Rep.* **2021**, *23*, 95. [CrossRef] [PubMed]
9. Webb, J.G.; Murdoch, D.J.; Boone, R.H.; Moss, R.; Attinger-Toller, A.; Blanke, P.; Cheung, A.; Hensey, M.; Leipsic, J.; Ong, K.; et al. Percutaneous transcatheter mitral valve replacement. *J. Am. Coll. Cardiol.* **2019**, *73*, 1239–1246. [CrossRef] [PubMed]
10. Garcia-Sayan, E.; Chen, T.; Khalique, O.K. Multimodality cardiac imaging for procedural planning and guidance of transcatheter mitral valve replacement and mitral paravalvular leak closure. *Front. Cardiovasc. Med.* **2021**, *8*, 582925. [CrossRef] [PubMed]
11. Kargoli, F.; Pagnesi, M.; Rahgozar, K.; Goldberg, Y.; Ho, E.; Chau, M.; Colombo, A.; Latib, A. Current devices and complications related to transcatheter mitral valve replacement: The bumpy road to the top. *Front. Cardiovasc. Med.* **2021**, *8*, 639058. [CrossRef] [PubMed]
12. Alperi, A.; Granada, J.F.; Bernier, M.; Dagenais, F.; Rodés-Cabau, J. Current status and future prospects of transcatheter mitral valve replacement: JACC state-of-the-art review. *J. Am. Coll. Cardiol.* **2021**, *77*, 3058–3078. [CrossRef]
13. Niikura, H.; Gössl, M.; Kshettry, V.; Olson, S.; Sun, B.; Askew, J.; Stanberry, L.; Garberich, R.; Tang, L.; Lesser, J.; et al. Causes and clinical outcomes of patients who are ineligible for transcatheter mitral valve replacement. *JACC Cardiovasc. Interv.* **2019**, *12*, 196–204. [CrossRef] [PubMed]

14. Urena, M.; Himbert, D.; Brochet, E.; Carrasco, J.L.; Iung, B.; Nataf, P.; Vahanian, A. Transseptal Transcatheter Mitral Valve Replacement Using Balloon-Expandable Transcatheter Heart Valves: A Step-by-Step Approach. *JACC Cardiovasc. Interv.* **2017**, *10*, 1905–1919. [CrossRef]
15. Little, S.H.; Bapat, V.; Blanke, P.; Guerrero, M.; Rajagopal, V.; Siegel, R. Imaging Guidance for Transcatheter Mitral Valve Intervention on Prosthetic Valves, Rings, and Annular Calcification. *JACC Cardiovasc. Imaging* **2021**, *14*, 22–40. [CrossRef] [PubMed]
16. Harloff, M.T.; Chowdhury, M.; Hirji, S.A.; Percy, E.D.; Yazdchi, F.; Shim, H.; Malarczyk, A.A.; Sobieszczyk, P.S.; Sabe, A.A.; Shah, P.B.; et al. A step-by-step guide to transseptal valve-in-valve transcatheter mitral valve replacement. *Ann. Cardiothorac. Surg.* **2021**, *10*, 113–121. [CrossRef] [PubMed]
17. Pulerwitz, T.C.; Khalique, O.K.; Leb, J.; Hahn, R.T.; Nazif, T.; Leon, M.B.; George, I.; Vahl, T.P.; D'Souza, B.; Bapat, V.N.; et al. Optimizing Cardiac CT Protocols for Comprehensive Acquisition Prior to Percutaneous MV and TV Repair/Replacement. *JACC Cardiovasc. Imaging* **2020**, *13*, 836–850. [CrossRef] [PubMed]
18. Reid, A.; Ben Zekry, S.; Turaga, M.; Tarazi, S.; Bax, J.J.; Wang, D.D.; Piazza, N.; Bapat, V.N.; Ihdayhid, A.R.; Cavalcante, J.L.; et al. Neo-LVOT and Transcatheter Mitral Valve Replacement: Expert Recommendations. *JACC Cardiovasc. Imaging* **2021**, *14*, 854–866. [CrossRef] [PubMed]
19. Babaliaros, V.C.; Lederman, R.J.; Gleason, P.T.; Khan, J.M.; Kohli, K.; Sahu, A.; Rogers, T.; Bruce, C.G.; Paone, G.; Xie, J.X.; et al. The Art of SAPIEN 3 Transcatheter Mitral Valve Replacement in Valve-in-Ring and Valve-in-Mitral-Annular-Calcification Procedures. *Cardiovasc. Interv.* **2021**, *14*, 2195–2214.
20. Guerrero, M.; Dvir, D.; Himbert, D.; Urena, M.; Eleid, M.; Wang, D.D.; Greenbaum, A.; Mahadevan, V.S.; Holzhey, D.; O'Hair, D.; et al. Transcatheter Mitral Valve Replacement in Native Mitral Valve Disease with Severe Mitral Annular Calcification: Results from the First Multicenter Global Registry. *JACC Cardiovasc. Interv.* **2016**, *9*, 1361–1371. [CrossRef] [PubMed]
21. Khan, J.M.; Babaliaros, V.C.; Greenbaum, A.B.; Foerst, J.R.; Yazdani, S.; McCabe, J.M.; Paone, G.; Eng, M.H.; Leshnower, B.G.; Gleason, P.T.; et al. Anterior Leaflet Laceration to Prevent Ventricular Outflow Tract Obstruction During Transcatheter Mitral Valve Replacement. *J. Am. Coll. Cardiol.* **2019**, *73*, 2521–2534. [CrossRef] [PubMed]
22. Case, B.C.; Khan, J.M.; Satler, L.F.; Ben-Dor, I.; Lederman, R.; Babaliaros, V.C.; Greenbaum, A.B.; Waksman, R.; Rogers, T. Tip-to-Base LAMPOON to Prevent Left Ventricular Outflow Tract Obstruction in Valve-in-Valve Transcatheter Mitral Valve Replacement. *JACC Cardiovasc. Interv.* **2020**, *13*, 1126–1128. [CrossRef] [PubMed]
23. Lisko, J.C.; Greenbaum, A.B.; Khan, J.M.; Kamioka, N.; Gleason, P.T.; Byku, I.; Condado, J.F.; Jadue, A.; Paone, G.; Grubb, K.J.; et al. Antegrade Intentional Laceration of the Anterior Mitral Leaflet to Prevent Left Ventricular Outflow Tract Obstruction: A Simplified Technique From Bench to Bedside. *Circ. Cardiovasc. Interv.* **2020**, *13*, e008903. [CrossRef] [PubMed]
24. Van Hemelrijck, M.; Taramasso, M.; Gökhan, G.; Maisano, F.; Mestres, C.A. Mitral anular calcification: Challenges and future perspectives. *Indian J. Thorac. Cardiovasc. Surg.* **2020**, *36*, 397–403. [CrossRef] [PubMed]
25. Urena, M.; Vahanian, A.; Brochet, E.; Ducrocq, G.; Lung, B.; Himbert, D. Current Indications for Transcatheter Mitral Valve Replacement Using Transcatheter Aortic Valves. *Circulation* **2021**, *143*, 178–196. [CrossRef] [PubMed]
26. Guerrero, M.; Salinger, M.; Pursnani, A.; Pearson, P.; Lampert, M.; Levisay, J.; Russell, H.; Feldman, T. Transseptal transcatheter mitral valve-in-valve: A step by step guide from preprocedural planning to postprocedural care. *Catheter. Cardiovasc. Interv.* **2018**, *92*, E185–E196. [CrossRef] [PubMed]
27. Vincent, F.; Spillemaeker, H.; Kyheng, M.; Belin-Vincent, C.; Delhaye, C.; Piérache, A.; Denimal, T.; Verdier, B.; Debry, N.; Moussa, M.; et al. Ultrasound Guidance to Reduce Vascular and Bleeding Complications of Percutaneous Transfemoral Transcatheter Aortic Valve Replacement: A Propensity Score-Matched Comparison. *J. Am. Heart Assoc.* **2020**, *9*, e014916. [CrossRef]
28. Alkhouli, M.; Rihal, C.S.; Holmes, D.R., Jr. Transseptal techniques for emerging structural heart interventions. *J. Am. Coll. Cardiol. Interv.* **2016**, *9*, 2465–2480. [CrossRef] [PubMed]
29. Yoon, S.-H.; Bleiziffer, S.; Latib, A.; Eschenbach, L.; Ancona, M.; Vincent, F.; Kim, W.-K.; Unbehaum, A.; Asami, M.; Dhoble, A.; et al. Predictors of Left Ventricular Outflow Tract Obstruction after Transcatheter Mitral Valve Replacement. *JACC Cardiovasc. Interv.* **2019**, *12*, 182–193. [CrossRef]
30. Yoon, S.H.; Whisenant, B.K.; Bleiziffer, S.; Delgado, V.; Dhoble, A.; Schofer, N.; Eschenbach, L.; Bansal, E.; Murdoch, D.J.; Ancona, M.; et al. Outcomes of transcatheter mitral valve replacement for degenerated bioprosthesis, failed annuloplasty rings, and mitral annular calcification. *Eur. Heart J.* **2019**, *40*, 441–451. [CrossRef] [PubMed]
31. Guerrero, M.; Urena, M.; Himbert, D.; Wang, D.D.; Eleid, M.; Kodali, S.; George, I.; Chakravarty, T.; Mathur, M.; Holzhey, D.; et al. 1-Year outcomes of transcatheter mitral valve replacement in patients with severe mitral annular calcification. *J. Am. Coll. Cardiol.* **2018**, *71*, 1841–1853. [CrossRef] [PubMed]
32. Guerrero, M.; Wang, D.D.; Eleid, M.F.; Pursnani, A.; Salinger, M.; Russell, H.M.; Kodali, S.K.; George, I.; Bapat, V.N.; Dangas, G.D.; et al. Prospective Study of TMVR Using Balloon-Expandable Aortic Transcatheter Valves in MAC. MITRAL Trial 1-Year Outcomes. *Cardiovasc. Interv.* **2021**, *14*, 830–845.
33. Blanke, P.; Dvir, D.; Cheung, A.; Ye, J.; Levine, R.A.; Precious, B.; Berger, A.; Stub, D.; Hague, C.; Murphy, D.; et al. A simplified Dshaped model of the mitral annulus to facilitate CT-based sizing before transcatheter mitral valve implantation. *J. Cardiovasc. Comput. Tomogr.* **2014**, *8*, 459–467. [CrossRef] [PubMed]

34. Guerrero, M.; Wang, D.D.; Pursnani, A.; Eleid, M.; Khalique, O.; Urena, M.; Salinger, M.; Kodali, S.; Kaptzan, T.; Lewis, B.; et al. A cardiac computed tomography-based score to categorize mitral annular calcification severity and predict valve embolization. *Cardiovasc. Imaging* **2020**, *13*, 1945–1957. [CrossRef] [PubMed]
35. Sorajja, P.; Gössl, M.; Babaliaros, V.; Rizik, D.; Conradi, L.; Bae, R.; Burke, R.F.; Schäfer, U.; Lisko, J.C.; Riley, R.D.; et al. Novel Transcatheter Mitral Valve Prothesis for Patients With Severe Mitral Annular Calcification. *J. Am. Coll. Cardiol.* **2019**, *74*, 1431–1440. [CrossRef]
36. Bapat, V.N.; Attia, R.; Thomas, M. Effect of valve design on the stent internal diameter of a bioprosthetic valve: A concept of true internal diameter and its implications for the valve-invalve procedure. *JACC Cardiovasc. Interv.* **2014**, *7*, 115–127. [CrossRef]
37. Play.google.com. Mitral Valve-in-Valve APP. 2021. Available online: https://play.google.com/store/apps/details?id=com.ubqo.vivmitral&hl=es_AR&gl=US (accessed on 10 December 2021).
38. App Store. Valve in Valve (Mitral). 2021. Available online: https://apps.apple.com/es/app/valve-in-valve-mitral/id703369667 (accessed on 10 December 2021).
39. El Sabbagh, A.; Al-Hijji, M.; Wang, D.D.; Eleid, M.; Urena, M.; Himbert, D.; Chakravarty, T.; Holzhey, D.; Pershad, A.; Fang, H.K.; et al. Predictors of Left Ventricular Outflow Tract Obstruction after Transcatheter Mitral Valve Replacement in Severe Mitral Annular Calcification: An Analysis of the Transcatheter Mitral Valve Replacement in Mitral Annular Calcification Global Registry. *Circ. Cardiovasc. Interv.* **2021**, *14*, e010854. [CrossRef] [PubMed]
40. Russo, G.; Gennari, M.; Gavazzoni, M.; Pedicino, D.; Pozzoli, A.; Taramasso, M.; Maisano, F. Transcatheter Mitral Valve Implantation: Current Status and Future Perspectives. *Circ. Cardiovasc. Interv.* **2021**, *14*, e010628. [CrossRef] [PubMed]
41. Hensey, M.; Brown, R.A.; Lal, S.; Sathananthan, J.; Ye, J.; Cheung, A.; Blanke, P.; Leipsic, J.; Moss, R.; Boone, R.; et al. Transcatheter Mitral Valve Replacement: An Update on Current Techniques, Technologies, and Future Directions. *JACC Cardiovasc. Interv.* **2021**, *14*, 489–500. [CrossRef] [PubMed]
42. Lutter, G.; Lozonschi, L.; Ebner, A.; Gallo, S.; Kall, C.M.Y.; Missov, E.; de Marchena, E. First-in-human off-pump transcatheter mitral valve replacement. *JACC Cardiovasc. Interv.* **2014**, *7*, 1077–1078. [CrossRef]
43. Duncan, A.; Daqa, A.; Yeh, J.; Davies, S.; Uebing, A.; Quarto, C.; Moat, N.; Alison, D.; Anan, D.; James, Y.; et al. Transcatheter mitral valve replacement: Long-term outcomes of first-in-man experience with an apically tethered device—A case series from a single centre. *EuroIntervention* **2017**, *13*, e1047–e1057. [CrossRef] [PubMed]
44. Sorajja, P.; Moat, N.; Badhwar, V.; Walters, D.; Paone, G.; Bethea, B.; Bae, R.; Dahle, G.; Mumtaz, M.; Grayburn, P.; et al. Initial feasibility study of a new transcatheter mitral prosthesis: The first 100 patients. *J. Am. Coll. Cardiol.* **2019**, *73*, 1250–1260. [CrossRef] [PubMed]
45. Lisko, J.C.; Greenbaum, A.B.; Guyton, R.A.; Kamioka, N.; Grubb, K.J.; Gleason, P.T.; Byku, I.; Condado, J.F.; Jadue, A.; Paone, G.; et al. Electrosurgical Detachment of MitraClips From the Anterior Mitral Leaflet Prior to Transcatheter Mitral Valve Implantation. *JACC Cardiovasc. Interv.* **2020**, *13*, 2361–2370. [CrossRef] [PubMed]
46. Zahr, F.; Song, H.K.; Chadderdon, S.M.; Gada, H.; Mumtaz, M.; Byrne, T.; Kirshner, M.; Bajwa, T.; Weiss, E.; Kodali, S.; et al. Thirty-Day Outcomes Following Transfemoral Transseptal Transcatheter Mitral Valve Replacement: Intrepid TMVR Early Feasibility Study Results. *JACC Cardiovasc. Interv.* **2021**. ahead of print. [CrossRef] [PubMed]

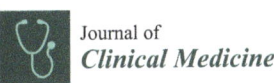

Review

The Use of BASILICA Technique to Prevent Coronary Obstruction in a TAVI-TAVI Procedure

Ana Paula Tagliari [1,2,3,*,†], Rodrigo Petersen Saadi [1,4,†], Eduardo Ferreira Medronha [3] and Eduardo Keller Saadi [1,2,3,4]

1. Postgraduate Program in Cardiology and Cardiovascular Science Universidade Federal do Rio Grande do Sul, Porto Alegre 90035-002, Brazil; rodrigosaadi@terra.com.br (R.P.S.); esaadi@terra.com.br (E.K.S.)
2. Cardiac Surgery Department, Hospital São Lucas da PUC/RS, Porto Alegre 90619-900, Brazil
3. Cardiac Surgery and Radiology Department, Hospital Mãe de Deus, Porto Alegre 90880-0481, Brazil; medronha@gmail.com
4. Cardiac Surgery Department, Hospital de Clínicas de Porto Alegre, Porto Alegre 90035-903, Brazil
* Correspondence: anapaulatagliari@gmail.com
† Shared co-first authorship.

Abstract: Transcatheter aortic valve implantation (TAVI) to manage structural bioprosthetic valve deterioration has been successful in mitigating the risk of a redo cardiac surgery. However, TAVI-in-TAVI is a complex intervention, potentially associated with feared complications such as coronary artery obstruction. Coronary obstruction risk is especially high when the previously implanted prosthesis had supra-annular leaflets and/or the distance between the prosthesis and the coronary ostia is short. The BASILICA technique (bioprosthetic or native aortic scallop intentional laceration to prevent iatrogenic coronary artery obstruction) was developed to prevent coronary obstruction during native or valve-in-valve interventions but has now also been considered for TAVI-in-TAVI interventions. Despite its utility, the technique requires a not so widely available toolbox. Herein, we discuss the TAVI-in-TAVI BASILICA technique and how to perform it using more widely available tools, which could spread its use.

Keywords: transcatheter aortic valve implantation; transcatheter aortic valve replacement; BASILICA; coronary artery obstruction

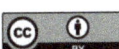

1. Introduction

The introduction of transcatheter aortic valve implantation (TAVI) in 2002, as an alternative to treat patients with severe aortic valve stenosis who previously had only surgery as an intervention option, represented a huge mark in the structural heart disease management revolution [1].

Recently, the American and European Guidelines for the management of valvular heart disease have recommended TAVI in several clinical scenarios provided that the anatomy is favorable for performing a transfemoral approach [2,3]. According to the American College of Cardiology (ACC) and American Heart Association (AHA) Guideline, TAVI may be considered in patients above 65 years and should be the first choice in those above 80 years [2]. To the European Society of Cardiology (ESC) and European Association for Cardio-Thoracic Surgery (EACTS) Guideline, TAVI should be chosen for those above 75 years and with high surgical risk (STS score or EuroScore $\geq$ 8) [3]. These changes in the last Guidelines, compared to the previous ones, were corroborated by important randomized clinical trials, whose results showed TAVI non-inferiority, or even superiority, compared to surgical aortic valve replacement (SAVR), in low-risk patients with a mean age of 73 and 74 years in the PARTNER 3 and EVOLUT Low-risk trials, respectively [4,5].

Taking into account the increasing number of low-risk patients undergoing TAVI and their long-life expectancy, one can assume that patients could outlive the bioprostheses' expected durability. Consequently, the number of repeated transcatheter interventions following the first TAVI, the so-called TAVI-in-TAVI procedure, is also expected to increase [6].

Even though less invasive, TAVI-in-TAVI is more challenging and carries a higher complication risk, mainly coronary artery obstruction, than TAVI in a native valve. In an attempt to reduce the risk of coronary artery obstruction during native or valve-in-valve interventions, the BASILICA technique (bioprosthetic or native aortic scallop intentional laceration to prevent iatrogenic coronary artery obstruction) was conceptualized [7]. However, the BASILICA employment during TAVI-in-TAVI lacks evidence.

Herein, we provide an updated and comprehensive literature review focused on TAVI-in-TAVI BASILICA, and we illustrate this concept with a case report.

2. TAVI-in-TAVI

TAVI-in-TAVI is defined as a second transcatheter heart valve (THV) deployment within a previously implanted bioprosthesis because of suboptimal device position and/or function, during or after the procedure [8].

In 2007, Ruiz C. et al. reported the first TAVI-in-TAVI performed three years earlier. At the index procedure, a patient with severe aortic regurgitation and moderate aortic stenosis was submitted to a CoreValve (Medtronic Inc., Minneapolis, MN, USA) implant. Due to the presence of severe aortic regurgitation immediately after the implant, a second CoreValve was required. Based on the success of this case, the authors suggested that the concept and durability of the TAVI-in-TAVI started to be demonstrated [9].

Nowadays, a second valve implantation is applied in a broad spectrum of acute or chronic scenarios [10]. The most common TAVI-in-TAVI indications are:

(a) As a bail-out approach: in an acute setting, as a rescue strategy undertaken due to unsuccessful or suboptimal implantation.
(b) Late THV failure: due to late structural valve deterioration (stenosis, regurgitation, or mixed disease).
(c) A combination of structural and non-structural valve dysfunction: a combination of paravalvular regurgitation (PVL) and bioprosthesis failure, which could require a combined approach, such as PVL closure and a new prosthesis implantation.

Although TAVI-in-TAVI can offer immediate rescue management, avoiding open cardiac surgery and cardiopulmonary bypass, this is not without inherent complication risks.

In 2014, Witkowsky A. et al. reviewed 43 articles reporting TAVI-in-TAVI cases. In most of them, TAVI-in-TAVI was used as a rescue intervention to manage suboptimal bioprosthesis function. Aortic regurgitation was the main reason for a second bioprosthesis implantation, and prosthesis malposition was the main underlying cause of TAVI failure (81%). The reported TAVI-in-TAVI success rate varied from 90% to 100%, and the 30-day mortality rate was 0–14.3% [11]. While in the PARTNER trial multiple valve implantation was required in 1–2% (Cohort B: 1.1%; Cohort A: 2%), Vrachatis DA et al. [12] reported that in the CoreValve U.S. Pivotal Trial multiple valves were implanted in 3.5–4.5% (Extreme Risk Cohort: 3.5%; High-Risk Cohort: 4.1%) [13–16]. Similarly, Makkar R.R. et al. described that, among 2554 consecutive patients reviewed from the PARTNER cohorts A and B and accompanying registries, TAVI-in-TAVI was required in about 2.5%. In most cases (89%), it was performed intra-procedurally. On multivariable analysis, TAVI-in-TAVI was an independent predictor of 1-year mortality (Hazard ratio (HR) 2.68, 95% Confidence Interval (CI) 1.34–5.36; $p = 0.0055$). The authors highlighted that these early results, which were largely derived from rescue TAVI-in-TAVI, should not be extrapolated to future populations, such as elective TAVI-in-TAVI for degenerated bioprosthesis [17].

A more detailed description of the most recent and relevant TAVI-in-TAVI studies is presented in Table 1.

Table 1. Most recent and relevant TAVI-in-TAVI studies.

Author and Year	Number of Patients	Recruitment	Follow-Up	Survival at 30 Days and 1 Year	Device Success **
Percy, ED. 2021 [18]	617	All Medicare beneficiaries who underwent TAVI from 2012 to 2017	1 year	94% at 30 days and 78% at 1 year	—
Attizzani, GF. 2021 [19]	292	All TVT Registry patients who underwent redo-TAVI with Evolut platform between April 2015 and March 2020	1 year	96.8% at 30 days and 82.3% at 1 year	94.5%
Landes, U. 2020 [20]	212	Redo-TAVI registry, 37 centers	30 days	94.6% and 98.5% for early and late valve dysfunction *	85.1%
Toggweiler, S. 2012 [21]	21	Three Canadian centers, between January 2005 and March 2011	1 year	85.7% at 30 days and 76% at 1 year	90%
Schmidt, T. 2016 [22]	19	Consecutive patients in 2 German centers, between October 2011 and November 2015	1 year	89% at 30 days and 67% at 1 year	89%
Tsuda, M. 2019 [23]	6	Osaka University Hospital, between October 2009 and June 2018	1 year	100% at 30 days and 83.3% at 1 year	83.3%

* The study considered early valve dysfunction when it occurred within the first year after first valve implantation, and late if after one year. ** According to VARC-2 criteria.

3. TAVI-in-TAVI Complications

Regarding TAVI-in-TAVI major concerns, bioprosthesis malpositioning and deformation, critical coronary flow obstruction, and residual transvalvular gradients are the three most relevant [24]. While coronary artery obstruction incidence is low (<1%) in native TAVI, this risk increases by 4 to 6 times (2.5–3.5%) in valve-in-valve intervention, and it has been associated with approximately 50% in-hospital mortality [24–26].

Coronary artery obstruction occurs when the THV displaces the underlying surgical or native aortic valve leaflets outward, obstructing the coronary ostia directly or by sequestering the sinus of Valsalva at the sinotubular junction (STJ) [27]. Consequently, patients with low coronary ostia and narrow sinus of Valsalva have a higher risk of coronary obstruction [28]. Komatsu I et al. stated that, based on the anatomical relationship of the aortic root to the coronary ostium, three types of coronary ostia and aortic valve complex size could be identified, as follow [28]:

(a) Type I: coronary ostium lies above the top of the deflected native or bioprosthetic aortic valve leaflet. In this case, the deflected leaflet will not be able to cover the flow to the coronary artery, even if the sinuses are extremely narrow.
(b) Type II: coronary ostium lies below the top of the deflected leaflet. In this case, the risk of coronary obstruction will depend on the capacity of the sinuses to accommodate the deflected leaflet. In type IIA, the sinus is wide and coronary obstruction will not occur. In type IIB, the sinus is effaced and coronary obstruction can happen after TAVI.
(c) Type III: implanted leaflets extend above the STJ when deflected, which is especially common in supra-annular THV. In type IIIA, both the sinuses and the STJ are wide and this condition may not be at risk for coronary obstruction. In type IIIB, either sinuses or STJ are narrow and coronary obstruction may occur. In type IIIC, non-effaced sinuses may obstruct the inflow to the coronaries if the leaflets can be deflected above the STJ level and positioned close to the aortic wall.

Therefore, anatomies at risk for coronary obstruction would include types IIB, IIIB, and IIIC, and these conditions may require coronary obstruction protection with the BASILICA technique. Coronary obstruction risk assessment also includes the VTC measurement (virtual THV to coronary ostium distance). In the case of a VTC less than 4 mm, the BASILICA technique should be considered. When the VTC is > 4 mm, the risk for STJ-inflow obstruction should be evaluated by analyzing STJ and commissures relationship. If the VTSTJ (virtual THV to STJ distance) is small, then the BASILICA should also be considered [28].

Alternative approaches to reduce the risk of coronary occlusion include coronary protection with a supportive coronary guidewire, undeployed balloon, chimney technique, or snorkel stents [7,29,30].

TAVI-in-TAVI on supra-annular devices is considered especially risky as the new THV tends to push the prior leaflets against the original frame that extends above the STJ, potentially blocking coronary blood flow and limiting catheter access [18].

Buzzatti N et al. stated that while after a native TAVI the coronary access can be maintained through the open-cell stent, after a TAVI-in-TAVI the stent frames of the two prostheses will overlap, and the new stent will push and spread the previous leaflets over the original stent, converting it into a "covered" stent up to the edge of the leaflets. Thus, stents frame overlaps and loss of free-flow may impair both coronary flow and cannulation. According to these authors, the anatomical and device-related factors predisposing to increased risk of impaired coronary access after TAVI-in-TAVI are: [31]

(a) STJ: represents the critical anatomical bottleneck regulating the access to the aortic root and coronary ostia; shorter and narrower STJ will leave less free space between the aortic wall and the edge of the "covered" old TAVI stent frame;
(b) Height of the leaflets of the original device: is the first determinant of the level below which the previous stent frame will not be crossable anymore after the implantation of a second device. Higher leaflets will more easily impinge on the STJ and impair catheter movement in the aortic root;
(c) Depth of device implantation: it will also modify the height of TAVI leaflets in respect to the aortic root, therefore possibly jeopardizing coronary access.

4. The BASILICA Technique

The BASILICA technique was first reported by Kan JM et al. in 2018. In this first report, the authors described that the procedure was performed on a compassionate basis in seven patients. Procedural success was achieved in all patients, with no hemodynamic compromise, no coronary obstruction, stroke, or any major complications [7].

BASILICA main objective is to intentionally lacerate the native or bioprosthetic leaflets to prevent critical coronary obstruction using catheter electrosurgery. Thus, BASILICA directly addresses the pathophysiology of coronary artery obstruction by lacerating the leaflet in front of a threatened coronary artery. After laceration, the sliced leaflet will splay and create a triangular space ("triangle of flow") that may permit blood flow towards the sinus and from it to the coronary artery [32].

In 2020, Kitamura et al. evaluated the feasibility of the BASILICA technique in patients with high risk of coronary obstruction. In this study, BASILICA was feasible in 95% of the cases and resulted in effective prevention of coronary obstruction in 90% of them. Complication rates were low, with no cases of major vascular complication, need for mechanical circulatory support, stroke, or mortality at 30 days. These results provide further evidence on the feasibility, efficacy, and relative safety of the BASILICA technique [33].

Westermann D et al. assessed BASILICA clinical outcome in a single-center cohort described as the Hamburg BASILICA experience. In this study, 15 consecutive high-surgical risk patients were enrolled and submitted to TAVI due to degeneration of stented (80.0%) or stentless (6.7%) bioprosthetic aortic valves, or native aortic stenosis (13.3%). Procedure feasibility was 86.7%, with no 30-day all-cause deaths or stroke [34].

In this same line, Tagliari et al. had described six cases of valve-in-valve BASILICA procedures. Median left and right coronary artery heights were 9.1 mm (6.2–10.3) and 12.4 mm (10–13.5), respectively, with a median VTC of 2.9 mm on the left and 4.6 mm on the right side. The success rate was 87.5%, and there were no intraprocedural complications, coronary obstruction, in-hospital death, valve complication, cardiovascular event, or pacemaker implantation [35].

Recently, the 1-year outcomes from the BASILICA trial were published. This study enrolled 30 patients (43% native and 57% bioprosthesis). The 30-day success rate was 93.3%, with a stroke rate of 10%, and 1 death. Between 30 days and 1 year, there were no additional strokes, no myocardial infarction, and two deaths (10% 1-year mortality). No patient needed repeat intervention for aortic valve or coronary disease. Despite these encouraging outcomes, the authors concluded that the "applicability of BASILICA for failed THV is potentially large, but early benchtop studies suggest that it may not be suitable in all TAVI-in-TAVI procedures because of THV design and randomness of commissural alignment" [36].

Investigating TAVI-in-TAVI BASILICA feasibility in a benchtop model, Khan JM et al. analyzed if leaflets from the four commonest THV (Evolut R, SAPIEN XT, SAPIEN 3, and Lotus) could be split longitudinally to mimic BASILICA laceration. After some tests, they observed that effective leaflet splay could be achieved in the older generation SAPIEN XT and Lotus valves, but the newer generation SAPIEN 3 and Evolut appeared to demonstrate less effective leaflet splay. The authors also commented that, even in the case of feasible BASILICA laceration, the new TAVI commissures might randomly align unfavorably and obstruct the splayed leaflet. Besides, if the new TAVI skirt is positioned too high, this might also obstruct the lacerated leaflet. Therefore, success or failure would depend on commissural alignment and depth of new TAVI device implantation [37].

There are several unique concerns when a TAVI-in-TAVI BASILICA is planned, such as to ensure that the guidewire does not traverse through the stent frame and stays within the previous THV and to avoid interaction of the wire loop with the lower skirt of the THV [38]. Another concern is the possibility that the outer TAVI leaflets could get pinned against their frame by the inner TAVI device and, thereby, failing to splay and allow coronary perfusion [27].

5. BASILICA Required Equipment

As described by Komatsu I et al. there are several not so commonly utilized equipment required to perform a BASILICA procedure, comprising a Snare system (Amplatz Gooseneck™), a 6 Fr multipurpose (MP) guide catheter, an Astato XS 20 300 cm guidewire (Asahi Intecc USA, Inc., Tustin, CA, USA), a PiggyBack® Wire Converter (Vascular Solutions, Minneapolis, MN, USA), an 8 Fr guide catheter (8 Fr AL3 or AL1/2/4 or EBU 3.5/4 for left cusp; 8 Fr MP or JR for right cusp), a 125 cm diagnostic 5 Fr internal mammary (IMA) catheter, an electrosurgical generator, surgical pencil, ground pad, scalpel blade, and mosquito clamps. For a rapid new THV deployment after leaflet laceration, a pigtail positioned in the left ventricle, inserted in parallel to the traversal guide, is also recommended. The snare size is determined by the perimeter-derived diameter of the LVOT at 5–10 mm below the annulus plane [28].

Even though this toolbox is highly recommended, it is not available in many countries and centers, precluding a widespread BASILICA employment. Searching solutions and similar equipment to replace the traditional ones, we describe the case report below. This case also corroborates TAVI-in-TAVI BASILICA feasibility since, to the best of our knowledge, it is the second case report describing a TAVI-in-TAVI BASILICA.

6. Case Report

6.1. History of Presentation

An 86-year-old woman was admitted to a tertiary hospital with severe refractory heart failure secondary to severe aortic stenosis and moderate aortic regurgitation (New York Heart Association functional class IV). The patient was stable up to two years ago when she became lost to follow up.

Her previous medical history included arterial hypertension, persistent atrial fibrillation on oral anticoagulant therapy (rivaroxaban 10 mg/day), previous smoking, chronic obstructive pulmonary disease, previous breast cancer, colonic angiodysplasia, and diverticular disease. Regarding previous cardiac interventions, the patients had received a permanent pacemaker 1 year before due to tachycardia-bradycardia syndrome and a TAVI (23 mm CoreValve) in 2012 to treat severe aortic stenosis. STS score was 8% and EuroScore II 14.9%.

6.2. Preoperative Investigation

Transthoracic echocardiogram (Figure 1) showed moderate aortic valve regurgitation and severe aortic stenosis. Aortic valve peak and mean gradients were 74 mmHg and 46 mmHg, respectively, with an effective orifice area of 0.7 cm^2 and a peak velocity of 4.3 m/s. Left ventricle ejection fraction was preserved (67%). In view of these findings, the diagnosis of structural bioprosthetic valve deterioration with severe BVF was stablished. Considering her high surgical risk and frailty condition, the heart team indicated a new transcatheter intervention (TAVI-in-TAVI).

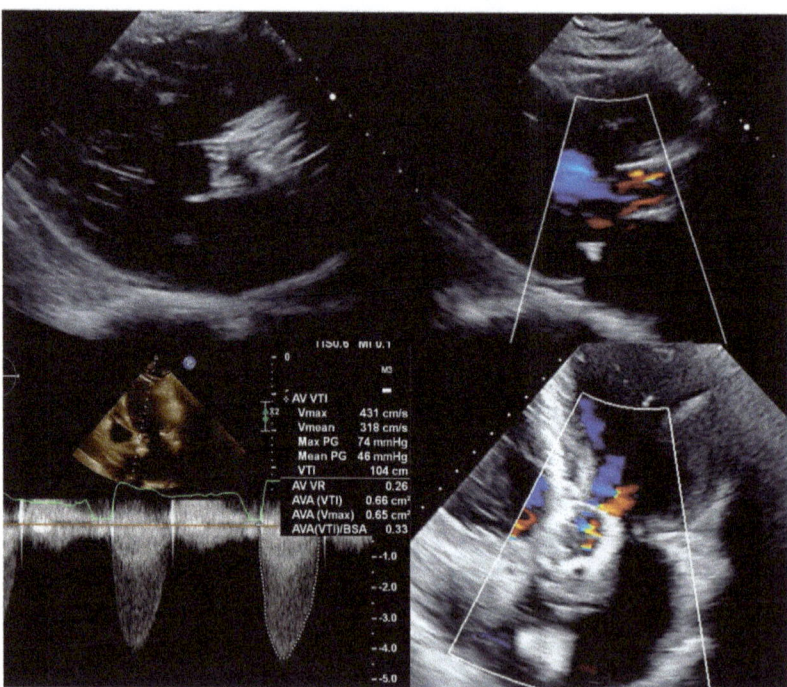

Figure 1. Transthoracic echocardiogram long-axis and 4-chamber views showing a degenerated CoreValve bioprosthesis with thickened leaflets, severe aortic stenosis, and moderate aortic regurgitation.

A computed tomography angiography (CT) showed a degenerated 23 mm CoreValve bioprosthesis and almost immobile leaflets. Both coronary arteries Ostia were originated below the top of the CoreValve leaflets' heigh: CoreValve leaflets' height = 26 mm; left coronary ostium height (from frame bottom to coronary ostium) = 19 mm; right coronary artery ostium height = 18 mm. The calculated VTC was around 3.8 mm on both sides. Therefore, both coronary arteries were at risk of sinus sequestration and flow obstruction (Figure 2).

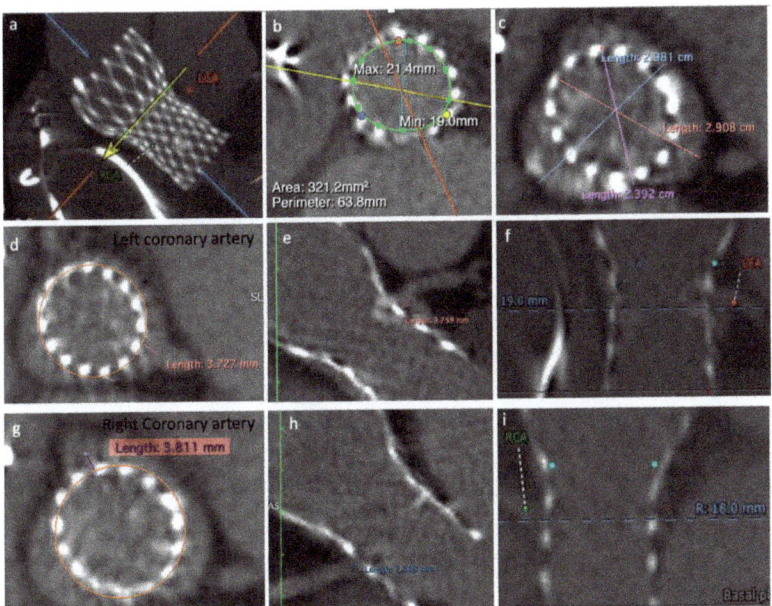

Figure 2. Computed tomography angiography images: (**a**) CoreValve structure, left coronary artery ostium (LCA) and right coronary artery ostium (RCA); (**b**) Calculated area and perimeter; (**c**) Sinus of Valsalva diameter; (**d,e**) left coronary cusp VTC; (**f**) LCA height related to the frame bottom; (**g,h**) right coronary cusp VTC; (**i**) RCA height related to the frame bottom.

Since on the right side, a combination of low coronary artery height and too narrow sinus of Valsalva was observed, a condition described as a relative contraindication to BASILICA (the skirt of a new THV itself could potentially occlude the newly formed "triangle of flow"), we decided to protect the right coronary with a supportive coronary guidewire and an undeployed balloon, and proceed with the BASILICA in the left leaflet.

Searching for previous TAVI-in-TAVI BASILICA cases, none but one was found. In that case, the patient was at risk for sinus sequestration and impeding coronary access; thus, a left cusp BASILICA followed by a SAPIEN 3 implantation within a degenerated 31 mm CoreValve was performed. Regarding equipment, the authors described having used standard BASILICA equipment [38].

6.3. Procedure

Under general anesthesia, transesophageal echocardiography (TEE) guidance and full systemic heparinization, we accessed the right radial artery as a route to insert a protective guidewire in the right coronary artery. A temporary pacemaker was inserted in the right ventricle through the right femoral venous access.

After these steps, both right and left femoral arteries were punctured. The right one was used as the main access (14 Fr sheath), while the left was the contralateral access (7 Fr sheath). Through the right side, a 5 Fr pigtail was positioned in the left ventricle aiming to allow a fast new THV deployment if hemodynamic instability occurred after leaflet laceration.

Through the contralateral access, a 6 Fr 20-mm snare (ONE Snare, Merit Medical Systems) inside a 6 Fr MP guiding catheter (Medtronic) was positioned in the LVOT, 5–10 mm below the CoreValve. Through the main access, an 8 Fr AL 2 catheter (guide catheter) with an extra-long 5 Fr × 125 cm JL 4.0 catheter (child catheter) was positioned directed to the left cusp mid base. Replacing the Astato and the PiggyBack® we used a 0.014 × 300 cm ProVia guidewire (Medtronic) insulated in a micro-guide catheter (FineCross MG 1.8/2.4 Fr × 150 cm, Terumo) (Figure 3).

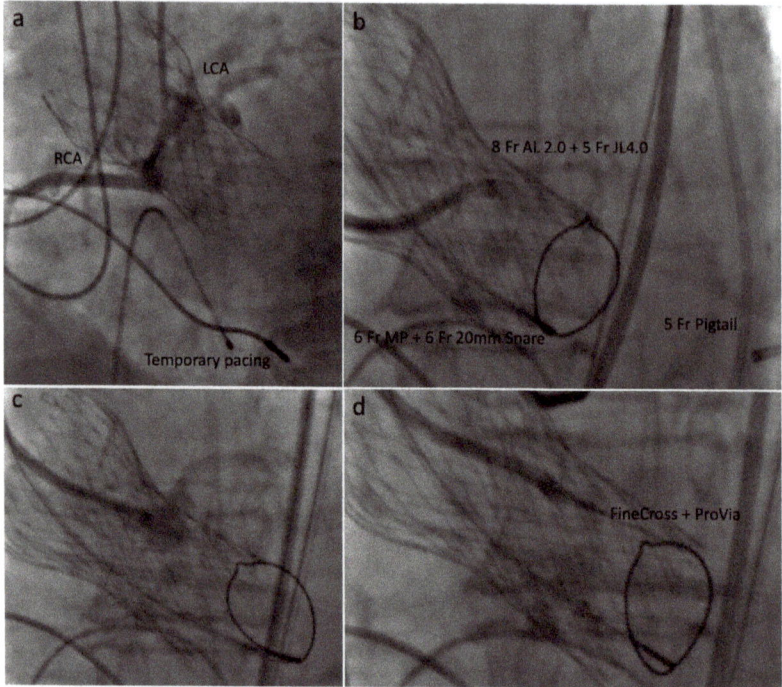

Figure 3. Intraprocedural steps: (**a**) Contrast injection showing right and left coronary ostia; (**b**) 8 Fr AL 2 catheter and 5 Fr × 125 cm JL 4.0 directed to the left leaflet mid base; (**c**) Contrast injection confirming proper position; (**d**) 0.014 × 300 cm ProVia guidewire and 1.8/2.6 Fr × 150 cm FineCross micro-catheter insertion.

After fluoroscopy and TEE had confirmed the proper position, the back of the ProVia guidewire was scraped and connected with an electrical pencil. The electrosurgical generator was set on 70 W "pure cut" mode for traversal. Electricity was applied, and the leaflet traversed by the guidewire, which was snared. Once snaring was achieved, a V-shape was performed in the middle part of the wire by denuding it approximately 10 mm in its inner curve. By pulling the snare, the V-shape was advanced until the traversed point. At this point, simultaneous 5% dextrose was injected into each guide catheter and leaflet laceration was performed using 100 W power. Successful leaflet laceration was confirmed and BASILICA equipment removed. The remaining steps for complete a 23 mm SAPIEN 3 valve deployment were performed in a standard fashion (Figures 4 and 5).

Final results showed proper SAPIEN 3 position, no PVL, no transvalvular aortic regurgitation, adequate gradients and coronary artery perfusion (Supplementary Figure S1). The patient remained stable during the whole procedure and presented no ECG change.

A summary of procedural steps and equipment used are presented in (Supplementary Table S1).

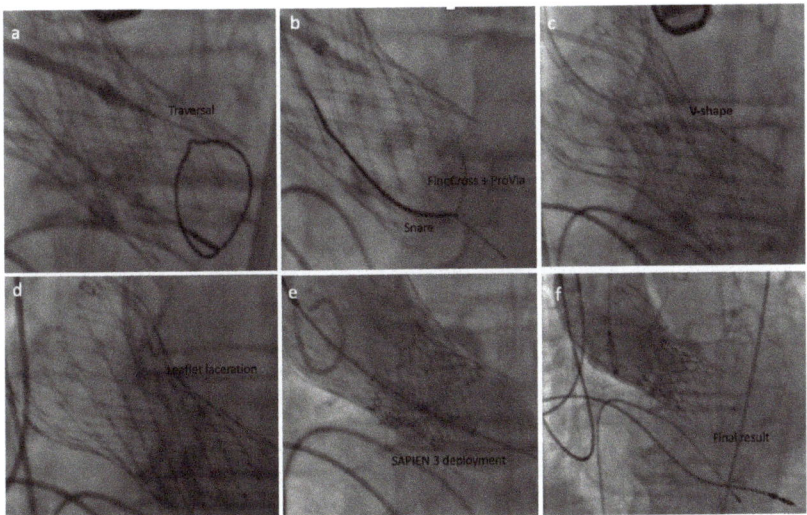

Figure 4. The BASILICA technique: (**a**) left coronary leaflet traversal; (**b**) guidewire snaring; (**c**) V-shape formation and delivery; (**d**) left coronary leaflet laceration; (**e**) SAPIEN 3 deployment; (**f**) final result assessment.

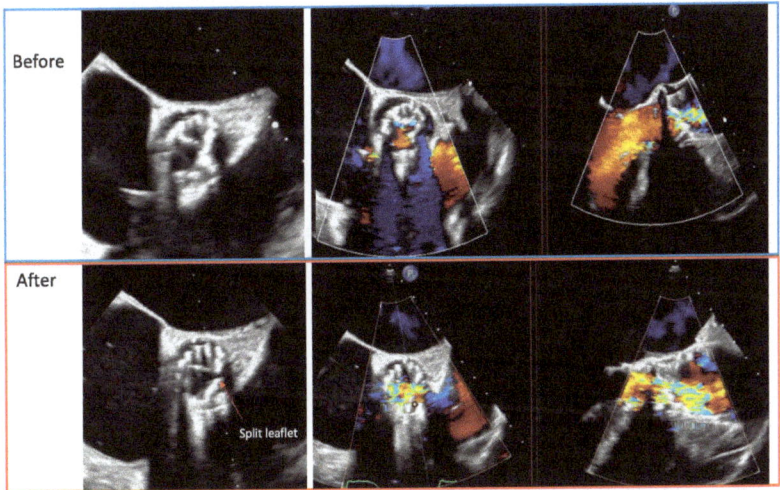

Figure 5. Transesophageal echocardiogram showing the left coronary leaflet before and after the laceration.

7. Discussion

In the last decades, the scientific community has seen a spreading application of transcatheter solutions to treat several structural heart valve diseases. Considering the rapid increase in the number of TAVI procedures, the need for subsequent reinterventions is expected to rise dramatically. In this setting, coronary artery access and coronary obstruction prevention become extremely relevant [6].

In order to facilitate future coronary access, approaches to achieve new THV commissural alignment have been recently described by Tang GHL and Tagliari AP et al. [39,40]. As we have previously described for the PORTICO platform, commissural alignment concept consists in finding a fluoroscopic projection where two native commissures are overlapped leaving the other one isolated. In a cusp overlap projection (RAO/CAUDAL), for instance, we know that two native commissures will be overlapped in the outer aorta curvature while the other one will remain isolated in the inner curvature. To achieve commissural alignment, we rotate the delivery system when it arrives in the descending aorta until the neo-commissures are displayed in the same way (two neo-commissures in the lateral aspect of the descending aorta and one isolated in the medial aspect of the descending aorta) [40]. Tang GHL et al. have suggested that with the EVOLUT platform a better commissural alignment can be achieved if we implant the delivery system with the flush port rotated from a 12 o'clock position to a 3 o'clock position [39].

It is relevant to highlight that during SAVR, commissural alignment is routinely achieved since native leaflets are resected, and surgeons align the commissural posts of bioprosthetic valves to native commissures to avoid coronary obstruction. However, SAVR following TAVI is an extremely risky procedure and with scarce data from large cohorts. Due to adhesions of the valve to the surrounding tissue, removing a THV poses a high risk, because it may disrupt the aortic root. Ando T et al. reported an in-hospital mortality for redo interventions of 7.6% (5.3% for redo TAVI or balloon valvuloplasty vs. 13.8% for redo SAVR, unadjusted p =0.10). Stroke, myocardial infarction, bleeding requiring transfusion, new pacemaker, and acute kidney injury rates were 4.7%, 2.6%, 9.3%, 10.0%, and 31.2%, respectively [41]. In this same line, Jawitz OK et al. pointed out that SAVR after a failure TAVI is a complex, technically demanding procedure, associated with long operative times, increased perioperative morbidity, and much higher than expected operative mortality when compared to redo SAVR. In this study, the authors included 123 patients (median age 77 years) from STS adult cardiac surgery database who underwent SAVR following TAVI between 2011 and 2015. The operative mortality rate was 17.1%, and the observed versus expected mortality ratios were heightened regardless of baseline mortality risk (low 5.48; intermediate 1.66; high 1.16) [42].

Alternatives for the treatment of acute coronary occlusion following TAVI include snaring and removal of the THV or referral for urgent surgery. The employment of chimney stenting is a more reproducible and straightforward approach, whose results were recently published by Mercanti F et al. In the Chimney Registry, 60 cases were examined. Procedural and in-hospital death occurred in three patients. During a median follow-up of 612 days (405–842 days), 2 cases of stent failure were reported (1 in-stent restenosis, 1 possible late stent thrombosis). Discussing these results, authors commented that the BASILICA technique has advantages over chimney stenting, including the avoidance of placing a coronary stent in the aorta and the consequent risk for reaccessing coronaries, restenosis, and thrombosis. Familiarity with both, BASILICA and chimney stenting, is advised for TAVI operators. However, the efficacy of chimney stenting relative to an alternative management strategy, such as BASILICA or elective deferral to conventional SAVR, is unknown [43].

Here we provided a comprehensive review of TAVI-in-TAVI and BASILICA technique employment, outcomes, and concerns, adding evidence to support the technique feasibility and effectiveness.

We reported a Sapien 3 valve implantation inside a degenerated CoreValve bioprosthesis performed together with the BASILICA technique in a patient with high-risk of coronary obstruction. BASILICA was employed to lacerate the left coronary leaflet using not previously described alternative equipment. This report contributes to supporting TAVI-in-TAVI BASILICA's feasibility and safety as a treatment option in patients at risk for coronary obstruction or sinus sequestration. Despite being just a case report, our article is the second one to report a successful TAVI-in-TAVI BASILICA.

There is no doubt that TAVI-in-TAVI BASILICA is an extremely complex and risky procedure, with a high chance of non-success due to several factors. However, when we face highly complex patients, with contraindication to open cardiac surgery, we need to find alternative solutions and push our limits. As said by Vavuranakis M et al. "various technical issues and complications urged pioneer "structuralists" to discover solutions" [44].

8. Conclusions

TAVI-in-TAVI is a growing field that offers a less invasive alternative to treat degenerated THV. However, the inherent TAVI-in-TAVI procedural risks, especially coronary artery obstruction, should be considered. Careful preprocedural planning and an integrated heart team approach are essential to a successful TAVI-in-TAVI procedure. TAVI-in-TAVI BASILICA is a promising new transcatheter solution but needs further studies to be validated.

Supplementary Materials: The following are available online at https://www.mdpi.com/article/10.3390/jcm10235534/s1. Figure S1: Transesophageal echocardiogram short and long axis views showing: (a) new implanted SAPIEN 3 with no residual aortic regurgitation or aortic stenosis; (b) color Doppler images. Table S1: TAVI-in-TAVI BASILICA equipment.

Author Contributions: Conceptualization, A.P.T., R.P.S., E.F.M., E.K.S.; data curation, A.P.T., R.P.S., E.F.M., E.K.S.; writing—original draft preparation, A.P.T., R.P.S., E.F.M., E.K.S.; writing—review and editing, A.P.T., R.P.S., E.F.M., E.K.S.; visualization, A.P.T., R.P.S., E.F.M., E.K.S.; supervision, E.K.S. All authors have read and agreed to the published version of the manuscript.

Funding: This research received no external funding.

Institutional Review Board Statement: Not applicable.

Informed Consent Statement: Written informed consent has been obtained from the patient to publish this paper.

Conflicts of Interest: Tagliari AP has received a Research Grant from Coordenação de Aperfeiçoamento de Pessoal de Nível Superior-Brasil (Capes)-Finance Code 001. Saadi EK is a consultant and Proctor for Medtronic, Abbott and Edwards and received speaker honoraria from Edwards and Medtronic.

References

1. Cribier, A.; Eltchaninoff, H.; Tron, C.; Bauer, F.; Agatiello, C.; Sebagh, L.; Bash, A.; Nusimovici, D.; Litzler, P.Y.; Bessou, J.P.; et al. Early experience with percutaneous transcatheter implantation of heart valve prosthesis for the treatment of end-stage inoperable patients with calcific aortic stenosis. *J. Am. Coll. Cardiol.* **2004**, *43*, 698–703. [CrossRef]
2. Otto, C.M.; Nishimura, R.A.; Bonow, R.O.; Carabello, B.A.; Erwin, J.P.; Gentile, F., III; Jneid, H.; Krieger, E.V.; Mack, M.; McLeod, C.; et al. 2020 ACC/AHA Guideline for the Management of Patients With Valvular Heart Disease: Executive Summary: A Report of the American College of Cardiology/American Heart Association Joint Committee on Clinical Practice Guidelines. *Circulation* **2021**, *143*, e35–e71. [CrossRef]
3. Vahanian, A.; Beyersdorf, F.; Praz, F.; Milojevic, M.; Baldus, S.; Bauersachs, J.; Capodanno, D.; Conradi, L.; De Bonis, M.; De Paulis, R.; et al. ESC/EACTS Scientific Document Group. 2021 ESC/EACTS Guidelines for the management of valvular heart disease. *Eur. Heart J.* **2021**, *60*, 727–800.
4. Mack, M.J.; Leon, M.B.; Thourani, V.H.; Makkar, R.; Kodali, S.K.; Russo, M.; Kapadia, S.R.; Malaisrie, S.C.; Cohen, D.J.; Pibarot, P.; et al. PARTNER 3 Investigators. Transcatheter Aortic-Valve Replacement with a Balloon-Expandable Valve in Low-Risk Patients. *N. Engl. J. Med.* **2019**, *380*, 1695–1705. [CrossRef]
5. Popma, J.J.; Deeb, G.M.; Yakubov, S.J.; Mumtaz, M.; Gada, H.; O'Hair, D.; Bajwa, T.; Heiser, J.C.; Merhi, W.; Kleiman, N.S.; et al. Evolut Low Risk Trial Investigators. Transcatheter Aortic-Valve Replacement with a Self-Expanding Valve in Low-Risk Patients. *N. Engl. J. Med.* **2019**, *380*, 1706–1715. [CrossRef] [PubMed]
6. Jędrzejczyk, S.; Scisło, P.; Grodecki, K.; Rymuza, B.; Kochman, J.; Huczek, Z. TAVI-in-TAVI—Is this the future? *Cardiol. J.* **2019**, *26*, 614–615. [CrossRef]
7. Khan, J.M.; Dvir, D.; Greenbaum, A.B.; Babaliaros, V.C.; Rogers, T.; Aldea, G.; Reisman, M.; Mackensen, G.B.; Eng, M.; Paone, G.; et al. Transcatheter Laceration of Aortic Leaflets to Prevent Coronary Obstruction during Transcatheter Aortic Valve Replacement: Concept to First-in-Human. *JACC Cardiovasc. Interv.* **2018**, *11*, 677–689. [CrossRef]
8. Kappetein, A.P.; Head, S.J.; Généreux, P.; Piazza, N.; van Mieghem, N.M.; Blackstone, E.H.; Brott, T.G.; Cohen, D.J.; Cutlip, D.E.; van Es, G.A.; et al. Updated standardized endpoint definitions for transcatheter aortic valve implantation: The Valve Academic Research Consortium-2 consensus document. *Eur. Heart J.* **2012**, *33*, 2403–2418. [CrossRef]
9. Ruiz, C.E.; Laborde, J.C.; Condado, J.F.; Chiam, P.T.; Condado, J.A. First percutaneous transcatheter aortic valve-in-valve implant with three year follow-up. *Catheter. Cardiovasc. Interv. Off. J. Soc. Card. Angiogr. Interv.* **2008**, *72*, 143–148. [CrossRef]
10. VARC-3 Writing Committee; Généreux, P.; Piazza, N.; Alu, M.C.; Nazif, T.; Hahn, R.T.; Pibarot, P.; Bax, J.J.; Leipsic, J.A.; Blanke, P.; et al. Valve Academic Research Consortium 3: Updated endpoint definitions for aortic valve clinical research. *Eur. Heart J.* **2021**, *42*, 1825–1857. [CrossRef]

11. Witkowski, A.; Jastrzebski, J.; Dabrowski, M.; Chmielak, Z. Second transcatheter aortic valve implantation for treatment of suboptimal function of previously implanted prosthesis: Review of the literature. *J. Interv. Cardiol.* **2014**, *27*, 300–307. [CrossRef]
12. Vrachatis, D.A.; Vavuranakis, M.; Tsoukala, S.; Giotaki, S.; Papaioannou, T.G.; Siasos, G.; Deftereos, G.; Giannopoulos, G.; Raisakis, K.; Tousoulis, D.; et al. TAVI: Valve in valve. A new field for structuralists? Literature review. *Hell. J. Cardiol.* **2020**, *61*, 148–153. [CrossRef] [PubMed]
13. Leon, M.B.; Smith, C.R.; Mack, M.; Miller, D.C.; Moses, J.W.; Svensson, L.G.; Tuzcu, E.M.; Webb, J.G.; Fontana, G.P.; Makkar, R.R.; et al. PARTNER Trial Investigators. Transcatheter aortic-valve implantation for aortic stenosis in patients who cannot undergo surgery. *N. Engl. J. Med.* **2010**, *363*, 1597–1607. [CrossRef] [PubMed]
14. Smith, C.R.; Leon, M.B.; Mack, M.J.; Miller, D.C.; Moses, J.W.; Svensson, L.G.; Tuzcu, E.M.; Webb, J.G.; Fontana, G.P.; Makkar, R.R.; et al. PARTNER Trial Investigators Transcatheter versus surgical aortic-valve replacement in high-risk patients. *N. Engl. J. Med.* **2011**, *364*, 2187–2198. [CrossRef]
15. Popma, J.J.; Adams, D.H.; Reardon, M.J.; Yakubov, S.J.; Kleiman, N.S.; Heimansohn, D.; Hermiller, J.; Hughes, G.C., Jr.; Harrison, J.K.; Coselli, J.; et al. CoreValve United States Clinical Investigators Transcatheter aortic valve replacement using a self-expanding bioprosthesis in patients with severe aortic stenosis at extreme risk for surgery. *J. Am. Coll. Cardiol.* **2014**, *63*, 1972–1981. [CrossRef] [PubMed]
16. Adams, D.H.; Popma, J.J.; Reardon, M.J. Transcatheter aortic-valve replacement with a self-expanding prosthesis. *N. Engl. J. Med.* **2014**, *371*, 967–968. [CrossRef]
17. Makkar, R.R.; Jilaihawi, H.; Chakravarty, T.; Fontana, G.P.; Kapadia, S.; Babaliaros, V.; Cheng, W.; Thourani, V.H.; Bavaria, J.; Svensson, L.; et al. Determinants and outcomes of acute transcatheter valve-in-valve therapy or embolization: A study of multiple valve implants in the U.S. PARTNER trial (Placement of AoRTic TraNscathetER Valve Trial Edwards SAPIEN Transcatheter Heart Valve). *J. Am. Coll. Cardiol.* **2013**, *62*, 418–430. [CrossRef]
18. Percy, E.D.; Harloff, M.T.; Hirji, S.; McGurk, S.; Yazdchi, F.; Newell, P.; Malarczyk, A.; Sabe, A.; Landes, U.; Webb, J.; et al. Nationally Representative Repeat Transcatheter Aortic Valve Replacement Outcomes: Report From the Centers for Medicare and Medicaid Services. *JACC Cardiovasc. Interv.* **2021**, *14*, 1717–1726. [CrossRef]
19. Atizzani, G.F.; Dallan, L.A.; Forrest, J.K.; Reardon, M.J.; Szeto, W.Y.; Liu, F.; Pelletier, M. Redo-transcatheter aortic valve replacement with the supra-annular, self-expandable Evolut platform: Insights from the Transcatheter valve Therapy Registry. *Catheterization and Cardiovascular Intervention* **2021**. Epub Ahead of Print.
20. Landes, U.; Webb, J.G.; De Backer, O.; Sondergaard, L.; Abdel-Wahab, M.; Crusius, L.; Kim, W.K.; Hamm, C.; Buzzatti, N.; Montorfano, M.; et al. Repeat Transcatheter Aortic Valve Replacement for Transcatheter Prosthesis Dysfunction. *J. Am. Coll. Cardiol.* **2020**, *75*, 1882–1893. [CrossRef] [PubMed]
21. Toggweiler, S.; Boone, R.H.; Rodés-Cabau, J.; Humphries, K.H.; Lee, M.; Nombela-Franco, L.; Bagur, R.; Willson, A.B.; Binder, R.K.; Gurvitch, R.; et al. Transcatheter aortic valve replacement: Outcomes of patients with moderate or severe mitral regurgitation. *J. Am. Coll. Cardiol.* **2012**, *59*, 2068–2074. [CrossRef]
22. Schmidt, T.; Frerker, C.; Alessandrini, H.; Schlüter, M.; Kreidel, F.; Schäfer, U.; Thielsen, T.; Kuck, K.H.; Jose, J.; Holy, E.; et al. Redo TAVI: Initial experience at two German centres. *EuroIntervv. J. EuroPCR Collab. Work. Group Interv. Cardiol. Eur. Soc. Cardiol.* **2016**, *12*, 875–882. [CrossRef]
23. Tsuda, M.; Mizote, I.; Ichibori, Y.; Mukai, T.; Maeda, K.; Onishi, T.; Kuratani, T.; Sawa, Y.; Sakata, Y. Outcomes of Redo Transcatheter Aortic Valve Implantation for Structural Valve Degeneration of Transcatheter Aortic Valve. *Circ. Rep.* **2019**, *1*, 142–148. [CrossRef] [PubMed]
24. Dvir, D. Treatment of Small Surgical Valves: Clinical Considerations for Achieving Optimal Results in Valve-in-Valve Procedures. *JACC Cardiovasc. Interv.* **2015**, *8*, 2034–2036. [CrossRef] [PubMed]
25. Ribeiro, H.B.; Webb, J.G.; Makkar, R.R.; Cohen, M.G.; Kapadia, S.R.; Kodali, S.; Tamburino, C.; Barbanti, M.; Chakravarty, T.; Jilaihawi, H.; et al. Predictive factors, management, and clinical outcomes of coronary obstruction following transcatheter aortic valve implantation: Insights from a large multicenter registry. *J. Am. Coll. Cardiol.* **2013**, *62*, 1552–1562. [CrossRef] [PubMed]
26. Ribeiro, H.B.; Rodés-Cabau, J.; Blanke, P.; Leipsic, J.; Kwan Park, J.; Bapat, V.; Makkar, R.; Simonato, M.; Barbanti, M.; Schofer, J.; et al. Incidence, predictors, and clinical outcomes of coronary obstruction following transcatheter aortic valve replacement for degenerative bioprosthetic surgical valves: Insights from the VIVID registry. *Eur. Heart J.* **2018**, *39*, 687–695. [CrossRef] [PubMed]
27. Lederman, R.J.; Babaliaros, V.C.; Rogers, T.; Khan, J.M.; Kamioka, N.; Dvir, D.; Greenbaum, A.B. Preventing Coronary Obstruction During Transcatheter Aortic Valve Replacement: From Computed Tomography to BASILICA. *JACC Cardiovasc. Interv.* **2019**, *12*, 1197–1216. [CrossRef]
28. Komatsu, I.; Mackensen, G.B.; Aldea, G.S.; Reisman, M.; Dvir, D. Bioprosthetic or native aortic scallop intentional laceration to prevent iatrogenic coronary artery obstruction. Part 1: How to evaluate patients for BASILICA. *EuroIntervv. J. EuroPCR Collab. Work. Group Interv. Cardiol. Eur. Soc. Cardiol.* **2019**, *15*, 47–54. [CrossRef] [PubMed]
29. Hidalgo, F.; Ojeda, S.; Romero, M. Chimney Stent Technique in a Valve-in-valve Procedure. *Rev. Esp. De Cardiol.* **2018**, *71*, 972. [CrossRef]
30. Romano, V.; Buzzatti, N.; Latib, A.; Colombo, A.; Montorfano, M. Chimney technique for coronary obstruction after aortic valve in valve: Pros and cons. *Eur. Heart J. Cardiovasc. Imaging* **2018**, *19*, 1194. [CrossRef]

31. Buzzatti, N.; Romano, V.; De Backer, O.; Soendergaard, L.; Rosseel, L.; Maurovich-Horvat, P.; Karady, J.; Merkely, B.; Ruggeri, S.; Prendergast, B.; et al. Coronary Access After Repeated Transcatheter Aortic Valve Implantation: A Glimpse Into the Future. *JACC Cardiovasc. Imaging* **2020**, *13 Pt 1*, 508–515. [CrossRef]
32. Komatsu, I.; Mackensen, G.B.; Aldea, G.S.; Reisman, M.; Dvir, D. Bioprosthetic or native aortic scallop intentional laceration to prevent iatrogenic coronary artery obstruction. Part 2: How to perform BASILICA. *EuroInterv. J. EuroPCR Collab. Work. Group Interv. Cardiol. Eur. Soc. Cardiol.* **2019**, *15*, 55–66. [CrossRef] [PubMed]
33. Kitamura, M.; Majunke, N.; Holzhey, D.; Desch, S.; Bani Hani, A.; Krieghoff, C.; Gutberlet, M.; Protsyk, V.; Ender, J.; Borger, M.A.; et al. Systematic use of intentional leaflet laceration to prevent TAVI-induced coronary obstruction: Feasibility and early clinical outcomes of the BASILICA technique. *EuroInterv. J. EuroPCR Collab. Work. Group Interv. Cardiol. Eur. Soc. Cardiol.* **2020**, *16*, 682–690. [CrossRef] [PubMed]
34. Westermann, D.; Ludwig, S.; Kalbacher, D.; Spink, C.; Linder, M.; Bhadra, O.D.; Nikorowitsch, J.; Waldschmidt, L.; Demal, T.; Voigtländer, L.; et al. Prevention of coronary obstruction in patients at risk undergoing transcatheter aortic valve implantation: The Hamburg BASILICA experience. *Clin. Res. Cardiol. Off. J. Ger. Card. Soc.* **2021**, *110*, 1693. [CrossRef]
35. Tagliari, A.P.; Miura, M.; Gavazzoni, M.; Haager, P.K.; Russo, G.; Pozzoli, A.; Zuber, M.; Jörg, L.; Rickli, H.; Gennari, M.; et al. Bioprosthetic or native aortic scallop intentional laceration to prevent iatrogenic coronary artery obstruction technique in transcatheter aortic valve-in-valve procedures: A single-center initial experience. *J. Cardiovasc. Med.* **2021**, *22*, 212–221. [CrossRef]
36. Khan, J.M.; Greenbaum, A.B.; Babaliaros, V.C.; Dvir, D.; Reisman, M.; McCabe, J.M.; Satler, L.; Waksman, R.; Eng, M.H.; Paone, G.; et al. BASILICA Trial: One-Year Outcomes of Transcatheter Electrosurgical Leaflet Laceration to Prevent TAVR Coronary Obstruction. *Circulation. Cardiovasc. Interv.* **2021**, *14*, e010238. [CrossRef] [PubMed]
37. Khan, J.M.; Bruce, C.G.; Babaliaros, V.C.; Greenbaum, A.B.; Rogers, T.; Lederman, R.J. TAVR Roulette: Caution Regarding BASILICA Laceration for TAVR-in-TAVR. *JACC Cardiovasc. Interv.* **2020**, *13*, 787–789. [CrossRef]
38. Sharma, R.K.; Tuttle, M.K.; Poulin, M.F.; Laham, R.J. CoreValve bioprosthesis dysfunction treated with a Sapien 3 valve-in-valve transcatheter aortic valve replacement and BASILICA technique. *Catheter. Cardiovasc. Interv. Off. J. Soc. Card. Angiogr. Interv.* **2021**, *98*, 403–406. [CrossRef]
39. Tang, G.; Zaid, S.; Fuchs, A.; Yamabe, T.; Yazdchi, F.; Gupta, E.; Ahmad, H.; Kofoed, K.F.; Goldberg, J.B.; Undemir, C.; et al. Alignment of Transcatheter Aortic-Valve Neo-Commissures (ALIGN TAVR): Impact on Final Valve Orientation and Coronary Artery Overlap. *JACC Cardiovasc. Interv.* **2020**, *13*, 1030–1042. [CrossRef]
40. Tagliari, A.P.; Vicentini, L.; Zimmermann, J.M.; Miura, M.; Ferrari, E.; Perez, D.; Haager, P.K.; Jörg, L.; Maisano, F.; Taramasso, M. Transcatheter aortic valve neo-commissure alignment with the Portico system. *EuroInterv. J. EuroPCR Collab. Work. Group Interv. Cardiol. Eur. Soc. Cardiol.* **2021**, *17*, e152–e155. [CrossRef]
41. Ando, T.; Adegbala, O.; Aggarwal, A.; Afonso, L.; Takagi, H.; Grines, C.L.; Briasoulis, A. Redo aortic valve intervention after transcatheter aortic valve replacement: Analysis of the nationwide readmission database. *Int. J. Cardiol.* **2021**, *325*, 115–120. [CrossRef]
42. Jawitz, O.K.; Gulack, B.C.; Grau-Sepulveda, M.V.; Matsouaka, R.A.; Mack, M.J.; Holmes, D.R., Jr.; Carroll, J.D.; Thourani, V.H.; Brennan, J.M. Reoperation After Transcatheter Aortic Valve Replacement: An Analysis of the Society of Thoracic Surgeons Database. *JACC Cardiovasc. Interv.* **2020**, *13*, 1515–1525. [CrossRef] [PubMed]
43. Mercanti, F.; Rosseel, L.; Neylon, A.; Bagur, R.; Sinning, J.M.; Nickenig, G.; Grube, E.; Hildick-Smith, D.; Tavano, D.; Wolf, A.; et al. Chimney Stenting for Coronary Occlusion During TAVR: Insights from the Chimney Registry. *JACC Cardiovasc. Interv.* **2020**, *13*, 751–761. [CrossRef] [PubMed]
44. Vavuranakis, M.; Vrachatis, D.A.; Siasos, G.; Aznaouridis, K.; Vaina, S.; Moldovan, C.; Kalogeras, K.; Kariori, M.; Bei, E.; Papaioannou, T.G.; et al. Managing complications in transcatheter aortic valve implantation. *Hell. J. Cardiol. HJC Hell. Kardiol. Ep.* **2015**, *56* (Suppl. A), 20–30.

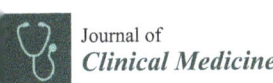

Journal of Clinical Medicine

Review

Vascular Complications in TAVR: Incidence, Clinical Impact, and Management

Markus Mach [1,*], Sercan Okutucu [2], Tillmann Kerbel [1], Aref Arjomand [3], Sefik Gorkem Fatihoglu [4], Paul Werner [1], Paul Simon [1] and Martin Andreas [1]

1. Department of Cardiac Surgery, Medical University Vienna, 1090 Vienna, Austria; tillmann.kerbel@meduniwien.ac.at (T.K.); paul.werner@meduniwien.ac.at (P.W.); paul.simon@meduniwien.ac.at (P.S.); martin.andreas@meduniwien.ac.at (M.A.)
2. Department of Cardiology, Memorial Ankara Hospital, 06520 Ankara, Turkey; sercan.okutucl@memorial.com.tr
3. Department of Cardiology, St. John of God Hospital, Geelong, VIC 3220, Australia; aref.arjomand@med.com
4. Department of Cardiology, Iskenderun State Hospital, 31240 Hatay, Turkey; sgfatihoglu@gmail.com
* Correspondence: markus.mach@meduniwien.ac.at; Tel.: +43-1-40400-52620

Abstract: Transcatheter aortic valve replacement (TAVR) has replaced surgical aortic valve replacement as the new gold standard in elderly patients with severe aortic valve stenosis. However, alongside this novel approach, new complications emerged that require swift diagnosis and adequate management. Vascular access marks the first step in a TAVR procedure. There are several possible access sites available for TAVR, including the transfemoral approach as well as transaxillary/subclavian, transcarotid, transapical, and transcaval. Most cases are primarily performed through a transfemoral approach, while other access routes are mainly conducted in patients not suitable for transfemoral TAVR. As vascular access is achieved primarily by large bore sheaths, vascular complications are one of the major concerns during TAVR. With rising numbers of TAVR being performed, the focus on prevention and successful management of vascular complications will be of paramount importance to lower morbidity and mortality of the procedures. Herein, we aimed to review the most common vascular complications associated with TAVR and summarize their diagnosis, management, and prevention of vascular complications in TAVR.

Keywords: transfemoral; transcatheter; aortic valve; vascular; complications; TAVR; TAVI

1. Introduction

Transcatheter aortic valve replacement (TAVR) has become the new standard of therapy for patients with severe aortic stenosis, and de facto replaced surgical aortic valve replacement (SAVR) when applicable [1,2]. Nevertheless, with the advent of this novel procedure, new complications emerged. Even though the first TAVR was performed via an antegrade transseptal approach, the transfemoral (TF) access is nowadays the most commonly used access strategy. It is applied in over 90% of all TAVR patients in most centers nowadays [1–3]. Vascular access is mainly achieved by puncturing the common femoral artery (CFA) and large bore sheaths that are advanced through retrograde access, and vascular complications are of particularly significant concern during TAVR. Alternative access strategies, via the apex or the ascending aorta as well as the transcarotid, transaxillary, or transcaval access, are performed in specific centers; however, they are not very widespread, primarily due to procedure-specific complexities. As the indication for TAVR is steadily moving towards lower-risk patients, an even stronger focus on the early diagnosis, adequate management, and prevention of these complications will be required for comparable results with SAVR. We hereby provide a broad overview of the most common vascular complications associated with TAVR, their effective management, and their prevention.

2. Materials and Methods

We performed a search of the PubMed database, Scopus, and the Web of Science using the keywords transcatheter aortic valve replacement (all fields) AND vascular (all fields) AND complications (all fields) (last update: 1 September 2021). There was no date or language restriction for our selection of publication. References of selected studies and all abstracts from cardiology congresses (American College of Cardiology, American Heart Association, European Society of Cardiology, PCR London Valves, and Transcatheter Cardiovascular Therapeutics) were searched for relevant data. Supplementary Figure S1 provides the PRISMA flowchart of studies included in this systematic review. Supplementary Table S1 provides an overview of vascular access complications and associated bleeding events in all studies analyzed in this review. The data were subdivided with respect to access routes, TAVR devices, and the application of VARC endpoint definitions. [1,2,4–50].

The manuscript aims to provide a concise and precise description of the experimental results, their interpretation, and the experimental conclusions that can be drawn.

3. Vascular Complications in TAVR

3.1. Incidence and Definition

The heterogenic group of intra-operative, as well as early postoperative, vascular complications are significantly associated with a higher rate of postinterventional morbidity and mortality, and it is alongside postinterventional pacemaker implantations as the most common type of complications after TAVR [47,51]. Especially in the early days of TAVR, vascular complications were relatively common, even though they varied widely around 2% and 30% due to unstandardized definitions of vascular complications [47,51]. Valve Academic Research Consortium (VARC) formulated standardized endpoint definitions for common adverse events after TAVR for better comparability between published data [52,53]. Three main subgroups were conceived as major vascular complications, minor vascular complications, and percutaneous closure device failure (Table 1) [53].

The PARTNER trial described vascular complications in almost a quarter of patients treated with TAVR, with a nearly even distribution of major (15.3%) and minor vascular complications (11.9%) using these definitions [47]. Genereux et al. reported a vascular complication rate of 11.9% in a meta-analysis with 3519 patients [54]. Current literature reporting outcomes, according to the updated standard VARC definitions, describe vascular complication rates ranging between 10% and 20% [51,55,56]. Comparing the relatively high vascular complication rates in the early days of TAVR, a significant decrease down to 4% and less can be observed in the recent literature [1,2,57–59]. However, vascular access complications are still quite common, with a major influence on adverse outcomes after TAVR [60]. Not only are they strongly correlated with increased hospitalization days, poorer quality of life outcomes, and 30-day and 1-year mortality, but also with bleeding complications, access site infections, and renal impairment leading to substantially increased procedural costs [51,61]. Observed 30-day mortality was significantly higher in patients with major vascular complications as opposed to those without vascular complications [51,61]. The PARTNER trial even demonstrated a four-fold increase in 30-day mortality in patients with major vascular access complications [47]. Notably, minor vascular complications have less impact on outcome and survival [62]. Endovascular experts or even vascular surgeons need to be firmly involved in heart team decisions and preoperative assessment to improve outcomes in TAVR patients and make this treatment applicable in young, low-risk patients. Vascular complications need to be diagnosed early and treated accordingly, but prevention will be pivotal for TAVR to be beneficial in younger patients with less surgical risk.

Table 1. Valve Academic Research Consortium-2 classification of vascular access site and access-related complications.

Complication	Definition
Major vascular complications	<ul><li>Any aortic dissection, aortic rupture, annulus rupture, left ventricle perforation, or new apical aneurysm/pseudoaneurysm;</li><li>Access site or access-related vascular injury (dissection, stenosis, perforation, rupture, arterio-venous fistula, pseudoaneurysm, hematoma, irreversible nerve injury, compartment syndrome, percutaneous closure device failure) leading to death, life-threatening or major bleeding *, visceral ischemia, or neurological impairment;</li><li>Distal embolization (non-cerebral) from a vascular source requiring surgery or resulting in amputation or irreversible end-organ damage;</li><li>The use of unplanned endovascular or surgical intervention associated with death, major bleeding, visceral ischemia, or neurological impairment;</li><li>Any new ipsilateral lower extremity ischemia documented by patient symptoms, physical exam, and/or decreased or absent blood flow on lower extremity angiogram;</li><li>Surgery for access site-related nerve injury or permanent access site-related nerve injury.</li></ul>
Minor vascular complications	<ul><li>Access site or access-related vascular injury (dissection, stenosis, perforation, rupture, arterio-venous fistula, pseudoaneurysm, hematomas, percutaneous closure device failure) not leading to death, life-threatening or major bleeding *, visceral ischemia, or neurological impairment;</li><li>Distal embolization treated with embolectomy and/or thrombectomy and not resulting in amputation or irreversible end-organ damage;</li><li>Any unplanned endovascular stenting or unplanned surgical intervention not meeting the criteria for a major vascular complication;</li><li>Vascular repair or the need for vascular repair (via surgery, ultrasound-guided compression, transcatheter embolization, or stent graft).</li></ul>
Percutaneous closure device failure	<ul><li>Failure of a closure device to achieve hemostasis at the arteriotomy site leading to alternative treatment (other than manual compression or adjunctive endovascular ballooning).</li></ul>

* Refers to VARC-2 bleeding definitions. Adapted and reproduced with permission from the copyright owner [63].

3.2. Risk Factors

Several procedural, as well as patient-related, factors contribute to the occurrence of vascular complications (Table 2). Female gender, peripheral vascular disease–especially in patients with a borderline femoral diameter and/or circumferential calcification patterns, a sheath-to-femoral-artery-ratio (SFAR) of less than 1.05 or a sheath diameter that exceeds the minimal femoral diameter, severe iliofemoral tortuosity patterns with an iliofemoral tortuosity score above 21.2, as well as operator experience and planned surgical cut-down are substantiated independent predictors of vascular complications [47,51,61,63–67]. High volume centers that can provide a sufficient learning curve to warrant adequate operator experience, meticulous patient selection as well as deliberate preoperative assessing measurements, and the use of low-profile sheaths (<19Fr) and valves of the newer generation substantially reduce the rate of such complications [61,68,69]. A further decline in vascular complication rates is expected due to the further development of vascular closure devices and smaller delivery systems.

Table 2. Risk factors associated with vascular complications.

Risk Factors	
Non-modifiable	• Gender (women men) • Age (older younger) • Obesity • Peripheral vascular disease (SFAR 1.05, circumferential/ horseshoe calcification) • Vascular tortuosity • Blood dyscrasia
Modifiable	• Puncture site (CFA SFA or EIA) • Sheath size (LPS HPS) • Puncture type (anterior wall only anterior + posterior wall; CFA only CFA + vein puncture) • Anticoagulation regime

SFAR—sheath-to-femoral-artery-ratio; CFA—common femoral artery; SFA—superficial femoral artery; EIA—external iliac artery; LPS—low-profile sheath; HPS—high profile sheath. Adapted and reproduced with permission from the copyright owner [20].

3.3. Access Techniques

Diligent preprocedural assessment of the access vessels is crucial to select the best strategy for the patient and to keep vascular complications at a bare minimum. Contrast-enhanced multidetector computed tomography (MDCT) helps assess iliofemoral vessel diameters, calcification load and pattern distribution, tortuosity, and skin-to-artery distance. In the earlier days of TAVR, operators would mainly rely on traditional anatomical landmark guidance (TALG) for a vascular puncture, using the inguinal ligament and the zone of maximal femoral pulsation as a reference. Arterial puncture 2–3 cm caudally to this point in a 30–45° angle targets the CFA over the femoral head that serves as a firm counter bearing during manual compression for hemostasis. A low puncture, especially distally to the femoral bifurcation, should be avoided as it bears a higher risk for pseudoaneurysm or arteriovenous fistula formation, dissection, rupture, or thrombus formation [70]. A high puncture penetrating the external iliac artery or inferior epigastric artery will likewise impede achieving hemostasis and result in an eighteen-fold increase of risk for retroperitoneal bleedings [71]. Noteworthy, the sole reliance on anatomical features such as the skin crease will lead to a low puncture in 72% of patients and the zone of maximal femoral pulsation to a high puncture in 93% of patients [72]. Another approach to locate the optimal zone for arterial puncture is ultrasound-guided access. Therefore, a linear ultrasound probe is used to determine the height of femoral bifurcation and to exclude anterior wall calcification in the puncture zone. Identification of the artery is facilitated by the possibility of compression of the femoral vein. Real-time needle guidance reduces the risk of a posterior wall or sidewall puncture. Compared to fluoroscopy guidance, the vascular complications, the risk of venous puncture, and the number of attempts of successful vessel access were significantly reduced [73]. Although no study demonstrated a clear benefit of ultrasound or fluoroscopy-guided femoral access over TALG as a default strategy, it is potentially helpful in high-risk patients with profound vascular calcification or a marked skin-to-artery distance [73–75]. In such cases, a fluoroscopic target zone for safe CFA puncture can be defined in anterior-posterior projection between the centerline of the femoral head and a caudal 14mm margin avoiding both the femoral bifurcation and retroperitoneal vessels (Figure 1). Road mapping using digital subtraction crossover angiography via contralateral CFA access is another useful technique to mitigate the risk of access complications. Initial vascular access is usually performed using a micro-puncture needle and a 4–5F sheath to avoid large-bore needle trauma in case of an unsuccessful puncture and can later be exchanged over a standard guidewire.

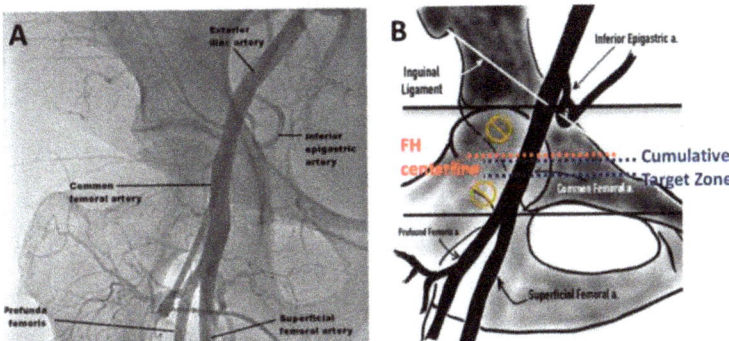

Figure 1. (**A**) Fluoroscopic and (**B**) schematic illustration of the ideal common femoral artery puncture site.

Even though percutaneous closure devices offer good postoperative results and sheath sizes became notably smaller over the years, the surgical access offers a controlled and safe access, whose benefits might be overlooked in patients that are at risk for vascular complications [76–79]. While some studies demonstrated that surgical access is comparably safe and cost-effective, other studies indicated specific advantages of a percutaneous approach, especially with regard to access site infections [76,79–82]. The surgical cut-down is performed via a 30–40mm transversal incision starting right distally of the inguinal ligament and laterally from the femoral artery to preserve lymphatic integrity. The subcutaneous tissue is carefully dissected, and the femoral artery is prepared to place a purse-string suture or two U-sutures in a non-calcified spot on the CFA. Vascular access is then gained via direct puncture under direct visual control. After sheath removal, the sutures are tied. A femoral patch angioplasty or interposition grafting is mainly used when direct vascular closure cannot be achieved.

The subclavian access is the most frequent alternative access strategy to the transfemoral access and is usually performed from the left side for better valve alignment. Even though transaxillary TAVR is commonly performed over surgical cut-down, a fully percutaneous approach is feasible with puncturing the proximal third of the axillary artery. A minimum vessel diameter of 6mm is recommended, but in cases with prior coronary bypass grafting using the ipsilateral internal mammary artery, the vessel diameter should exceed 7 mm. Increased angulation at the aorto-subclavian junction favors kinking of the sheath or delivery system. Ectatic and severally calcified arteries should be avoided due to the increased risk for vascular complications that can be challenging to control [83].

Transcarotid (TC) TAVR has the main advantage of the short distance to the native aortic valve and the anatomically facilitated coaxial alignment; however, this access strategy is not widely performed due to its proximity to nerval structures and the respiratory tract, as well as its risk of stroke, even though experienced centers report similar stroke and vascular complication rates as via a transfemoral approach. TC-TAVR is usually performed under local anesthesia and cerebral near-infrared spectroscopy. A complete Circle of Willis is a prerequisite for the safety of this approach [84,85].

Depending on the anatomical position of the aorta, the transaortic access is performed either through a right anterior mini-thoracotomy in case of a right-sided ascending aorta or patent bypass grafts or through a median hemi-sternotomy in case of deep intrathoracic location or severe lung disease [86]. A minimum puncture to native aortic annulus distance of 8 mm for the Edwards Sapien 3 valve and 6mm for the Medtronic CoreValve is required [37,87]. Compared to the transapical approach, patients treated with transaortic TAVR are not at risk of ventricular scarring and subsequent development of apical pseudoaneurysm. Fiorina et al. demonstrated lower overall vascular complication rates predominantly driven by minor vascular complication transaortic TAVR patients compared to transaxillary TAVR patients [88]. However, direct comparisons to other access strategies are scarce, and observational studies and meta-analyses suggest similar mortality rates and vascular complications when compared to the transfemoral access [87,89–92].

The transapical access is performed over an anterolateral intercostal incision, puncturing the left ventricle at the apex cordis. Sufficient myocardial thickness and frailty must be considered, as apex closure can be cumbersome in patients with a tenuous free wall of the left ventricle. Hence, procedure-specific access complications such as left ventricular pseudoaneurysm formation and tamponade may occur. Even though access complications rates are low, it has been indicated that the transapical access is an independent predictor of higher postinterventional mortality [93–95].

If there is a lack of alternative access sites, transcaval access can be performed via femoral venous access. At the level of the inferior vena cava, an arteriovenous fistula is created by the application of electrocautery over a coronary guidewire. The transcatheter valve implantation is then carried out in a standard fashion, and the fistula is closed with an Amplatzer P.D.A. occlude or a similar device. There are limited outcome data, but with major vascular complications ranging between 11% and 28% and major or life-threatening bleeding rates between 13% and 28%, a significant learning curve must be considered as well as operator and center experience [96].

3.4. Guidewires, Catheters, and Sheaths

3.4.1. Guidewires

Different guidewires need to be used during TAVR, but all usually come at a 0.0035" diameter and an exchange length of 260 cm or more. They typically consist of a solid proximal core for adequate support and push-ability that is tapered towards the soft atraumatic tip, ensuring shape-ability and steerability. Some will have either hydrophilic coating, for increased lubricity and easier tracking to minimize vessel trauma, or hydrophobic coating, for a better tactile response. A wide range of wires are used and differ between institutions but most commonly include catheters of the Amplatz family (Boston Scientific, Marlborough, MA, USA), the Back-up Meier wire (Boston Scientific, Marlborough, MA, USA), the Lunderqvist Extra stiff (Cook Medical, Bloomington, IN, USA), and the Safari wire (Medtronic Inc). The Safari wire is pre-shaped with a distal exaggerated J curve, but other wires may need to be bent manually, with the rigid portion forming a part of the J curve. This will ensure good wire support and, more importantly, reduce the risk of vascular or left ventricular perforation. The flexural modulus describes the bending stiffness of wires in gigapascals (GPa) and was introduced by Harrison et al. to provide objective comparability between different products, as market terminology can be misleading [97]. High wire stiffness can be beneficial in cases with severe vascular tortuosity, but such wires require cautious handling.

3.4.2. Catheters

A novel method to ensure safe passage of delivery systems in borderline-sized iliofemoral vessels is the use of intravascular lithotripsy. For this purpose, specifically designed catheter systems are used to disrupt intimal and medial calcifications through controlled microfractures and microdissections, thereby achieving an increase in vascular compliance. These catheter systems were evaluated in the DISRUPT-PAD I and II trials in patients with calcified femoropopliteal vascular lesions and demonstrated a surprisingly low incidence of vascular complications requiring intervention (1.7%) without displaying an increased rate of embolic debris in distal embolic filters [98,99].

Registry data of 42 patients with peripheral artery disease and otherwise prohibitive transfemoral access pathways showed that these intravascular lithotripsy catheters allowed safe transfemoral passage of TAVR delivery systems in more than 90% of all patients [100,101]. Within this small cohort, no iliofemoral dissections or perforations requiring intervention were reported, with only one patient (2.4%) demonstrating a pseudoaneurysm and another (2.4%) requiring endarterectomy [101].

3.4.3. Sheaths

The insertion of larger sheaths in the CFA strongly correlates with higher vascular complication rates [102]. However, sheath size depends on the size and type of the implanted device. As such, a minimal femoral vessel diameter of 5.5 mm or a SFAR of less than 1.05 is recommended for transfemoral TAVR [51]. Due to ongoing developments of valve delivery systems, initial sheath sizes of 24 Fr and 26 Fr of the first generation of the Edwards Sapien valves and 25 Fr for the Medtronic CoreValve newer generation valves require 14Fr to 16Fr sheaths for balloon-expandable valves and 14Fr sheaths for self-expanding valves.

Three sheath designs need to be mentioned due to their innovative design. The eSheath (Edwards LifeSciences, Irvine, CA, USA) is a transiently expandable sheath with a length of 26 cm and has a 14Fr profile for the Sapien 3 valve. The sheath expands approximately 2 mm during valve passage and then returns to its original diameter. The sheathless EnVeo-R delivery system with its built-in 14Fr InLine sheath (Medtronic, Minneapolis, MN, United States) currently offers the lowest profile on the market. The SoloPath sheath (Terumo Medical Corporation, Irvine, CA, USA) is a 35 cm tapered balloon-expandable hydrophilic sheath. Its distal end is folded over a pre-mounted inflatable balloon dilatation catheter that can expand the sheath to 19Fr. Once the balloon is removed, the sheath will maintain its expanded shape and can return to its original size once the balloon is deflated. This design decreases vascular friction and trauma during sheath insertion in patients with borderline-sized femoral vessels. A single-arm study with 90 patients demonstrated the safety and efficacy of the Solopath sheath even in patients with a SFAR of greater than 1.05. Compared to patients with a SFAR of less than 1.05, no difference in procedural success and overall vascular or bleeding complications had been observed [103]. As low-profile sheaths (<19Fr) cause less vascular and bleeding complications [102], there is no evidence yet on the actual clinical benefit of expandable sheaths over fixed diameter. And even though smaller vessels can be tackled with such sheaths, valve passage through the sheath may not be feasible in all cases.

3.5. Hemostasis Methods

Transfemoral TAVR in its initial phase was predominantly performed via surgical cut-down, which is still a viable option in situations with morbidly obese patients, significant anterior calcification of the access vessel, alternative access sites (e.g., the subclavian access), and surgically experienced centers [80,104–106]. Even though reported outcomes demonstrate less vascular and bleeding complications, the reduction in sheath size and the increased use and evolution of pre-closure devices and techniques lead to the predominant use of a fully percutaneous access technique. Hemostasis after sheath removal is mainly achieved using suture-mediated closure devices such as the Prostar XL or Perclose ProGlide closure devices (Abbott Vascular Devices, Redwood City, CA, USA). A reduction in vascular access and bleeding complications had been demonstrated in several studies [81,82]. Even though these devices are indicated for closure of 10F (Prostar XL) and 8F (Perclose ProGlide) arteriotomy sites, if deployed before the initial sheath insertion—as in the "preclose" technique—generally, good hemostasis can be achieved [107,108]. The sutures are placed before large-bore sheaths are inserted, tied manually, and approximated with the help of knot pushers at the end of the procedure, once the sheath and the 0.0035″ guidewire are consecutively removed. A single Prostar XL device can close arteriotomies up to 19Fr using the pre-closure technique. If two devices are deployed at a 45° angle, sufficient closure of larger arteriotomy sites up to 24Fr can be achieved [109]. Similarly, such a "double preclose technique" can be applied using two Perclose ProGlide devices deployed at a 30–35° angle to create an interrupted x-figure suture for closing larger arteriotomy sites. This technique has proven to be effective and efficient with a low incidence of early and late closure site complications, as well as reduced hospital stay [104,110].

The MANTA VCD consists of a toggle placed within the vessel and a bovine collagen plug situated outside the artery. Both components are connected and pushed together, fixating each other on the internal and external vessel wall, leading to arteriotomy closure. Both device parts are completely resolvable within 6 months. The device got the C.E. mark for vascular closure for sheath sizes up to 22 French. Retrospective studies that compared MANTA to ProStarXL revealed comparable rates of vascular complications but significantly lower bleeding rates after MANTA application. A hybrid closure technique using both a suture (ProGlide) and a collagen (Angio-Seal) mediated closure device has been proposed with good results, having a high success rate (98%) and low vascular complications [111].

Even though some centers propagate the use of an ipsilateral double arterial access to reduce the use of contrast agents, most centers prefer an ancillary arterial at the contralateral side [112]. Both access strategies can be used to ensure vascular closure after sheath removal and control potential access site complications. However, contralateral access allows the application of the crossover balloon occlusion technique (CBOT). Therefore, an angioplasty balloon is inflated above the access site prior to sheath removal to temporarily reduce blood flow and, subsequently, blood pressure at the access site. This technique ensures safe and successful closure in patients undergoing TAVR with large bore-sheaths up to 24Fr. In unfavorable contralateral femoral anatomy, a transradial crossover approach can be used as a reasonable alternative [113].

3.6. Diagnosis and Management of Specific Vascular Complications

Most commonly, vascular access is gained over the CFA. Therefore, vessel dissection, rupture, access site hematoma, and the formation of pseudoaneurysms are all possible complications during or after TAVR. General measures such as blood volume substitution or medical resuscitation need to be promptly available. Other possible causes for a hemodynamic decline, such as coronary artery obstruction or valve function impairment, should be excluded immediately when suspected. In any case, both endovascular and surgical treatment must always be available to ensure a maximum safe environment for any patient treated with TAVR. Diagnostic crossover angiography to assess aortic or iliofemoral vascular complication after sheath removal is routinely advocated in most centers and is considered best clinical practice. This diagnostic maneuver is not only performed for early detection of vascular complication—arguably the most critical factor for optimal management—but also allows rapid vascular access through the placement of a crossover wire from the contralateral CFA. An overview of common vascular complications and their management is depicted in Table 3.

Table 3. Management of vascular complications.

Location	Management
Aortic complications	
Aortic rupture	Open surgical repair
	Aortic occlusion balloon and cardiopulmonary bypass to stabilize
Aortic dissection	Surgical and endovascular repair
	Medical management
Iliofemoral complications	
	Immediate reversal of anticoagulation
Arterial perforation	Prolonged balloon angioplasty or, less commonly, covered stent-graft implantation from a contralateral or ipsilateral CFA access
Arterial dissection	Flow-limiting, prolonged balloon angioplasty or covered stent-graft implantation from a contralateral or ipsilateral CFA access
Arterial stenosis, thrombosis, and occlusion	Thrombectomy or balloon angioplasty
Pseudoaneurysm	Size <3.0–3.5 cm: observation
	Size >3.0–3.5 cm or expanding: thrombin injection
Hematoma	Conservative, manual compression, prolonged balloon angioplasty from contralateral CFA access

Adapted and reproduced with permission from the copyright owner [66].

3.6.1. Aortic Dissection or Rupture

These complications occur quite rarely, but dissection and rupture of the aorta and especially the aortic annulus are catastrophic and immediately life-threatening complications. Even though the incidence with less than 2% is relatively low, the clinical impact is quite devastating, with mortality rates of up to 50% for aortic dissections [51,105,110,114]. The aortic root and ascending aorta can be injured by the expanding balloons, valves, or the delivery system itself. At the same time, catheters or guidewires can lead to injury of the intima leading to acute or subacute aortic dissection of Stanford type A. Typically, this mechanism occurs during valvuloplasty or valve implantation, especially in the case of device migration during the expansion phase (Figure 2). The dissection of the descending aorta without the involvement of the ascending aorta, as in a Stanford type B dissection, is an even rarer entity limited to single case reports and is mainly caused due to tip injury of the sheath at the time of delivery system introduction and advancement [115]. Patients may present with acute or subacute chest or abdominal pain or neurological or hemodynamic changes, depending on the location and limitations of the dissection. Most centers still rely on periprocedural transesophageal echo (TEE) during TAVR, even if transfemoral TAVR is increasingly performed under local anesthesia without TEE nowadays. Hence, periprocedural TEE and/or angiography may expedite such diagnosis if suspected early. Postprocedural CT-angiography (CTA) is commonly performed for affirmation. As Stanford type B dissections can be treated medically by limiting systolic arterial pressures to 100–110 mmHg and keeping M.A.P. over 70 mmHg, endovascular treatment with TEVAR may be necessary in some cases. Stanford type A dissections, on the other side, mandate immediate surgical treatment. Rupture of the aortic annulus that requires similar to aortic dissection surgical repair is mainly caused by oversizing of the valvuloplasty balloon or prosthesis in the presence of severe annular calcification extending in the muscular region of the LVOT (between right-to-left coronary cusp commissure and the left fibrous trigone), and especially in cases with an isolated bulky calcification of a single cusp [116]. A large multicenter study demonstrated that a higher annular calcification score was associated with landing zone rupture compared to patients with lower scores (181 ± 211 vs. 22 ± 37; $p\ 0.001$) [117]. Several other MDCT related parameters, including leaflet asymmetry defined as

$$\sqrt{[(non\ coronary\ leaflet\ area - right\ coronary\ leaflet\ area)2 + (right\ coronary\ leaflet\ area - left\ coronaryy\ leaflet\ area)2]}$$

or the annular cover index defined as

$$\left[prosthesis\ nominal\ area - \frac{annular\ area}{prostehsis\ nomina\ area} \times 100 \right]$$

might add incremental predictive value during risk stratification in patients with a high risk for landing zone rupture. Valves that generate high radial forces, as well as post-dilatation in patients with THV valves implanted with >20% area oversizing, should be avoided in such cases [118].

Risky situations potentially occur when the valvuloplasty balloon recoils into the left ventricle during full expansion. Annular rupture occurs at rates around 1% and results in rapid development of hemopericardium and pericardial tamponade. Delayed clinical manifestations are rare but possible in slow-progressing or contained ruptures. MDCT-based assessment of aortic annulus dimension in conjunction with adapted sizing guidelines may reduce the incidence of severe oversizing [119,120]. The imminent importance of "heart team" on-site must be stressed again, as only immediate surgical intervention will control these life-threatening complications. Rupture of the descending or abdominal aorta can be managed by immediate balloon occlusion followed by either surgical or endovascular repair using covered stent-grafts.

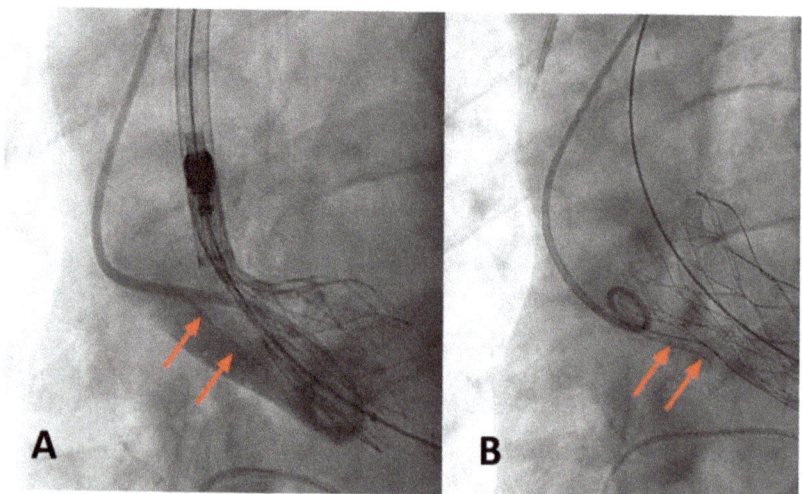

Figure 2. (**A**,**B**) Fluoroscopic evidence of dissection in the ascending aorta during THV deployment with red arrows indicating the dissection flap.

3.6.2. Iliofemoral Dissection or Rupture

The incidence of dissection of the CFA or iliac arteries ranges between 1.6% and 21.4% for a complete percutaneous transfemoral approach and between 2% and 7% for a surgical cut-down approach [51,61,68,107,121]. Dissections occur most likely in the external iliac artery during any phase between the initial vascular access and advancement of the delivery system, and they may not be observed until sheath withdrawal. Retrograde or contralateral antegrade control angiography prior to completion of TAVR usually reveals vascular access injuries, possibly leading to limb ischemia depending on the grade of vascular blood flow limitation, subsequent thrombus formation, and thromboembolic events. Postinterventional vascular Doppler, CTA, or angiography should be performed in case of acute onset of leg or back pain, clinical signs of ischemia, or hemodynamic deterioration. In case of compromised blood flow, angioplasty with prolonged balloon inflation alone may suffice for intima-media re-apposition. However, extensive dissection may require uncovered or even covered stent implantation or surgical treatment [68,107,121,122]. Asymptomatic small dissections without flow-limitation can be treated conservatively but need to be followed up closely.

Potentially fatal iliofemoral rupture is observed in 0.7% to up to 9.3% of TAVR procedures. Similar to iliofemoral dissections, lower incidence rates are displayed in more recent publications due to the introduction of low-profile sheath systems and sheathless delivery systems [68,107,121,122]. It is mainly detected after sheath withdrawal, as it usually seals the tear during the valve implantation [123,124]. Especially large bore sheath withdrawal from small, calcified vessels can be critical as it can lead to arterial avulsion [121,125]. The patient's clinical status can deteriorate rapidly in case of extensive rupture and gradually over hours if small tears remain undetected. However, extraluminal contrast accumulation during final access site angiography is a clear indicator. Immediate sealing of the tear should be performed, either through the reintroduction of the sheath or contralateral balloon occlusion. Bleeding from smaller tears can resolve after a couple of minutes after occlusion and anticoagulation reversal. However, larger vessel injuries warrant immediate covered stent-graft implantation, surgical patch-repair, or interposition-grafting [123].

3.6.3. Access Site Bleeding and Hematoma

Access site hematomas are relatively common, with reported incidences between 2.2 and 12.5%. Still, a steady decline can be observed due to increasing operator experience, use of low-profile sheaths, and advances in vascular closure techniques [51,104,126]. They appear either immediately reversal or gradually over hours to days of TAVR, despite manual compression and anticoagulation. They are generally benign and with spontaneous resolution over weeks, but they are associated with a prolonged hospital stay, secondary infection, need for blood transfusion, and increased mortality [127]. Diagnosed primarily during clinical examination, hematomas can be treated conservatively in most cases. Manual compression and anticoagulation reversal should be performed if oozing or active bleeding from the puncture site is apparent. Similar to small vascular tears, endovascular treatment involving prolonged balloon occlusion and self-expanding stent implantation can be indicated. Infrequently, large hematoma compressing nerval structures need to be evacuated surgically.

Retroperitoneal hemorrhage or hematoma can be due to aortic, iliac, inferior epigastric, or femoral injury and very often lead to nonspecific symptoms of groin, flank, or back pain with or without hemodynamic changes. If retroperitoneal hematomas are radiologically confirmed by CT or angiography, and with an overall incidence of up to 2.2%, most can be managed by transfusion of coagulation factors or red blood cell units [53,104,107]. In case of overt bleeding, coil embolization of small, ruptured vessels and covert stent-graft implantation or surgical repair in larger ruptures are indicated, depending on the size and location of the bleeding [53,104,107,126].

3.6.4. Access Site Pseudoaneurysm

Pseudoaneurysm (PSA) formation results in 2–6% of TAVR cases due to contained rupture with extravascular arterial bleeding into a pseudo-capsule [128]. Mostly diagnosed as a pulsatile mass in the groin during the clinical examination or Doppler ultrasound, a systolic bruit can be heard during auscultation. Several risk factors, such as advanced age, frailty, high B.M.I., current anticoagulation medication, the use of high-profile sheaths, high or low puncture, arterial and venous puncture, severe vascular calcification, and failed manual compression, can promote PSA formation [129]. Spontaneous PSA thrombosis is common in small pseudoaneurysm (3.0–3.5 cm) and patients without the necessity of anticoagulation [130,131]. A larger PSA leads to progressing discomfort, local infection, septic embolism, and rupture [131]. With a success rate of 97%, ultrasound-guided thrombin injection is favored over ultrasound-guided compression [132,133]. Incremental doses of 0.2–0.4 mL are injected until flow within the PSA ceases. Complication such as infection or thromboembolism is observed in less than 1% of cases [129]. Larger pseudoaneurysm unfavorable for thrombin injection require interventional or surgical occlusion (Figure 3). Similar to cut down for transfemoral TAVR, the CFA is approached, while sparing the PSA as much as possible, and clamped after heparin administration. Subsequently, the PSA is opened, and the puncture site is closed with either single sutures or a patch-plasty.

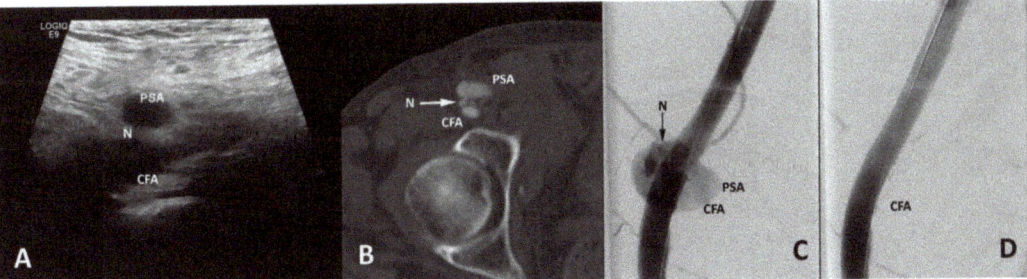

Figure 3. (**A**) Sonographic, (**B**) computer-tomographic, and (**C**) fluoroscopic evidence of pseudoaneurysm formation (PSA) with a short, broad neck (N) in the common femoral artery (CFA) after transfemoral THV implantation. (**D**) Pseudoaneurysm exclusion by endovascular implantation of a balloon-expandable covered stent graft (8 × 50 mm Gore® Viabahn®).

3.6.5. Access Site Infection

The rate of access site infections ranges up to 6.3% in transfemoral cases and are more often reported after surgical cut-down than complete percutaneous access [51,126]. Partner 1A reported access site infections of 2% with no difference in sternal wound infection rates after SAVR [48]. Preventive measures include the administration of broad-spectrum antibiotics thorough prepping and draping prior to and after the procedure. Superficial infections respond well to local or systemic therapy if treated early. Infections involving periarterial tissue can lead to sepsis and substantially increase the risk of mortality [51,126]. Surgical debridement and V.A.C.© therapy (vacuum-assisted closure; Kinetic Concepts; KCI Medical, San Antonio, TX, USA) are the main therapeutic treatment options for deep wound infections.

3.6.6. Closure Device Failure

Closure device failure is described in 4.4 to 8.7% of cases and can cause arterial dissection, rupture, and vascular constriction or occlusion [51,104,107]. In case of insufficient hemostasis, treatment options are not different from access site oozing. Manual compression alone is sufficient in most cases. If limb ischemia is suspected, vascular Doppler, CTA, or angiography are appropriate to verify unrestricted blood flow. Angioplasty or stent implantation may be indicated in case of severe vascular stenosis or bleeding (Figure 4).

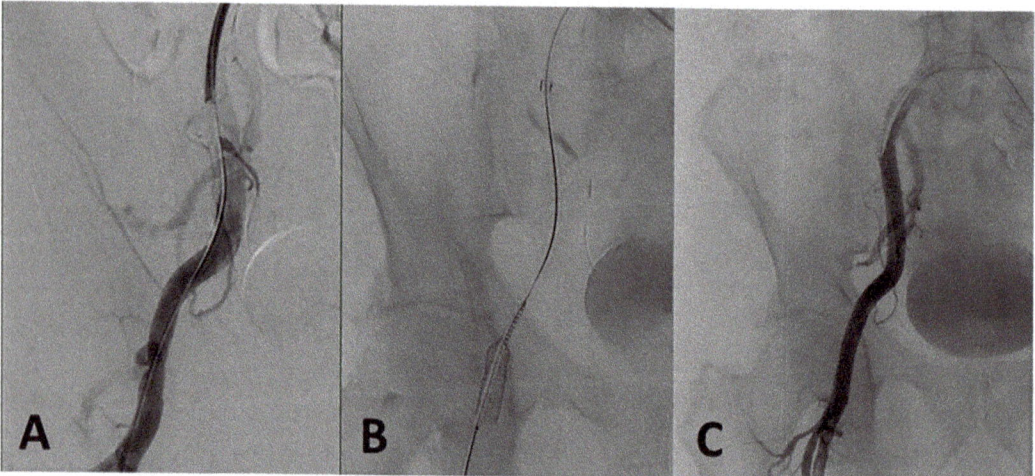

Figure 4. (**A**) Vascular closure device failure after TAVI with consecutive stenosis and bleeding of the right common femoral artery. (**B**) Endovascular treatment of the right common femoral artery with a self-expanding covered stent graft (9 × 50 mm Gore® Viabahn®). (**C**) Control angiography shows unobstructed outflow without extravasation.

3.6.7. Vascular Complications Associated with Non-Transfemoral Access

Access complications during TA-TAVR are rare but potentially fatal complications. Bleeding from the puncture site, or myocardial tears during access site closure, are the most frequent complications observed. As TAVR is usually performed in elderly patients, myocardial tissue can be rather soft and frail. Patients with a dilated left ventricle and a thin free wall are at particular risk. Apical hypokinesis can be observed during follow-up and is caused by myocardial scarring or close puncture to the left anterior descending artery, with closing suture limiting myocardial blood flow [93,134,135]. These complications can lead to ventricular aneurysm formation over time. Rib retraction and intercostal nerve damage can cause chronic chest pain at the access site and are less frequently observed when elastic soft tissue retractors are used instead of mechanical rib spreaders [134–136].

Vascular complications during or after transaxillary TAVR are limited to small series or single case reports. The pattern of vascular complications is similar to that seen with transfemoral access; however, achieving hemostasis with manual compression is rather difficult due to the lack of a supporting structure to buttress against during compression. Therefore, a low threshold towards endovascular stent implantation seems advisable, especially since closure device failure rates of 29.2% have been reported by Schäfer et al. Of note, the same study suggested the use of the ProGlide over the ProStar closure system since all closure device failures were related to the ProStar use. However, the outcome depends largely on the experience of the Heart Team [137].

As predominantly elderly patients are treated with transaortic TAVR, the ascending aorta may be soft and fragile, leading to tearing suture lines and a cumbersome arterial closure. Typical complications for the median hemi-sternotomy or anterior-lateral thoracotomy are deep sternal wound infections, mediastinitis, and right internal mammary artery injury. Very rarely, lacerations of the right ventricle during mini-thoracotomy and PSA formation of an intercostal artery after hemi-sternotomy has been described [76,138].

3.6.8. Prevention Measures

With vascular access complications having a major impact on the outcome and mortality after TAVR, no effort must be spared to limit the risk of adverse events to a minimum. Thorough preoperative risk assessment involves detailed radiological and clinical preprocedural work-up. Multimodality imaging is pivotal for a tailor-made and patient-orientated approach warranting the safest access based on the individual vessel condition. CTA prior to the procedure is the foundation of an in-depth analysis of the patient's anatomy and an integral part of risk stratification [139]. It is not only necessary for annular sizing and valve selection but also vital for access site analysis. Vessel diameters, calcification patterns, and tortuosity are integral to access site selection [67]. The International Society of Cardiovascular Computed Tomography (SCCT) has formulated recommendations in aortic valve and access site assessment prior to TAVR (Table 4) [140].

Table 4. SSCT expert consensus on CT evaluation before TAVR.

Recommendations for assessment of access route by CT before TAVR
• CT imaging should be performed for vascular access assessment (pelvic arteries and aorta) when not contraindicated.
• CT examinations should be performed with iodinated contrast medium.
• Manual multiplanar reformation or semi-automated centerline reconstruction should be used to achieve cross-sectional visualization to measure vessel dimensions. From these reconstructed images, the minimal luminal diameter along the course of the vascular access should be determined.
• Qualitative assessment of vascular tortuosity should be performed.
• Qualitative assessment of vascular calcification should be performed.
• Consideration of varied thresholds of vessel size (sheath/femoral artery ratio) should be contemplated, depending on the presence and extent of vascular calcification.
• The left ventricle should be evaluated for the presence of thrombus and, if a transapical access route is planned, for geometry and position of the apex.
Recommendations for assessment of the aorta before TAVR
• The entire aorta should be imaged and evaluated, unless a transapical access is planned.
• Severe elongation and kinking of the aorta, dissection, and obstructions caused by thrombus or other material should be reported.

Adapted and reproduced with permission from the copyright owner [140].

4. Conclusions

With TAVR now being an integral part of modern valvular interventions, the procedure has undergone an incredible evolution since first performed two decades ago. With the possibility to choose between many different access sites, ongoing technological advances in the valve design, sheath technology, and growing expertise, the rates of vascular access complications will continue their persistent decline. Even though TAVR is steadily gaining in simplicity and manual ease, we must not cease to focus on diligent vascular access and closure techniques, but, even more importantly, we must focus on preventive measures. Optimizing the strategies for vascular access in every individual patient, further miniaturizing sheath diameters and developing improved vascular closure devices will be mandatory to enhance the safety of transcatheter valve therapies.

Supplementary Materials: The following are available online at https://www.mdpi.com/article/10.3390/jcm10215046/s1, Figure S1: Preferred Reporting Items for Systematic Reviews and Met-Analysis (PRISMA)-flowchart, Table S1: Vascular access and access-site related bleeding complications reported for TAVR.

Author Contributions: Conceptualization, M.M. and S.O.; methodology, M.M. and S.O.; formal analysis, M.M. and S.O.; writing—original draft preparation, M.M., S.O. and A.A.; writing—review and editing, M.A., P.S., P.W., S.G.F. and T.K.; visualization, S.G.F.; All authors have read and agreed to the published version of the manuscript.

Funding: This research received no external funding.

Institutional Review Board Statement: Not applicable.

Informed Consent Statement: Not applicable.

Data Availability Statement: The datasets for this study will be available from the corresponding author upon reasonable request.

Acknowledgments: The authors would like to thank Francesco Maisano, Maurizio Taramasso, Carlos Mestres, Assoc. Martin Andreas, other C.A.S.—Aortic Valve Structural Interventions faculty and participants for enabling positive research and academic environment during the writing process of this manuscript.

Conflicts of Interest: M. Mach has received a research grant from Edwards Lifesciences, JenaValve, and Symetis. M. Andreas is a proctor for Edwards Lifesciences and Abbott Laboratories and an adviser to Medtronic. All other authors have reported that they have no relationships relevant to the content.

References

1. Mack, M.J.; Leon, M.B.; Thourani, V.H.; Makkar, R.; Kodali, S.K.; Russo, M.; Kapadia, S.R.; Malaisrie, S.C.; Cohen, D.J.; Pibarot, P.; et al. Transcatheter Aortic-Valve Replacement with a Balloon-Expandable Valve in Low-Risk Patients. *N. Engl. J. Med.* **2019**, *380*, 1695–1705. [CrossRef] [PubMed]
2. Popma, J.J.; Deeb, G.M.; Yakubov, S.J.; Mumtaz, M.; Gada, H.; O'Hair, D.; Bajwa, T.; Heiser, J.C.; Merhi, W.; Kleiman, N.S.; et al. Transcatheter Aortic-Valve Replacement with a Self-Expanding Valve in Low-Risk Patients. *N. Engl. J. Med.* **2019**, *380*, 1706–1715. [CrossRef]
3. Walther, T.; Hamm, C.W.; Schuler, G.; Berkowitsch, A.; Kotting, J.; Mangner, N.; Mudra, H.; Beckmann, A.; Cremer, J.; Welz, A.; et al. Perioperative Results and Complications in 15,964 Transcatheter Aortic Valve Replacements: Prospective Data from the GARY Registry. *J. Am. Coll. Cardiol.* **2015**, *65*, 2173–2180. [CrossRef]
4. van Wiechen, M.P.; Tchétché, D.; Ooms, J.F.; Hokken, T.W.; Kroon, H.; Ziviello, F.; Ghattas, A.; Siddiqui, S.; Laperche, C.; Spitzer, E.; et al. Suture- or Plug-Based Large-Bore Arteriotomy Closure: A Pilot Randomized Controlled Trial. *JACC Cardiovasc. Interv.* **2021**, *14*, 149–157. [CrossRef]
5. Akodad, M.; Roubille, F.; Marin, G.; Lattuca, B.; Macia, J.C.; Delseny, D.; Gandet, T.; Robert, P.; Schmutz, L.; Piot, C.; et al. Myocardial Injury after Balloon Predilatation Versus Direct Transcatheter Aortic Valve Replacement: Insights from the DIRECTAVI Trial. *J. Am. Heart Assoc.* **2020**, *9*, e018405. [CrossRef] [PubMed]
6. Yong, G.; Walton, T.; Ng, M.; Gurvitch, R.; Worthley, S.; Whitbourn, R.; Jepson, N.; Bhindi, R.; Shang, K.; Sinhal, A. Performance and Safety of Transfemoral TAVI with SAPIEN XT in Australian Patients with Severe Aortic Stenosis at Intermediate Surgical Risk: SOLACE-AU Trial. *Heart Lung Circ.* **2020**, *29*, 1839–1846. [CrossRef] [PubMed]
7. Makkar, R.R.; Cheng, W.; Waksman, R.; Satler, L.F.; Chakravarty, T.; Groh, M.; Abernethy, W.; Russo, M.J.; Heimansohn, D.; Hermiller, J.; et al. Self-expanding intra-annular versus commercially available transcatheter heart valves in high and extreme risk patients with severe aortic stenosis (PORTICO IDE): A randomised, controlled, non-inferiority trial. *Lancet* **2020**, *396*, 669–683. [CrossRef]

8. Waksman, R.; Craig, P.E.; Torguson, R.; Asch, F.M.; Weissman, G.; Ruiz, D.; Gordon, P.; Ehsan, A.; Parikh, P.; Bilfinger, T.; et al. Transcatheter Aortic Valve Replacement in Low-Risk Patients with Symptomatic Severe Bicuspid Aortic Valve Stenosis. *JACC Cardiovasc. Interv.* **2020**, *13*, 1019–1027. [CrossRef]
9. Lanz, J.; Kim, W.K.; Walther, T.; Burgdorf, C.; Möllmann, H.; Linke, A.; Redwood, S.; Thilo, C.; Hilker, M.; Joner, M.; et al. Safety and efficacy of a self-expanding versus a balloon-expandable bioprosthesis for transcatheter aortic valve replacement in patients with symptomatic severe aortic stenosis: A randomised non-inferiority trial. *Lancet* **2019**, *394*, 1619–1628. [CrossRef]
10. Khan, J.M.; Greenbaum, A.B.; Babaliaros, V.C.; Rogers, T.; Eng, M.H.; Paone, G.; Leshnower, B.G.; Reisman, M.; Satler, L.; Waksman, R.; et al. The BASILICA Trial: Prospective Multicenter Investigation of Intentional Leaflet Laceration to Prevent TAVR Coronary Obstruction. *JACC Cardiovasc. Interv.* **2019**, *12*, 1240–1252. [CrossRef] [PubMed]
11. Toutouzas, K.; Benetos, G.; Voudris, V.; Drakopoulou, M.; Stathogiannis, K.; Latsios, G.; Synetos, A.; Antonopoulos, A.; Kosmas, E.; Iakovou, I.; et al. Pre-Dilatation Versus No Pre-Dilatation for Implantation of a Self-Expanding Valve in All Comers Undergoing TAVR: The DIRECT Trial. *JACC Cardiovasc. Interv.* **2019**, *12*, 767–777. [CrossRef]
12. Barbanti, M.; van Mourik, M.S.; Spence, M.S.; Iacovelli, F.; Martinelli, G.L.; Muir, D.F.; Saia, F.; Bortone, A.S.; Densem, C.G.; van der Kley, F.; et al. Optimising patient discharge management after transfemoral transcatheter aortic valve implantation: The multicentre European FAST-TAVI trial. *EuroIntervention* **2019**, *15*, 147–154. [CrossRef] [PubMed]
13. Beve, M.; Auffret, V.; Belhaj Soulami, R.; Tomasi, J.; Anselmi, A.; Roisne, A.; Boulmier, D.; Bedossa, M.; Leurent, G.; Donal, E.; et al. Comparison of the Transarterial and Transthoracic Approaches in Nontransfemoral Transcatheter Aortic Valve Implantation. *Am. J. Cardiol.* **2019**, *123*, 1501–1509. [CrossRef] [PubMed]
14. Feldman, T.E.; Reardon, M.J.; Rajagopal, V.; Makkar, R.R.; Bajwa, T.K.; Kleiman, N.S.; Linke, A.; Kereiakes, D.J.; Waksman, R.; Thourani, V.H.; et al. Effect of Mechanically Expanded vs Self-Expanding Transcatheter Aortic Valve Replacement on Mortality and Major Adverse Clinical Events in High-Risk Patients with Aortic Stenosis: The REPRISE III Randomized Clinical Trial. *JAMA* **2018**, *319*, 27–37. [CrossRef] [PubMed]
15. Yamawaki, M.; Araki, M.; Ito, T.; Honda, Y.; Tokuda, T.; Ito, Y.; Ueno, H.; Mizutani, K.; Tabata, M.; Higashimori, A.; et al. Ankle-brachial pressure index as a predictor of the 2-year outcome after transcatheter aortic valve replacement: Data from the Japanese OCEAN-TAVI Registry. *Heart Vessel.* **2018**, *33*, 640–650. [CrossRef] [PubMed]
16. Denegri, A.; Nietlispach, F.; Kottwitz, J.; Suetsch, G.; Haager, P.; Rodriguez, H.; Taramasso, M.; Obeid, S.; Maisano, F. Real-world procedural and 30-day outcome using the Portico transcatheter aortic valve prosthesis: A large single center cohort. *Int. J. Cardiol.* **2018**, *253*, 40–44. [CrossRef]
17. Seeger, J.; Gonska, B.; Rottbauer, W.; Wöhrle, J. New generation devices for transfemoral transcatheter aortic valve replacement are superior compared with last generation devices with respect to VARC-2 outcome. *Cardiovasc. Interv. Ther.* **2018**, *33*, 247–255. [CrossRef] [PubMed]
18. Hengstenberg, C.; Chandrasekhar, J.; Sartori, S.; Lefevre, T.; Mikhail, G.; Meneveau, N.; Tron, C.; Jeger, R.; Kupatt, C.; Vogel, B.; et al. Impact of pre-existing or new-onset atrial fibrillation on 30-day clinical outcomes following transcatheter aortic valve replacement: Results from the BRAVO 3 randomized trial. *Catheter. Cardiovasc. Interv.* **2017**, *90*, 1027–1037. [CrossRef] [PubMed]
19. Reardon, M.J.; Van Mieghem, N.M.; Popma, J.J.; Kleiman, N.S.; Søndergaard, L.; Mumtaz, M.; Adams, D.H.; Deeb, G.M.; Maini, B.; Gada, H.; et al. Surgical or Transcatheter Aortic-Valve Replacement in Intermediate-Risk Patients. *N. Engl. J. Med.* **2017**, *376*, 1321–1331. [CrossRef]
20. Popma, J.J.; Reardon, M.J.; Khabbaz, K.; Harrison, J.K.; Hughes, G.C.; Kodali, S.; George, I.; Deeb, G.M.; Chetcuti, S.; Kipperman, R.; et al. Early Clinical Outcomes After Transcatheter Aortic Valve Replacement Using a Novel Self-Expanding Bioprosthesis in Patients with Severe Aortic Stenosis Who Are Suboptimal for Surgery: Results of the Evolut R U.S. Study. *JACC Cardiovasc. Interv.* **2017**, *10*, 268–275. [CrossRef]
21. Takimoto, S.; Saito, N.; Minakata, K.; Shirai, S.; Isotani, A.; Arai, Y.; Hanyu, M.; Komiya, T.; Shimamoto, T.; Goto, T.; et al. Favorable Clinical Outcomes of Transcatheter Aortic Valve Implantation in Japanese Patients—First Report from the Post Approval K-TAVI Registry. *Circ. J.* **2017**, *81*, 103–109. [CrossRef] [PubMed]
22. Lansky, A.J.; Brown, D.; Pena, C.; Pietras, C.G.; Parise, H.; Ng, V.G.; Meller, S.; Abrams, K.J.; Cleman, M.; Margolis, P.; et al. Neurologic Complications of Unprotected Transcatheter Aortic Valve Implantation (from the Neuro-TAVI Trial). *Am. J. Cardiol.* **2016**, *118*, 1519–1526. [CrossRef] [PubMed]
23. Seeger, J.; Gonska, B.; Rodewald, C.; Rottbauer, W.; Wöhrle, J. Impact of suture mediated femoral access site closure with the Prostar XL compared to the ProGlide system on outcome in transfemoral aortic valve implantation. *Int. J. Cardiol.* **2016**, *223*, 564–567. [CrossRef]
24. Manoharan, G.; Linke, A.; Moellmann, H.; Redwood, S.; Frerker, C.; Kovac, J.; Walther, T. Multicentre clinical study evaluating a novel resheathable annular functioning self-expanding transcatheter aortic valve system: Safety and performance results at 30 days with the Portico system. *EuroIntervention* **2016**, *12*, 768–774. [CrossRef] [PubMed]
25. Wöhrle, J.; Gonska, B.; Rodewald, C.; Seeger, J.; Scharnbeck, D.; Rottbauer, W. Transfemoral aortic valve implantation with the repositionable Lotus valve for treatment of patients with symptomatic severe aortic stenosis: Results from a single-centre experience. *EuroIntervention* **2016**, *12*, 760–767. [CrossRef]
26. Leon, M.B.; Smith, C.R.; Mack, M.J.; Makkar, R.R.; Svensson, L.G.; Kodali, S.K.; Thourani, V.H.; Tuzcu, E.M.; Miller, D.C.; Herrmann, H.C.; et al. Transcatheter or Surgical Aortic-Valve Replacement in Intermediate-Risk Patients. *N. Engl. J. Med.* **2016**, *374*, 1609–1620. [CrossRef] [PubMed]

27. Wöhrle, J.; Gonska, B.; Rodewald, C.; Seeger, J.; Scharnbeck, D.; Rottbauer, W. Transfemoral Aortic Valve Implantation with the New Edwards Sapien 3 Valve for Treatment of Severe Aortic Stenosis-Impact of Valve Size in a Single Center Experience. *PLoS ONE* **2016**, *11*, e0151247. [CrossRef]
28. Webb, J.G.; Doshi, D.; Mack, M.J.; Makkar, R.; Smith, C.R.; Pichard, A.D.; Kodali, S.; Kapadia, S.; Miller, D.C.; Babaliaros, V.; et al. A Randomized Evaluation of the SAPIEN XT Transcatheter Heart Valve System in Patients with Aortic Stenosis Who Are Not Candidates for Surgery. *JACC Cardiovasc. Interv.* **2015**, *8*, 1797–1806. [CrossRef] [PubMed]
29. Binder, R.K.; Stortecky, S.; Heg, D.; Tueller, D.; Jeger, R.; Toggweiler, S.; Pedrazzini, G.; Amann, F.W.; Ferrari, E.; Noble, S.; et al. Procedural Results and Clinical Outcomes of Transcatheter Aortic Valve Implantation in Switzerland: An Observational Cohort Study of Sapien 3 Versus Sapien XT Transcatheter Heart Valves. *Circ. Cardiovasc. Interv.* **2015**, *8*, e002653. [CrossRef] [PubMed]
30. Manoharan, G.; Walton, A.S.; Brecker, S.J.; Pasupati, S.; Blackman, D.J.; Qiao, H.; Meredith, I.T. Treatment of Symptomatic Severe Aortic Stenosis with a Novel Resheathable Supra-Annular Self-Expanding Transcatheter Aortic Valve System. *JACC Cardiovasc. Interv.* **2015**, *8*, 1359–1367. [CrossRef] [PubMed]
31. Abramowitz, Y.; Chakravarty, T.; Jilaihawi, H.; Kashif, M.; Zadikany, R.; Lee, C.; Matar, G.; Cheng, W.; Makkar, R.R. Comparison of Outcomes of Transcatheter Aortic Valve Implantation in Patients ≥ 90 Years versus. *Am. J. Cardiol.* **2015**, *116*, 1110–1115. [CrossRef] [PubMed]
32. Bosmans, J.; Bleiziffer, S.; Gerckens, U.; Wenaweser, P.; Brecker, S.; Tamburino, C.; Linke, A. The Incidence and Predictors of Early- and Mid-Term Clinically Relevant Neurological Events after Transcatheter Aortic Valve Replacement in Real-World Patients. *J. Am. Coll. Cardiol.* **2015**, *66*, 209–217. [CrossRef]
33. Wendt, D.; Al-Rashid, F.; Kahlert, P.; Eißmann, M.; El-Chilali, K.; Jánosi, R.A.; Pasa, S.; Tsagakis, K.; Liakopoulos, O.; Erbel, R.; et al. Low Incidence of Paravalvular Leakage with the Balloon-Expandable Sapien 3 Transcatheter Heart Valve. *Ann. Thorac. Surg.* **2015**, *100*, 819–825; discussion 825–816. [CrossRef] [PubMed]
34. Castellant, P.; Didier, R.; Bezon, E.; Couturaud, F.; Eltchaninoff, H.; Iung, B.; Donzeau-Gouge, P.; Chevreul, K.; Fajadet, J.; Leprince, P.; et al. Comparison of Outcome of Transcatheter Aortic Valve Implantation with Versus without Previous Coronary Artery Bypass Grafting (from the FRANCE 2 Registry). *Am. J. Cardiol.* **2015**, *116*, 420–425. [CrossRef]
35. Baumbach, A.; Mullen, M.; Brickman, A.M.; Aggarwal, S.K.; Pietras, C.G.; Forrest, J.K.; Hildick-Smith, D.; Meller, S.M.; Gambone, L.; den Heijer, P.; et al. Safety and performance of a novel embolic deflection device in patients undergoing transcatheter aortic valve replacement: Results from the DEFLECT I study. *EuroIntervention* **2015**, *11*, 75–84. [CrossRef] [PubMed]
36. Fearon, W.F.; Kodali, S.; Doshi, D.; Fischbein, M.P.; Yeung, A.C.; Tuzcu, E.M.; Rihal, C.S.; Babaliaros, V.; Zajarias, A.; Herrmann, H.C.; et al. Outcomes after transfemoral transcatheter aortic valve replacement: A comparison of the randomized PARTNER (Placement of AoRTic TraNscathetER Valves) trial with the NRCA (Nonrandomized Continued Access) registry. *JACC Cardiovasc. Interv.* **2014**, *7*, 1245–1251. [CrossRef] [PubMed]
37. Reardon, M.J.; Adams, D.H.; Coselli, J.S.; Deeb, G.M.; Kleiman, N.S.; Chetcuti, S.; Yakubov, S.J.; Heimansohn, D.; Hermiller, J., Jr.; Hughes, G.C.; et al. Self-expanding transcatheter aortic valve replacement using alternative access sites in symptomatic patients with severe aortic stenosis deemed extreme risk of surgery. *J. Thorac. Cardiovasc. Surg.* **2014**, *148*, 2869–2876. [CrossRef]
38. Watanabe, Y.; Hayashida, K.; Takayama, M.; Mitsudo, K.; Nanto, S.; Takanashi, K.; Komiya, T.; Kuratani, T.; Tobaru, T.; Goto, K.; et al. First direct comparison of clinical outcomes between European and Asian cohorts in transcatheter aortic valve implantation: The Massy study group vs. the PREVAIL JAPAN trial. *J. Cardiol.* **2015**, *65*, 112–116. [CrossRef] [PubMed]
39. Stabile, E.; Pucciarelli, A.; Cota, L.; Sorropago, G.; Tesorio, T.; Salemme, L.; Popusoi, G.; Ambrosini, V.; Cioppa, A.; Agrusta, M.; et al. SAT-TAVI (single antiplatelet therapy for TAVI) study: A pilot randomized study comparing double to single antiplatelet therapy for transcatheter aortic valve implantation. *Int. J. Cardiol.* **2014**, *174*, 624–627. [CrossRef]
40. Abdel-Wahab, M.; Mehilli, J.; Frerker, C.; Neumann, F.J.; Kurz, T.; Tölg, R.; Zachow, D.; Guerra, E.; Massberg, S.; Schäfer, U.; et al. Comparison of balloon-expandable vs self-expandable valves in patients undergoing transcatheter aortic valve replacement: The CHOICE randomized clinical trial. *JAMA* **2014**, *311*, 1503–1514. [CrossRef] [PubMed]
41. Adams, D.H.; Popma, J.J.; Reardon, M.J.; Yakubov, S.J.; Coselli, J.S.; Deeb, G.M.; Gleason, T.G.; Buchbinder, M.; Hermiller, J., Jr.; Kleiman, N.S.; et al. Transcatheter aortic-valve replacement with a self-expanding prosthesis. *N. Engl. J. Med.* **2014**, *370*, 1790–1798. [CrossRef] [PubMed]
42. Sawa, Y.; Saito, S.; Kobayashi, J.; Niinami, H.; Kuratani, T.; Maeda, K.; Kanzaki, H.; Komiyama, N.; Tanaka, Y.; Boyle, A.; et al. First clinical trial of a self-expandable transcatheter heart valve in Japan in patients with symptomatic severe aortic stenosis. *Circ. J.* **2014**, *78*, 1083–1090. [CrossRef] [PubMed]
43. Popma, J.J.; Adams, D.H.; Reardon, M.J.; Yakubov, S.J.; Kleiman, N.S.; Heimansohn, D.; Hermiller, J., Jr.; Hughes, G.C.; Harrison, J.K.; Coselli, J.; et al. Transcatheter aortic valve replacement using a self-expanding bioprosthesis in patients with severe aortic stenosis at extreme risk for surgery. *J. Am. Coll. Cardiol.* **2014**, *63*, 1972–1981. [CrossRef] [PubMed]
44. Seco, M.; Martinez, G.; Bannon, P.G.; Cartwright, B.L.; Adams, M.; Ng, M.; Wilson, M.K.; Vallely, M.P. Transapical aortic valve implantation—An Australian experience. *Heart Lung Circ.* **2014**, *23*, 462–468. [CrossRef] [PubMed]
45. Czerwińska-Jelonkiewicz, K.; Michałowska, I.; Witkowski, A.; Dąbrowski, M.; Księżycka-Majczyńska, E.; Chmielak, Z.; Kuśmierski, K.; Hryniewiecki, T.; Demkow, M.; Stępińska, J. Vascular complications after transcatheter aortic valve implantation (TAVI): Risk and long-term results. *J. Thromb. Thrombolysis* **2014**, *37*, 490–498. [CrossRef]

46. Holper, E.M.; Kim, R.J.; Mack, M.; Brown, D.; Brinkman, W.; Herbert, M.; Stewart, W.; Vance, K.; Bowers, B.; Dewey, T. Randomized trial of surgical cutdown versus percutaneous access in transfemoral TAVR. *Catheter. Cardiovasc. Interv.* **2014**, *83*, 457–464. [CrossRef] [PubMed]
47. Généreux, P.; Webb, J.G.; Svensson, L.G.; Kodali, S.K.; Satler, L.F.; Fearon, W.F.; Davidson, C.J.; Eisenhauer, A.C.; Makkar, R.R.; Bergman, G.W.; et al. Vascular complications after transcatheter aortic valve replacement: Insights from the PARTNER (Placement of AoRTic TraNscathetER Valve) trial. *J. Am. Coll. Cardiol.* **2012**, *60*, 1043–1052. [CrossRef]
48. Smith, C.R.; Leon, M.B.; Mack, M.J.; Miller, D.C.; Moses, J.W.; Svensson, L.G.; Tuzcu, E.M.; Webb, J.G.; Fontana, G.P.; Makkar, R.R.; et al. Transcatheter versus surgical aortic-valve replacement in high-risk patients. *N. Engl. J. Med.* **2011**, *364*, 2187–2198. [CrossRef] [PubMed]
49. Leon, M.B.; Smith, C.R.; Mack, M.; Miller, D.C.; Moses, J.W.; Svensson, L.G.; Tuzcu, E.M.; Webb, J.G.; Fontana, G.P.; Makkar, R.R.; et al. Transcatheter aortic-valve implantation for aortic stenosis in patients who cannot undergo surgery. *N. Engl. J. Med.* **2010**, *363*, 1597–1607. [CrossRef] [PubMed]
50. Bleizffer, S.; Ruge, H.; Mazzitelli, D.; Schreiber, C.; Hutter, A.; Krane, M.; Bauernschmitt, R.; Lange, R. Valve implantation on the beating heart: Catheter-assisted surgery for aortic stenosis. *Dtsch. Arztebl. Int.* **2009**, *106*, 235–241. [CrossRef]
51. Hayashida, K.; Lefevre, T.; Chevalier, B.; Hovasse, T.; Romano, M.; Garot, P.; Mylotte, D.; Uribe, J.; Farge, A.; Donzeau-Gouge, P.; et al. Transfemoral aortic valve implantation new criteria to predict vascular complications. *JACC Cardiovasc. Interv.* **2011**, *4*, 851–858. [CrossRef]
52. Leon, M.B.; Piazza, N.; Nikolsky, E.; Blackstone, E.H.; Cutlip, D.E.; Kappetein, A.P.; Krucoff, M.W.; Mack, M.; Mehran, R.; Miller, C.; et al. Standardized endpoint definitions for transcatheter aortic valve implantation clinical trials: A consensus report from the Valve Academic Research Consortium. *Eur. Heart J.* **2011**, *32*, 205–217. [CrossRef] [PubMed]
53. Kappetein, A.P.; Head, S.J.; Genereux, P.; Piazza, N.; van Mieghem, N.M.; Blackstone, E.H.; Brott, T.G.; Cohen, D.J.; Cutlip, D.E.; van Es, G.A.; et al. Updated standardized endpoint definitions for transcatheter aortic valve implantation: The Valve Academic Research Consortium-2 consensus document. *Eur. Heart J.* **2012**, *33*, 2403–2418. [CrossRef] [PubMed]
54. Genereux, P.; Head, S.J.; Van Mieghem, N.M.; Kodali, S.; Kirtane, A.J.; Xu, K.; Smith, C.; Serruys, P.W.; Kappetein, A.P.; Leon, M.B. Clinical outcomes after transcatheter aortic valve replacement using valve academic research consortium definitions: A weighted meta-analysis of 3519 patients from 16 studies. *J. Am. Coll. Cardiol.* **2012**, *59*, 2317–2326. [CrossRef] [PubMed]
55. Gurvitch, R.; Toggweiler, S.; Willson, A.B.; Wijesinghe, N.; Cheung, A.; Wood, D.A.; Ye, J.; Webb, J.G. Outcomes and complications of transcatheter aortic valve replacement using a balloon expandable valve according to the Valve Academic Research Consortium (VARC) guidelines. *EuroIntervention* **2011**, *7*, 41–48. [CrossRef] [PubMed]
56. Van Mieghem, N.M.; Tchetche, D.; Chieffo, A.; Dumonteil, N.; Messika-Zeitoun, D.; van der Boon, R.M.; Vahdat, O.; Buchanan, G.L.; Marcheix, B.; Himbert, D.; et al. Incidence, predictors, and implications of access site complications with transfemoral transcatheter aortic valve implantation. *Am. J. Cardiol.* **2012**, *110*, 1361–1367. [CrossRef]
57. Holmes, D.R., Jr.; Nishimura, R.A.; Grover, F.L.; Brindis, R.G.; Carroll, J.D.; Edwards, F.H.; Peterson, E.D.; Rumsfeld, J.S.; Shahian, D.M.; Thourani, V.H.; et al. Annual Outcomes with Transcatheter Valve Therapy: From the STS/ACC TVT Registry. *J. Am. Coll. Cardiol.* **2015**, *66*, 2813–2823. [CrossRef]
58. Beurtheret, S.; Karam, N.; Resseguier, N.; Houel, R.; Modine, T.; Folliguet, T.; Chamandi, C.; Com, O.; Gelisse, R.; Bille, J.; et al. Femoral versus Nonfemoral Peripheral Access for Transcatheter Aortic Valve Replacement. *J. Am. Coll. Cardiol.* **2019**, *74*, 2728–2739. [CrossRef]
59. Abdelaziz, H.K.; Megaly, M.; Debski, M.; Rahbi, H.; Kamal, D.; Saad, M.; Wiper, A.; More, R.; Roberts, D.H. Meta-Analysis Comparing Percutaneous to Surgical Access in Trans-Femoral Transcatheter Aortic Valve Implantation. *Am. J. Cardiol.* **2020**, *125*, 1239–1248. [CrossRef]
60. Reidy, C.; Sophocles, A.; Ramakrishna, H.; Chadimi, K.; Patel, P.A.; Augoustides, J.G. Challenges after the first decade of transcatheter aortic valve replacement: Focus on vascular complications, stroke, and paravalvular leak. *J. Cardiothorac. Vasc. Anesth.* **2013**, *27*, 184–189. [CrossRef]
61. Toggweiler, S.; Gurvitch, R.; Leipsic, J.; Wood, D.A.; Willson, A.B.; Binder, R.K.; Cheung, A.; Ye, J.; Webb, J.G. Percutaneous aortic valve replacement: Vascular outcomes with a fully percutaneous procedure. *J. Am. Coll. Cardiol.* **2012**, *59*, 113–118. [CrossRef] [PubMed]
62. Steinvil, A.; Leshem-Rubinow, E.; Halkin, A.; Abramowitz, Y.; Ben-Assa, E.; Shacham, Y.; Bar-Dayan, A.; Keren, G.; Banai, S.; Finkelstein, A. Vascular complications after transcatheter aortic valve implantation and their association with mortality reevaluated by the valve academic research. consortium definitions. *Am. J. Cardiol.* **2015**, *115*, 100–106. [CrossRef] [PubMed]
63. Humphries, K.H.; Toggweiler, S.; Rodes-Cabau, J.; Nombela-Franco, L.; Dumont, E.; Wood, D.A.; Willson, A.B.; Binder, R.K.; Freeman, M.; Lee, M.K.; et al. Sex differences in mortality after transcatheter aortic valve replacement for severe aortic stenosis. *J. Am. Coll. Cardiol.* **2012**, *60*, 882–886. [CrossRef] [PubMed]
64. Kadakia, M.B.; Herrmann, H.C.; Desai, N.D.; Fox, Z.; Ogbara, J.; Anwaruddin, S.; Jagasia, D.; Bavaria, J.E.; Szeto, W.Y.; Vallabhajosyula, P.; et al. Factors associated with vascular complications in patients undergoing balloon-expandable transfemoral transcatheter aortic valve replacement via open versus percutaneous approaches. *Circ. Cardiovasc. Interv.* **2014**, *7*, 570–576. [CrossRef] [PubMed]

65. Lange, R.; Bleiziffer, S.; Piazza, N.; Mazzitelli, D.; Hutter, A.; Tassani-Prell, P.; Laborde, J.C.; Bauernschmitt, R. Incidence and treatment of procedural cardiovascular complications associated with trans-arterial and trans-apical interventional aortic valve implantation in 412 consecutive patients. *Eur. J. Cardiothorac. Surg.* **2011**, *40*, 1105–1113. [CrossRef] [PubMed]
66. Sardar, M.R.; Goldsweig, A.M.; Abbott, J.D.; Sharaf, B.L.; Gordon, P.C.; Ehsan, A.; Aronow, H.D. Vascular complications associated with transcatheter aortic valve replacement. *Vasc. Med.* **2017**, *22*, 234–244. [CrossRef]
67. Mach, M.; Poschner, T.; Hasan, W.; Szalkiewicz, P.; Andreas, M.; Winkler, B.; Geisler, S.; Geisler, D.; Rudziński, P.N.; Watzal, V.; et al. Iliofemoral tortuosity score predicts access and bleeding complications during transfemoral transcatheter aortic valve replacement. *Eur. J. Clin. Investig.* **2021**, *51*, e13491. [CrossRef]
68. Ducrocq, G.; Francis, F.; Serfaty, J.M.; Himbert, D.; Maury, J.M.; Pasi, N.; Marouene, S.; Provenchere, S.; Iung, B.; Castier, Y.; et al. Vascular complications of transfemoral aortic valve implantation with the Edwards SAPIEN prosthesis: Incidence and impact on outcome. *EuroIntervention* **2010**, *5*, 666–672. [CrossRef]
69. Mussardo, M.; Latib, A.; Chieffo, A.; Godino, C.; Ielasi, A.; Cioni, M.; Takagi, K.; Davidavicius, G.; Montorfano, M.; Maisano, F.; et al. Periprocedural and short-term outcomes of transfemoral transcatheter aortic valve implantation with the Sapien XT as compared with the Edwards Sapien valve. *JACC Cardiovasc. Interv.* **2011**, *4*, 743–750. [CrossRef]
70. Kim, D.; Orron, D.E.; Skillman, J.J.; Kent, K.C.; Porter, D.H.; Schlam, B.W.; Carrozza, J.; Reis, G.J.; Baim, D.S. Role of superficial femoral artery puncture in the development of pseudoaneurysm and arteriovenous fistula complicating percutaneous transfemoral cardiac catheterization. *Catheter. Cardiovasc. Diagn.* **1992**, *25*, 91–97. [CrossRef]
71. Ellis, S.G.; Bhatt, D.; Kapadia, S.; Lee, D.; Yen, M.; Whitlow, P.L. Correlates and outcomes of retroperitoneal hemorrhage complicating percutaneous coronary intervention. *Catheter. Cardiovasc. Interv.* **2006**, *67*, 541–545. [CrossRef] [PubMed]
72. Yoo, B.S.; Yoon, J.; Ko, J.Y.; Kim, J.Y.; Lee, S.H.; Hwang, S.O.; Choe, K.H. Anatomical consideration of the radial artery for transradial coronary procedures: Arterial diameter, branching anomaly and vessel tortuosity. *Int. J. Cardiol.* **2005**, *101*, 421–427. [CrossRef]
73. Seto, A.H.; Abu-Fadel, M.S.; Sparling, J.M.; Zacharias, S.J.; Daly, T.S.; Harrison, A.T.; Suh, W.M.; Vera, J.A.; Aston, C.E.; Winters, R.J.; et al. Real-time ultrasound guidance facilitates femoral arterial access and reduces vascular complications: FAUST (Femoral Arterial Access with Ultrasound Trial). *JACC Cardiovasc. Interv.* **2010**, *3*, 751–758. [CrossRef]
74. Turi, Z.G. Fluoroscopy guided vascular access: Asking the right question, but getting the wrong answer? *Catheter. Cardiovasc. Interv.* **2009**, *74*, 540–542. [CrossRef] [PubMed]
75. Schnyder, G.; Sawhney, N.; Whisenant, B.; Tsimikas, S.; Turi, Z.G. Common femoral artery anatomy is influenced by demographics and comorbidity: Implications for cardiac and peripheral invasive studies. *Catheter. Cardiovasc. Interv.* **2001**, *53*, 289–295. [CrossRef]
76. Bruschi, G.; de Marco, F.; Botta, L.; Cannata, A.; Oreglia, J.; Colombo, P.; Barosi, A.; Colombo, T.; Nonini, S.; Paino, R.; et al. Direct aortic access for transcatheter self-expanding aortic bioprosthetic valves implantation. *Ann. Thorac. Surg.* **2012**, *94*, 497–503. [CrossRef]
77. Barbanti, M.; Capranzano, P.; Ohno, Y.; Gulino, S.; Sgroi, C.; Immè, S.; Tamburino, C.; Cannata, S.; Patanè, M.; Di Stefano, D.; et al. Comparison of suture-based vascular closure devices in transfemoral transcatheter aortic valve implantation. *EuroIntervention* **2015**, *11*, 690–697. [CrossRef] [PubMed]
78. Dimitriadis, Z.; Scholtz, W.; Börgermann, J.; Wiemer, M.; Piper, C.; Vlachojannis, M.; Gummert, J.; Horstkotte, D.; Ensminger, S.; Faber, L.; et al. Impact of closure devices on vascular complication and mortality rates in TAVI procedures. *Int. J. Cardiol.* **2017**, *241*, 133–137. [CrossRef]
79. Hernández-Enriquez, M.; Andrea, R.; Brugaletta, S.; Jiménez-Quevedo, P.; Hernández-García, J.M.; Trillo, R.; Larman, M.; Fernández-Avilés, F.; Vázquez-González, N.; Iñiguez, A.; et al. Puncture versus Surgical Cutdown Complications of Transfemoral Aortic Valve Implantation (from the Spanish TAVI Registry). *Am. J. Cardiol.* **2016**, *118*, 578–584. [CrossRef]
80. Mach, M.; Wilbring, M.; Winkler, B.; Alexiou, K.; Kappert, U.; Delle-Karth, G.; Grabenwöger, M.; Matschke, K. Cut-down outperforms complete percutaneous transcatheter valve implantation. *Asian Cardiovasc. Thorac. Ann.* **2018**, *26*, 107–113. [CrossRef]
81. Nakamura, M.; Chakravarty, T.; Jilaihawi, H.; Doctor, N.; Dohad, S.; Fontana, G.; Cheng, W.; Makkar, R.R. Complete percutaneous approach for arterial access in transfemoral transcatheter aortic valve replacement: A comparison with surgical cut-down and closure. *Catheter. Cardiovasc. Interv.* **2014**, *84*, 293–300. [CrossRef]
82. Kawashima, H.; Watanabe, Y.; Kozuma, K.; Nara, Y.; Hioki, H.; Kataoka, A.; Yamamoto, M.; Takagi, K.; Araki, M.; Tada, N.; et al. Propensity-matched comparison of percutaneous and surgical cut-down approaches in transfemoral transcatheter aortic valve implantation using a balloon-expandable valve. *EuroIntervention* **2017**, *12*, 1954–1961. [CrossRef] [PubMed]
83. Petronio, A.S.; De Carlo, M.; Bedogni, F.; Maisano, F.; Ettori, F.; Klugmann, S.; Poli, A.; Marzocchi, A.; Santoro, G.; Napodano, M.; et al. 2-year results of CoreValve implantation through the subclavian access: A propensity-matched comparison with the femoral access. *J. Am. Coll. Cardiol.* **2012**, *60*, 502–507. [CrossRef]
84. Mylotte, D.; Sudre, A.; Teiger, E.; Obadia, J.F.; Lee, M.; Spence, M.; Khamis, H.; Al Nooryani, A.; Delhaye, C.; Amr, G.; et al. Transcarotid Transcatheter Aortic Valve Replacement: Feasibility and Safety. *JACC Cardiovasc. Interv.* **2016**, *9*, 472–480. [CrossRef]
85. Debry, N.; Delhaye, C.; Azmoun, A.; Ramadan, R.; Fradi, S.; Brenot, P.; Sudre, A.; Moussa, M.D.; Tchetche, D.; Ghostine, S.; et al. Transcarotid Transcatheter Aortic Valve Replacement: General or Local Anesthesia. *JACC Cardiovasc. Interv.* **2016**, *9*, 2113–2120. [CrossRef]

86. Latsios, G.; Gerckens, U.; Grube, E. Transaortic transcatheter aortic valve implantation: A novel approach for the truly "no-access option" patients. *Catheter. Cardiovasc. Interv.* **2010**, *75*, 1129–1136. [CrossRef]
87. Bapat, V.; Khawaja, M.Z.; Attia, R.; Narayana, A.; Wilson, K.; Macgillivray, K.; Young, C.; Hancock, J.; Redwood, S.; Thomas, M. Transaortic Transcatheter Aortic valve implantation using Edwards Sapien valve: A novel approach. *Catheter. Cardiovasc. Interv.* **2012**, *79*, 733–740. [CrossRef] [PubMed]
88. Fiorina, C.; Bruschi, G.; Testa, L.; De Carlo, M.; De Marco, F.; Coletti, G.; Bonardelli, S.; Adamo, M.; Curello, S.; Scioti, G.; et al. Transaxillary versus transaortic approach for transcatheter aortic valve implantation with CoreValve Revalving System: Insights from multicenter experience. *J. Cardiovasc. Surg.* **2017**, *58*, 747–754. [CrossRef] [PubMed]
89. Hayashida, K.; Romano, M.; Lefevre, T.; Chevalier, B.; Farge, A.; Hovasse, T.; Le Houerou, D.; Morice, M.C. The transaortic approach for transcatheter aortic valve implantation: A valid alternative to the transapical access in patients with no peripheral vascular option. A single center experience. *Eur. J. Cardiothorac. Surg.* **2013**, *44*, 692–700. [CrossRef]
90. Lardizabal, J.A.; O'Neill, B.P.; Desai, H.V.; Macon, C.J.; Rodriguez, A.P.; Martinez, C.A.; Alfonso, C.E.; Bilsker, M.S.; Carillo, R.G.; Cohen, M.G.; et al. The transaortic approach for transcatheter aortic valve replacement: Initial clinical experience in the United States. *J. Am. Coll. Cardiol.* **2013**, *61*, 2341–2345. [CrossRef]
91. Thourani, V.H.; Gunter, R.L.; Neravetla, S.; Block, P.; Guyton, R.A.; Kilgo, P.; Lerakis, S.; Devireddy, C.; Leshnower, B.; Mavromatis, K.; et al. Use of transaortic, transapical, and transcarotid transcatheter aortic valve replacement in inoperable patients. *Ann. Thorac. Surg.* **2013**, *96*, 1349–1357. [CrossRef]
92. Webb, J.G.; Altwegg, L.; Boone, R.H.; Cheung, A.; Ye, J.; Lichtenstein, S.; Lee, M.; Masson, J.B.; Thompson, C.; Moss, R.; et al. Transcatheter aortic valve implantation: Impact on clinical and valve-related outcomes. *Circulation* **2009**, *119*, 3009–3016. [CrossRef] [PubMed]
93. Walther, T.; Thielmann, M.; Kempfert, J.; Schroefel, H.; Wimmer-Greinecker, G.; Treede, H.; Wahlers, T.; Wendler, O. PREVAIL TRANSAPICAL: Multicentre trial of transcatheter aortic valve implantation using the newly designed bioprosthesis (SAPIEN-XT) and delivery system (ASCENDRA-II). *Eur. J. Cardiothorac. Surg.* **2012**, *42*, 278–283; discussion 283. [CrossRef]
94. Holzhey, D.M.; Hansig, M.; Walther, T.; Seeburger, J.; Misfeld, M.; Linke, A.; Borger, M.A.; Mohr, F.W. Transapical aortic valve implantation—The Leipzig experience. *Ann. Cardiothorac. Surg.* **2012**, *1*, 129–137. [CrossRef] [PubMed]
95. Toppen, W.; Suh, W.; Aksoy, O.; Benharash, P.; Bowles, C.; Shemin, R.J.; Kwon, M. Vascular Complications in the Sapien 3 Era: Continued Role of Transapical Approach to Transcatheter Aortic Valve Replacement. *Semin. Thorac. Cardiovasc. Surg.* **2018**, *30*, 144–149. [CrossRef]
96. Greenbaum, A.B.; Babaliaros, V.C.; Chen, M.Y.; Stine, A.M.; Rogers, T.; O'Neill, W.W.; Paone, G.; Thourani, V.H.; Muhammad, K.I.; Leonardi, R.A.; et al. Transcaval Access and Closure for Transcatheter Aortic Valve Replacement: A Prospective Investigation. *J. Am. Coll. Cardiol.* **2017**, *69*, 511–521. [CrossRef] [PubMed]
97. Harrison, G.J.; How, T.V.; Vallabhaneni, S.R.; Brennan, J.A.; Fisher, R.K.; Naik, J.B.; McWilliams, R.G. Guidewire stiffness: What's in a name? *J. Endovasc. Ther.* **2011**, *18*, 797–801. [CrossRef] [PubMed]
98. Brodmann, M.; Werner, M.; Brinton, T.J.; Illindala, U.; Lansky, A.; Lansky, M.R.; Lansky, A. Safety and performance of lithoplasty for treatment of calcified peripheral artery lesions. *J. Am. Coll. Cardiol.* **2017**, *70*, 908–910. [CrossRef]
99. Brodmann, M.; Werner, M.; Holden, A.; Tepe, G.; Scheinert, D.; Schwindt, A.; Wolf, F.; Jaff, M.; Lansky, A.; Zeller, T. Primary outcomes and mechanism of action of intravascular lithotripsy in calcified, femoropopliteal lesions: Results of Disrupt PAD II. *Catheter. Cardiovasc. Interv.* **2019**, *93*, 335–342. [CrossRef]
100. Di Mario, C.; Chiriatti, N.; Stolcova, M.; Meucci, F.; Squillantini, G. Lithoplasty- assisted transfemoral aortic valve implantation. *Eur. Heart J.* **2018**. [CrossRef]
101. Di Mario, C.; Goodwin, M.; Ristalli, F.; Ravani, M.; Meucci, F.; Stolcova, M.; Sardella, G.; Salvi, N.; Bedogni, F.; Berti, S.; et al. A prospective registry of intravascular lithotripsy-enabled vascular access for transfemoral transcatheter aortic valve replacement. *JACC Cardiovasc. Interv.* **2019**, *12*, 502–504. [CrossRef]
102. Barbanti, M.; Binder, R.K.; Freeman, M.; Wood, D.A.; Leipsic, J.; Cheung, A.; Ye, J.; Tan, J.; Toggweiler, S.; Yang, T.H.; et al. Impact of low-profile sheaths on vascular complications during transfemoral transcatheter aortic valve replacement. *EuroIntervention* **2013**, *9*, 929–935. [CrossRef]
103. Millan, X.; Azzalini, L.; Khan, R.; Cournoyer, D.; Dorval, J.F.; Ibrahim, R.; Bonan, R.; Asgar, A.W. Efficacy of a balloon-expandable vascular access system in transfemoral TAVI patients. *Catheter. Cardiovasc. Interv.* **2016**, *88*, 1145–1152. [CrossRef]
104. Tchetche, D.; Dumonteil, N.; Sauguet, A.; Descoutures, F.; Luz, A.; Garcia, O.; Soula, P.; Gabiache, Y.; Fournial, G.; Marcheix, B.; et al. Thirty-day outcome and vascular complications after transarterial aortic valve implantation using both Edwards Sapien and Medtronic CoreValve bioprostheses in a mixed population. *EuroIntervention* **2010**, *5*, 659–665. [CrossRef]
105. Thomas, M.; Schymik, G.; Walther, T.; Himbert, D.; Lefevre, T.; Treede, H.; Eggebrecht, H.; Rubino, P.; Michev, I.; Lange, R.; et al. Thirty-day results of the SAPIEN aortic Bioprosthesis European Outcome (SOURCE) Registry: A European registry of transcatheter aortic valve implantation using the Edwards SAPIEN valve. *Circulation* **2010**, *122*, 62–69. [CrossRef]
106. Spitzer, S.G.; Wilbring, M.; Alexiou, K.; Stumpf, M.; Kappert, U.; Matschke, K. Surgical cut-down or percutaneous access-which is best for less vascular access complications in transfemoral TAVI? *Catheter. Cardiovasc. Interv.* **2016**, *88*, E52–E58. [CrossRef]
107. Sharp, A.S.; Michev, I.; Maisano, F.; Taramasso, M.; Godino, C.; Latib, A.; Denti, P.; Dorigo, E.; Giacomini, A.; Iaci, G.; et al. A new technique for vascular access management in transcatheter aortic valve implantation. *Catheter. Cardiovasc. Interv.* **2010**, *75*, 784–793. [CrossRef] [PubMed]

108. Kahlert, P.; Al-Rashid, F.; Plicht, B.; Konorza, T.; Neumann, T.; Thielmann, M.; Wendt, D.; Erbel, R.; Eggebrecht, H. Suture-mediated arterial access site closure after transfemoral aortic valve implantation. *Catheter. Cardiovasc. Interv.* **2013**, *81*, E139–E150. [CrossRef]
109. Hayashida, K.; Lefevre, T.; Chevalier, B.; Hovasse, T.; Romano, M.; Garot, P.; Mylotte, D.; Uribe, J.; Farge, A.; Donzeau-Gouge, P.; et al. True percutaneous approach for transfemoral aortic valve implantation using the Prostar XL device: Impact of learning curve on vascular complications. *JACC Cardiovasc. Interv.* **2012**, *5*, 207–214. [CrossRef] [PubMed]
110. Grube, E.; Schuler, G.; Buellesfeld, L.; Gerckens, U.; Linke, A.; Wenaweser, P.; Sauren, B.; Mohr, F.W.; Walther, T.; Zickmann, B.; et al. Percutaneous aortic valve replacement for severe aortic stenosis in high-risk patients using the second- and current third-generation self-expanding CoreValve prosthesis: Device success and 30-day clinical outcome. *J. Am. Coll. Cardiol.* **2007**, *50*, 69–76. [CrossRef] [PubMed]
111. van Wiechen, M.P.; Ligthart, J.M.; Van Mieghem, N.M. Large-bore Vascular Closure: New Devices and Techniques. *Interv. Cardiol.* **2019**, *14*, 17–21. [CrossRef] [PubMed]
112. Frerker, C.; Schewel, D.; Kuck, K.H.; Schafer, U. Ipsilateral arterial access for management of vascular complication in transcatheter aortic valve implantation. *Catheter. Cardiovasc. Interv.* **2013**, *81*, 592–602. [CrossRef] [PubMed]
113. Curran, H.; Chieffo, A.; Buchanan, G.L.; Bernelli, C.; Montorfano, M.; Maisano, F.; Latib, A.; Maccagni, D.; Carlino, M.; Figini, F.; et al. A comparison of the femoral and radial crossover techniques for vascular access management in transcatheter aortic valve implantation: The Milan experience. *Catheter. Cardiovasc. Interv.* **2014**, *83*, 156–161. [CrossRef] [PubMed]
114. Laborde, J.C.; Brecker, S.J.; Roy, D.; Jahangiri, M. Complications at the time of transcatheter aortic valve implantation. *Methodist DeBakey Cardiovasc. J.* **2012**, *8*, 38–41. [CrossRef] [PubMed]
115. Nagasawa, A.; Shirai, S.; Hanyu, M.; Arai, Y.; Kamioka, N.; Hayashi, M. Descending aortic dissection injured by tip of the sheath during transcatheter aortic valve implantation. *Cardiovasc. Interv. Ther.* **2016**, *31*, 122–127. [CrossRef]
116. Hansson, N.C.; Nørgaard, B.L.; Barbanti, M.; Nielssen, N.N.E.; Yang, T.H.; Tamburino, C.; Dvir, D.; Jilaihawi, H.; Blanke, P.; Makkar, R.R.; et al. The impact of calcium volume and distribution in aortic root injury related to balloon-expandable transcatheter aortic valve replacement. *J. Cardiovasc. Comput. Tomogr.* **2015**, *9*, 382–392. [CrossRef]
117. .Barbanti, M.; Yang, T.H.; Rodès Cabau, J.; Tamburino, C.; Wood, D.A.; Jilaihawi, H.; Blanke, P.; Makkar, R.R.; Latib, A.; Colombo, A.; et al. Anatomical and procedural features associated with aortic root rupture during balloon-expandable transcatheter aortic valve replacement. *Circulation* **2013**, *128*, 244–253. [CrossRef] [PubMed]
118. Tzamtzis, S.; Viquerat, J.; Yap, J.; Mullen, M.J.; Burriesci, G. Numerical analysis of the radial force produced by the Medtronic-CoreValve and Edwards-SAPIEN after transcatheter aortic valve implantation (TAVI). *Med. Eng. Phys.* **2013**, *35*, 125–130. [CrossRef] [PubMed]
119. Hiltrop, N.; Adriaenssens, T.; Dymarkowski, S.; Herijgers, P.; Dubois, C. Aortic Annulus Rupture during TAVI: A Therapeutic Dilemma in the Inoperable Patient. *J. Heart Valve Dis.* **2015**, *24*, 436–438. [PubMed]
120. Hayashida, K.; Bouvier, E.; Lefevre, T.; Hovasse, T.; Morice, M.C.; Chevalier, B.; Romano, M.; Garot, P.; Farge, A.; Donzeau-Gouge, P.; et al. Potential mechanism of annulus rupture during transcatheter aortic valve implantation. *Catheter. Cardiovasc. Interv.* **2013**, *82*, E742–E746. [CrossRef]
121. Eltchaninoff, H.; Prat, A.; Gilard, M.; Leguerrier, A.; Blanchard, D.; Fournial, G.; Iung, B.; Donzeau-Gouge, P.; Tribouilloy, C.; Debrux, J.L.; et al. Transcatheter aortic valve implantation: Early results of the FRANCE (FRench Aortic National CoreValve and Edwards) registry. *Eur. Heart J.* **2011**, *32*, 191–197. [CrossRef]
122. Tsetis, D. Endovascular treatment of complications of femoral arterial access. *Cardiovasc. Interv. Radiol.* **2010**, *33*, 457–468. [CrossRef]
123. Masson, J.B.; Al Bugami, S.; Webb, J.G. Endovascular balloon occlusion for catheter-induced large artery perforation in the catheterization laboratory. *Catheter. Cardiovasc. Interv.* **2009**, *73*, 514–518. [CrossRef] [PubMed]
124. Dahdouh, Z.; Roule, V.; Grollier, G. Life-threatening iliac artery rupture during transcatheter aortic valve implantation (TAVI): Diagnosis and management. *Heart* **2013**, *99*, 1217–1218. [CrossRef] [PubMed]
125. Masson, J.B.; Kovac, J.; Schuler, G.; Ye, J.; Cheung, A.; Kapadia, S.; Tuzcu, M.E.; Kodali, S.; Leon, M.B.; Webb, J.G. Transcatheter aortic valve implantation: Review of the nature, management, and avoidance of procedural complications. *JACC Cardiovasc. Interv.* **2009**, *2*, 811–820. [CrossRef] [PubMed]
126. Van Mieghem, N.M.; Nuis, R.J.; Piazza, N.; Apostolos, T.; Ligthart, J.; Schultz, C.; de Jaegere, P.P.; Serruys, P.W. Vascular complications with transcatheter aortic valve implantation using the 18 Fr Medtronic CoreValve System: The Rotterdam experience. *EuroIntervention* **2010**, *5*, 673–679. [CrossRef]
127. Yatskar, L.; Selzer, F.; Feit, F.; Cohen, H.A.; Jacobs, A.K.; Williams, D.O.; Slater, J. Access site hematoma requiring blood transfusion predicts mortality in patients undergoing percutaneous coronary intervention: Data from the National Heart, Lung, and Blood Institute Dynamic Registry. *Catheter. Cardiovasc. Interv.* **2007**, *69*, 961–966. [CrossRef] [PubMed]
128. Tonnessen, B.H. Iatrogenic injury from vascular access and endovascular procedures. *Perspect. Vasc. Surg. Endovasc. Ther.* **2011**, *23*, 128–135. [CrossRef]
129. Stone, P.A.; Campbell, J.E.; AbuRahma, A.F. Femoral pseudoaneurysms after percutaneous access. *J. Vasc. Surg.* **2014**, *60*, 1359–1366. [CrossRef]

130. Kresowik, T.F.; Khoury, M.D.; Miller, B.V.; Winniford, M.D.; Shamma, A.R.; Sharp, W.J.; Blecha, M.B.; Corson, J.D. A prospective study of the incidence and natural history of femoral vascular complications after percutaneous transluminal coronary angioplasty. *J. Vasc. Surg.* **1991**, *13*, 328–333; discussion 333–325. [CrossRef]
131. Toursarkissian, B.; Allen, B.T.; Petrinec, D.; Thompson, R.W.; Rubin, B.G.; Reilly, J.M.; Anderson, C.B.; Flye, M.W.; Sicard, G.A. Spontaneous closure of selected iatrogenic pseudoaneurysms and arteriovenous fistulae. *J. Vasc. Surg.* **1997**, *25*, 803–808; discussion 808–809. [CrossRef]
132. Lonn, L.; Olmarker, A.; Geterud, K.; Risberg, B. Prospective randomized study comparing ultrasound-guided thrombin injection to compression in the treatment of femoral pseudoaneurysms. *J. Endovasc. Ther.* **2004**, *11*, 570–576. [CrossRef]
133. Stone, P.; Lohan, J.A.; Copeland, S.E.; Hamrick, R.E., Jr.; Tiley, E.H., 3rd; Flaherty, S.K. Iatrogenic pseudoaneurysms: Comparison of treatment modalities, including duplex-guided thrombin injection. *West Va. Med. J.* **2003**, *99*, 230–232.
134. Dvir, D.; Assali, A.; Porat, E.; Kornowski, R. Distal left anterior descending coronary artery obstruction: A rare complication of transapical aortic valve implantation. *J. Invasive Cardiol.* **2011**, *23*, E281–E283.
135. Nielsen, H.H.; Klaaborg, K.E.; Nissen, H.; Terp, K.; Mortensen, P.E.; Kjeldsen, B.J.; Jakobsen, C.J.; Andersen, H.R.; Egeblad, H.; Krusell, L.R.; et al. A prospective, randomised trial of transapical transcatheter aortic valve implantation vs. surgical aortic valve replacement in operable elderly patients with aortic stenosis: The STACCATO trial. *EuroIntervention* **2012**, *8*, 383–389. [CrossRef]
136. Himbert, D.; Descoutures, F.; Al-Attar, N.; Iung, B.; Ducrocq, G.; Detaint, D.; Brochet, E.; Messika-Zeitoun, D.; Francis, F.; Ibrahim, H.; et al. Results of transfemoral or transapical aortic valve implantation following a uniform assessment in high-risk patients with aortic stenosis. *J. Am. Coll. Cardiol.* **2009**, *54*, 303–311. [CrossRef]
137. Schafer, U.; Deuschl, F.; Schofer, N.; Frerker, C.; Schmidt, T.; Kuck, K.H.; Kreidel, F.; Schirmer, J.; Mizote, I.; Reichenspurner, H.; et al. Safety and efficacy of the percutaneous transaxillary access for transcatheter aortic valve implantation using various transcatheter heart valves in 100 consecutive patients. *Int. J. Cardiol.* **2017**, *232*, 247–254. [CrossRef] [PubMed]
138. Etienne, P.Y.; Papadatos, S.; El Khoury, E.; Pieters, D.; Price, J.; Glineur, D. Transaortic transcatheter aortic valve implantation with the Edwards SAPIEN valve: Feasibility, technical considerations, and clinical advantages. *Ann. Thorac. Surg.* **2011**, *92*, 746–748. [CrossRef]
139. Holmes, D.R., Jr.; Mack, M.J.; Kaul, S.; Agnihotri, A.; Alexander, K.P.; Bailey, S.R.; Calhoon, J.H.; Carabello, B.A.; Desai, M.Y.; Edwards, F.H.; et al. 2012 ACCF/AATS/SCAI/STS expert consensus document on transcatheter aortic valve replacement: Developed in collaboration with the American Heart Association, American Society of Echocardiography, European Association for Cardio-Thoracic Surgery, Heart Failure Society of America, Mended Hearts, Society of Cardiovascular Anesthesiologists, Society of Cardiovascular Computed Tomography, and Society for Cardiovascular Magnetic Resonance. *J. Thorac. Cardiovasc. Surg.* **2012**, *144*, e29–e84. [CrossRef]
140. Achenbach, S.; Delgado, V.; Hausleiter, J.; Schoenhagen, P.; Min, J.K.; Leipsic, J.A. SCCT expert consensus document on computed tomography imaging before transcatheter aortic valve implantation (TAVI)/transcatheter aortic valve replacement (TAVR). *J. Cardiovasc. Comput. Tomogr.* **2012**, *6*, 366–380. [CrossRef] [PubMed]

MDPI
St. Alban-Anlage 66
4052 Basel
Switzerland
Tel. +41 61 683 77 34
Fax +41 61 302 89 18
www.mdpi.com

Journal of Clinical Medicine Editorial Office
E-mail: jcm@mdpi.com
www.mdpi.com/journal/jcm

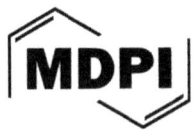

www.ingramcontent.com/pod-product-compliance
Lightning Source LLC
LaVergne TN
LVHW070653100526
838202LV00013B/955